Gentleman's Guide

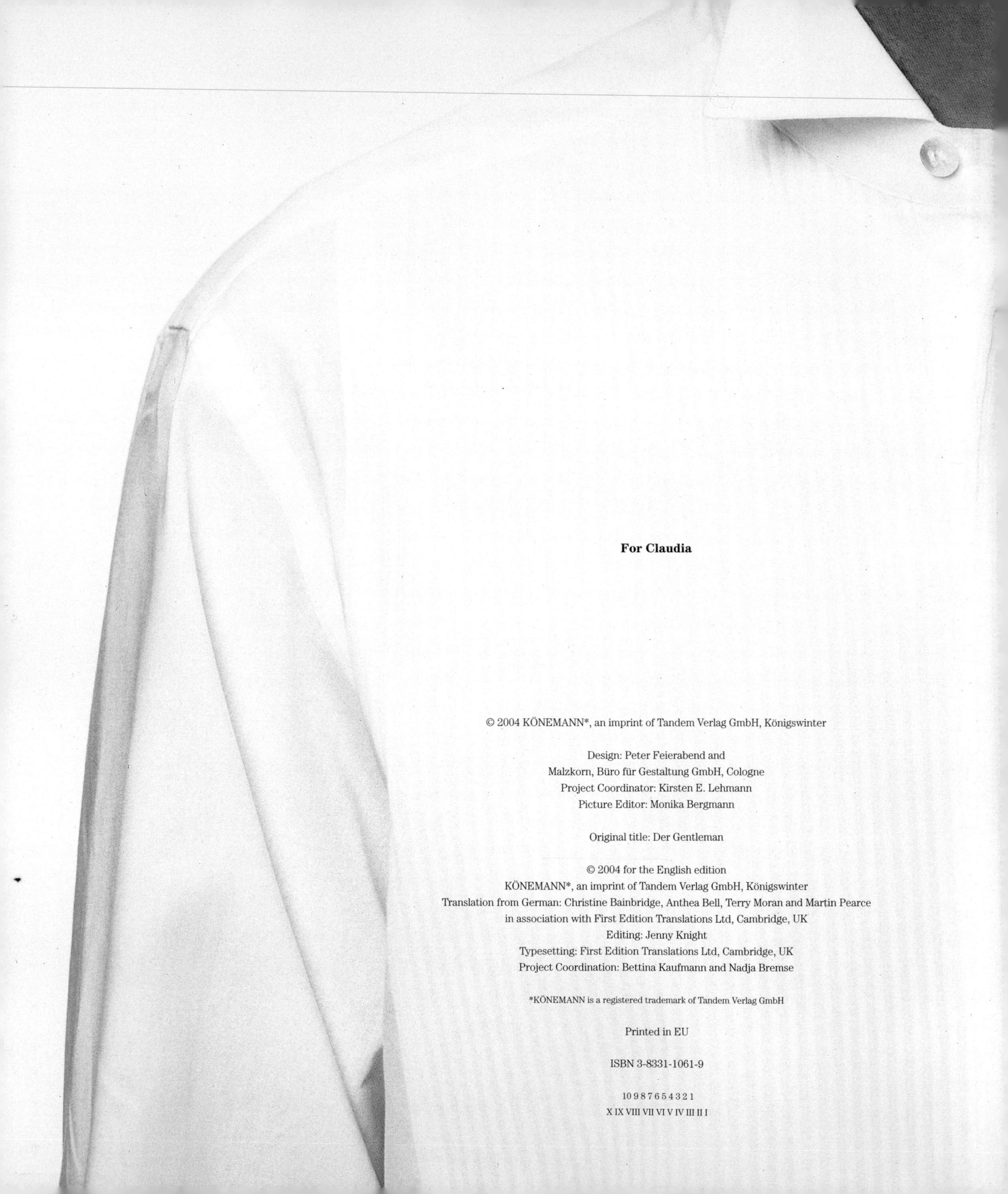

For Claudia

© 2004 KÖNEMANN*, an imprint of Tandem Verlag GmbH, Königswinter

Design: Peter Feierabend and
Malzkorn, Büro für Gestaltung GmbH, Cologne
Project Coordinator: Kirsten E. Lehmann
Picture Editor: Monika Bergmann

Original title: Der Gentleman

© 2004 for the English edition
KÖNEMANN*, an imprint of Tandem Verlag GmbH, Königswinter
Translation from German: Christine Bainbridge, Anthea Bell, Terry Moran and Martin Pearce
in association with First Edition Translations Ltd, Cambridge, UK
Editing: Jenny Knight
Typesetting: First Edition Translations Ltd, Cambridge, UK
Project Coordination: Bettina Kaufmann and Nadja Bremse

*KÖNEMANN is a registered trademark of Tandem Verlag GmbH

Printed in EU

ISBN 3-8331-1061-9

10 9 8 7 6 5 4 3 2 1
X IX VIII VII VI V IV III II I

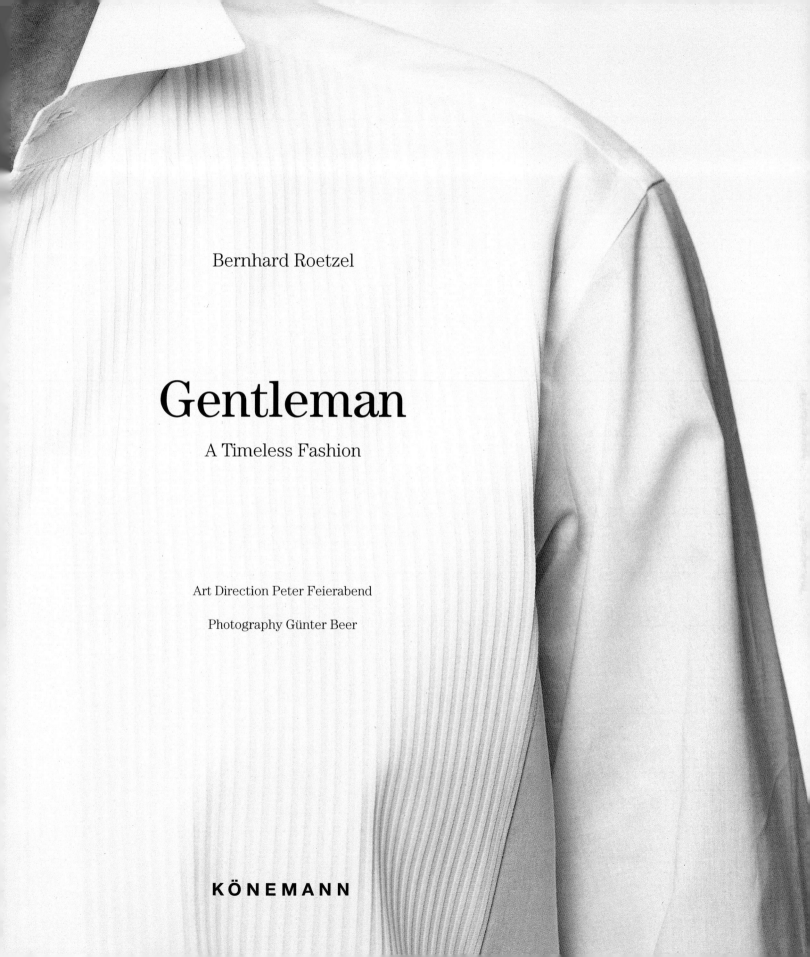

Bernhard Roetzel

Gentleman

A Timeless Fashion

Art Direction Peter Feierabend

Photography Günter Beer

KÖNEMANN

Foreword of an Englishman 8 | 9

The Gentleman's Visiting Card 10 | 11

The Beard 12 | 13

Shaving at Home 14 | 15
At the Barber's 16
A Good Wet Shave 17
The Electric Shaver 18 | 19
Different Men, Different Beards 20
Caring for Beards and Mustaches 21
Timeless Fragrances 22 | 23
The Perfumer's ABC 24 | 25

The Hair 26 | 27

The Joys of Visiting the Hairdresser 28 | 29
What Should I Put on My Hair? 30 | 31
The Right Way to Wash Hair 32 | 33
Hairstyles with Character 34 | 35
The Toupee: For and Against 36
The Fake Hair of the Stars 37
Chest Hair 37
The Royal Hairbrush 38
The Manicure 39

Underwear 40 | 41

The Most Important Question of All 42 | 43
Variations Underneath 44 | 45
A Fly-Away Success 46 | 47

The Shirt 48 | 49

A Gentleman's Shirt 50
Good Shirts at a Glance 51
Collar Shapes 52 | 53
Cotton 54 | 55
The Stuff that Shirts are Made of 56 | 57
Folding Your Shirt 57
Jermyn Street 58 | 59
The Best English Shirtmakers 60 | 61
How a Custom-Made Shirt is Created 62 | 63
Checks for the Weekend 64
The Brooks Brothers Shirt 65
The Right Shirt – the Right Fit 66 | 67
Washing and Ironing –
the Fundamentals of Shirt Care 68 | 69

The Necktie 70 | 71

From Neckcloth to Ornamental Neckwear 72
Stars of the Stripes 73
A Good Necktie 74
Woolen Neckties 75
The Best of the Best 76
A Great Success from the Grande Nation 77
The Origins of Silk 78
Making a Necktie 79
The Master of the Custom-Made Necktie 80
The Business Necktie 81
The Four-in-Hand 82
How to Tie a Necktie 83
The Windsor Knot 83
The Bow Tie 84 | 85
Tying a Bow Tie 86
The Cravat 87

The Suit   88 | 89

Style in the Suit 90 | 91
Button Undone 91
The Mecca of the Custom-made Suit 92-95
The English Suit 96
Patterns and Fabrics 97
A Suit from Gieves and Hawkes 98-101
Chester Barrie 102 | 103
Three Savile Row Customers 104
The King of Style 105
The Right Kind of Tweed Suit 106 | 107
The Italian Suit 108
Who's Who in Italy 109
Brioni – veni, vidi, vici 110 | 111
Classics of Fashion 112
The Hall of Fame 113
The Summer Suit 114 | 115
Brooks Brothers – New York Classics 116 | 117

Smart Casual   118 | 119

The Sports Jacket 120 | 121
Needle and Thread 122 | 123
Tweed Plus 124 | 125
Two Tweed Jackets 126 | 127
Today's Sports Jacket 128
An Eye for Detail 128 | 129
Fabrics for Trousers to Go
with the Sports Jacket 130 | 131
The Gray Eminence 132 | 133
Khaki Couture 134
Shorts 135
The Right Sort of Jeans 136 | 137
The Cut 138 | 139
How Trousers Got their Cuffs 139

The Waist Area 140
The Trousers in Detail 140 | 141
Other Countries, Other Trousers 141
All about Suspenders 142 | 143
The Right Belt 144 | 145
The Blazer – a Living Legend 146 | 147
Blazer and Trousers 148 | 149

Shoes   150 | 151

Good shoes 152-155
John Lobb 156 | 157
Formal shoes
with closed lacing 158 | 159
Formal shoes
with open lacing 160 | 161
Loafers 162 | 163
Moccasins Italian Style 164 | 165
Monkstraps – the Shoes
with Buckles 166
The Other Word for Weatherproof 167
Leather Does not always Mean Leather 168 | 169
The Center of the Shoe World 170 | 171
The Shoemaker's Tools 172 | 173
How a Shoe Takes Shape 174-177
The Other Word for Cordovan 178 | 179
Suede Shoes 180 | 181
American Classics – Saddle Shoes 182
Slippers 183
Shoes with Knobs on 184 | 185
Raincoats for Shoes 185
Socks – Getting the Combination Right 186 | 187
Shoes and the Rest 188 | 189

Overcoats & Jackets   190 | 191

Overcoat Culture 192 | 193
Essential Overcoats 194-197
For the Officer in the Gentleman 198
The Duffel Coat 199
The Barbour Phenomenon 200
The Story of the Waxed Jacket 201
The Barbour in Detail 202 | 203
The Top Six 203
Short is All Right 204 | 205

The Hat   206 | 207

The Hat Past and Present 208 | 209
The Bowler 210 | 211
Courage to Wear Hats 212 | 213
Who Wears Hats? 214 | 215
The Panama 216 | 217

Accessories   218 | 219

Those little differences 220 | 221
The Everyday Ballast 222 | 223
One has it – but where? 224 | 225
What does it tell us? 226 | 227
The best watches in the world 228 | 229
All About the Watch 230 | 231
Less is More 232 | 233
Preface to Tobacco 234 | 235
The Cigarette 236 | 237
The Pipe 238 | 239
Classic Pipe Squad 240 | 241
The Manufacture 241
The Cigar 242 | 243
The Sizes 244 | 245
The Bar in the Pocket 246 | 247
The Cuff Link 248 | 249
Our Daily Companion 250 | 251
The Original 252 | 253
Traveling in Style 254 | 255
For the Short Trip 256 | 257
The Knack with the Jacket 258
The Right Way to Pack a Suitcase 259
The Walking Cane 260
The Lap Robe 261
No Fear of Rain 262 | 263
The Other Word in Umbrellas 264 | 265
Glasses 266 | 267
Not only when the Sun Shines 268 | 269
The Handkerchief 270 | 271
From Hand to Breast Pocket 272 | 273
The Right Combination 274 | 275
The Glove 276 | 277
Scarf Refinement 278 | 279

Knitwear   280 | 281

In the Beginning Was the Sweater 282 | 283
From Sheep to Wool 284 | 285
Classic Knitwear 286 | 287
Between England and France 288
The Guernsey in Detail 289
From Fine to Chunky Knit 290 | 291
Correct Coordination 292 | 293
For Cold Winter Days 294 | 295
The Other Craze 296 | 297

Sporting Life   298 | 299

Why Sport? 300 | 301
Hunting, Riding, Fishing… 302 | 303
Shooting – the Outfit 304 | 305
The Real Thing 306 | 307
The pocketknife 307
Riding – the Outfit 308 | 309
Spectating in Style 310 | 311
Fishing – the Outfit 312 | 313
Hole in One 314 | 315
The Crocodile 316 | 317
The Other Polo Shirt 317
Water Sports – the Outfit 318 | 319

Formal Dress   320 | 321

White or black? 322 | 323
The Tuxedo – and What Goes With It 324 | 325
Black & White 325
White Tie 326 | 327
A Jacket for Smoking 328
Available to Rent… 328
The Right Shoes 329
Morning Dress 330 | 331

Home Comfort   332 | 333

A Hint of Decadence 334 | 335
Breakfast with Style 336 | 337
A Souvenir from the Colonies 338 | 339
Home Comfort 340 | 341

Appendix   342 | 343

Looking after your Wardrobe 344-347
    The Suit 344
    The Necktie 346
    Shoes 346 | 347
    Shoe Repair 347
Glossary 348-352
Bibliography – a Selection 353
Acknowledgments 353
Index 354-357
Picture Credits 360

Foreword of an Englishman

There is an old proverb that defines genius as "an infinite capacity for taking pains," and the same description would serve to define a gentleman. The real gentleman is one who leaves nothing to chance. It is not enough to make sure one's clothes are smart, of the finest cut and quality, and in immaculate order. There is one's physical appearance to consider. Does one need a visit to one's barber for a haircut or for that professional shave that leaves all do-it-yourself shaves looking – and feeling – inadequate? Is one's umbrella rolled as tight as could be?

A gentleman has to attend to these and many other matters the moment he has breakfasted (in pyjamas and slippers and dressing gown, on kippers or kidneys or kedgeree), and then shaved, bathed and dressed. For one does not carry around a sackful of accoutrements all day. Ladies may be permitted their handbags full of potions and elixirs, paints and powders, so that they may refresh their beauty as and when required. A gentleman, however, takes care that he leaves his house, flat chambers or club splendidly attired for the whole day. From morn till night, the carnation in one's buttonhole must never droop, one's delicately waxed and trimmed moustache must never need first aid, the gleam in one's eye must never dim.

There was an English comedian in the 1930s who described himself as "Billy Bennett – Almost a Gentleman." The concept is outrageous. One cannot be almost a gentleman. One either is, or one isn't. Standards are set, and must be kept up. It is better not to try to appear to be a gentleman if one is likely to fail to make the grade.

The 18th century political philosopher, Edmund Burke, once remarked in a letter to a friend: "a king may create a nobleman, but he cannot create a gentleman." Indeed, all the wealth and power in the world cannot create a gentleman. But if one honestly endeavours to become one and succeeds…! Ah, then a precious and delightful world is open to one – a world which few are permitted to inhabit. And then one realises that being a gentleman is not simply about how one looks – though that is an essential prerequisite. It is also about how one behaves.

For a gentleman is always thoroughly decent, always instinctively does the right thing. When one is a gentleman, one makes sure all the women and children are safely in the lifeboats while one goes down with the ship. One never maltreats a horse or betrays a friend. One knows when a lady desires company and when she wishes to be left alone. One would always rather have a glass of good champagne than a magnum of plonk. One is always polite, even in the face of arrogant rudeness on the part of lesser mortals.

One word of warning … it is possible to overdo the dressing-up side of being a gentleman. Bertrand Russell (himself too eccentric and uncaring of his appearance ever to be rated a gentleman) once said of Anthony Eden that Eden was "not a gentleman; he dresses too well." Eden was a dashing young man in the 1930s, the darling of the Conservative Party in Britain, and Foreign Secretary to Churchill in the 1950s. He was always to be seen in immaculately pressed pin stripe trousers, black jacket and waistcoat, stiff white collar and neatly knotted tie, crowned with the smart black hat that bore his name. Eden was a fashion setter, but in Russell's eyes, Eden's dress code outstripped his moral code.

Those who study Bernhard Roetzel's wonderful book need have no worries. Here is all one needs to assume the mantle that epitomises civilized man. Here is richness indeed – for here is the gentleman's handbook.

Nick Yapp

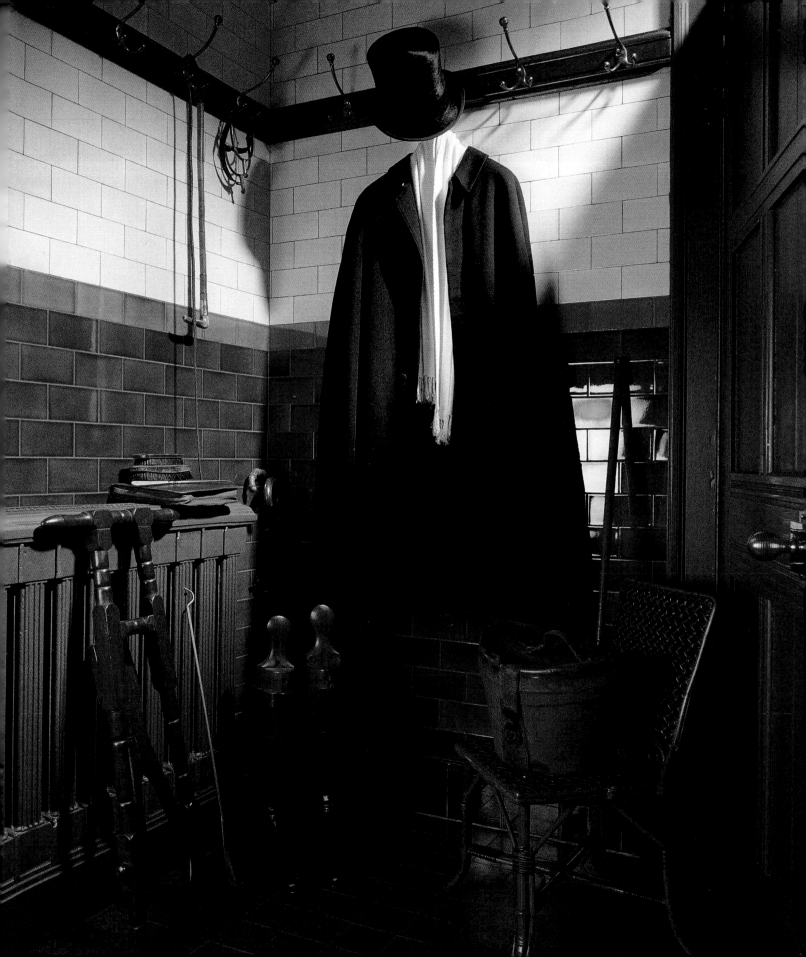

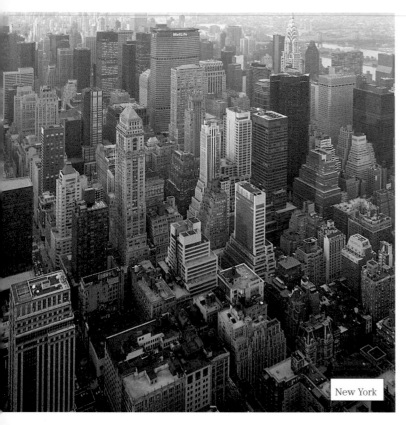

New York

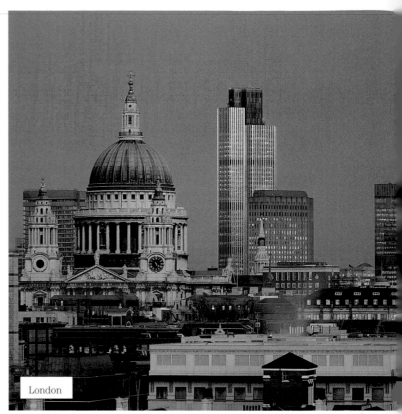

London

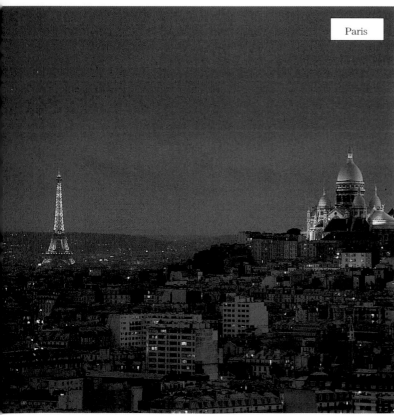

Paris

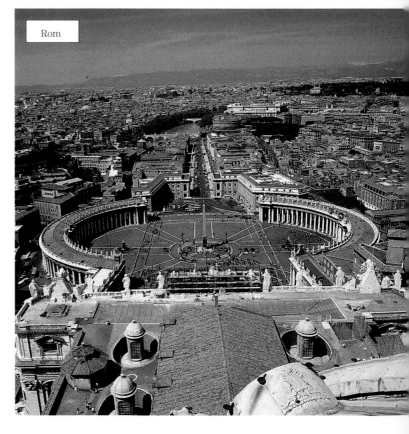

Rom

The Gentleman's Visiting Card

One thing should be clear: clothes do not make a man a gentleman; and, by the same token, a real gentleman is always a gentleman, even without his clothes. However, it would be a mistake to conclude from this that our appearance is not important. Clothes are the visiting card of a personality, and should therefore be chosen to match it.

This book is an attempt to provide a comprehensive description of the proper style of attire for a gentleman. By this we mean a dress code that has its roots in England, and that is accepted around the world today as classic style. Anyone who dresses as described in this book can be sure that he will look well-dressed, whether he is in London, Paris, Brussels, Düsseldorf, Rome, Milan, New York, or Tokyo.

Dressing like a gentleman means mixing tailored garments and mass products, exclusiveness and modest practicality. A pair of Levi's jeans with a tailored, made-to-measure tweed jacket is just as acceptable a weekend outfit as good-value boat shoes from Sperry with chinos by Polo Ralph Lauren and a blazer from Gieves and Hawkes.

Dressing like a gentleman is therefore not to be equated with a stubborn conservatism. Innovations which prove their worth and look good gradually find acceptance in the international style canon of London, Milan, and New York. Jeans are an example. Although it took a while, these blue cotton trousers eventually established themselves, and are now familiar and accepted leisurewear items almost everywhere. Or there is the Husky jacket, which was invented at the beginning of the 1960s but only became well known around the world in the 1980s. Or Diego Della Valle's Tod's shoes, which have only been on the market since 1979.

Combining pieces of clothing and accessories of the most varied origins to assemble a harmonic, interesting whole demands a thorough knowledge of the history of the individual garments. Naturally, this knowledge may also lead to the quite conscious creation of new and unusual combinations, which may occasionally even be the products of intuition and chance. But someone who does not wish to rely on these imponderables should learn about the individual components of his wardrobe. Only by doing so will he eventually understand how to wear them properly.

Of course, it is not by chance that English clothes and English style are discussed so much in this book.

London became the leading fashion center in Europe as early as the eighteenth century, especially since important new ideas kept coming from the British Isles. While the French aristocracy lived at the royal court, their English counterparts spent a great deal of time on their country estates. Their favorite pastime was fox hunting, and this required a completely new style of dress. The knee-length coat was a hindrance when riding, so it was cut shorter and shorter. The vest became shorter to match, and the pants tighter. This new look was taken up throughout Europe: in France the English frock coat became the fraque, and in Germany the Frack, while la Grande Nation corrupted "riding coat" into redingote.

Only at the end of the nineteenth century was the color finally driven out of the suit that evolved during the eighteenth century, and consisted of a frock coat, vest, and pants. In view of the muddy roads of the time and the city air filled with soot and smoke by innumerable coal fires, this trend was thoroughly practical. Only in the country was there a contrast to the gray and black of the city. The colors of nature the nobility saw on their country estates were reproduced in hunting and riding clothes. Unknown trendsetters who wanted to be able to wear comfortable riding jackets in the city as well came up with the idea of having them made of dark materials. Ultimately, it is this development we have to thank for the cut of the modern suit, with its short jacket. In consequence, the modern man who finds a dark suit stiff and formal may console himself with the knowledge that, in a sense, it is the dark version of a leisure outfit.

But there is also another lesson to be drawn: dressing like a gentleman costs not only time, but money as well. An investment in a good garment generally entails further expenditure. Someone who is wearing a pair of genuinely good shoes for the first time will automatically cast a critical eye over the rest of his clothes. And as a consequence the need for a good suit arises almost of necessity. This, in its turn, demands good shirts and ties.

It is a process which usually takes several years, and it is better that way. A wardrobe must grow like the decoration of an apartment. This is a highly individual process, which can, and should, lead each of us to a unique style. As has already been mentioned, clothes are the visiting card of a personality.

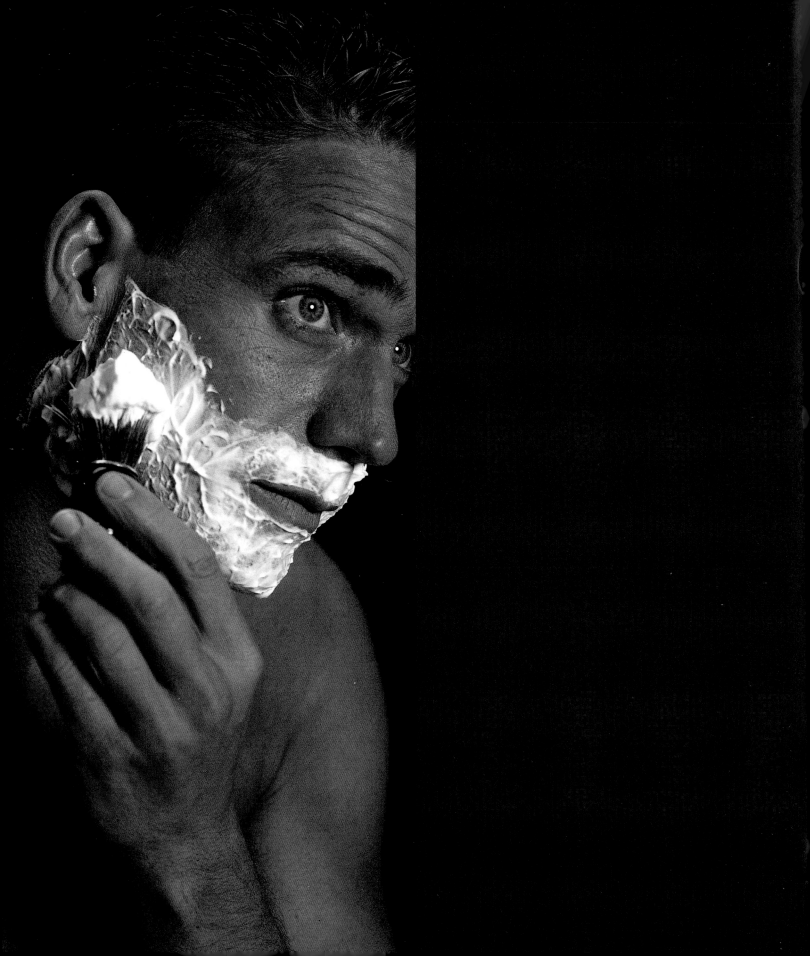

The Beard

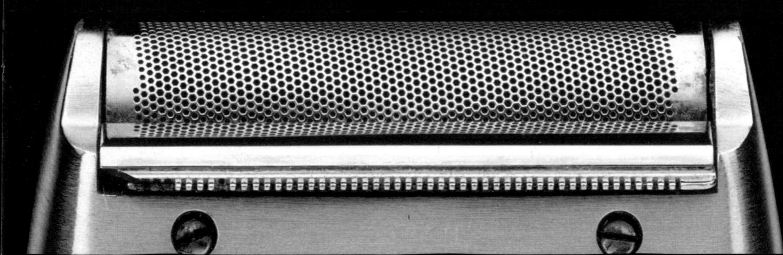

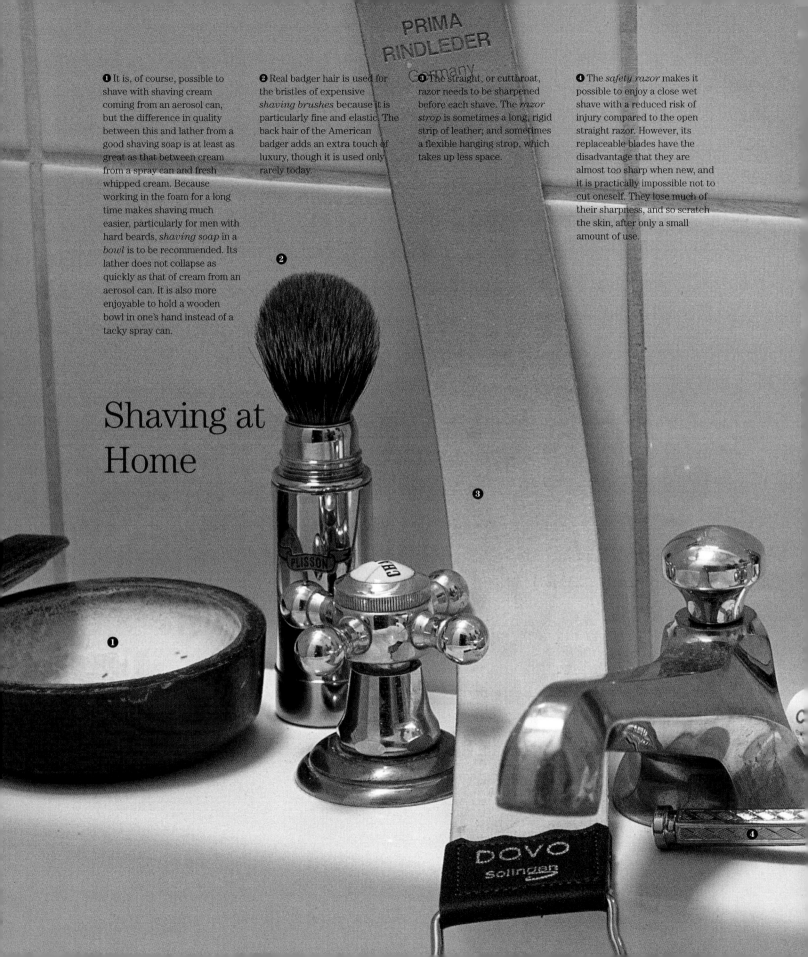

❶ It is, of course, possible to shave with shaving cream coming from an aerosol can, but the difference in quality between this and lather from a good shaving soap is at least as great as that between cream from a spray can and fresh whipped cream. Because working in the foam for a long time makes shaving much easier, particularly for men with hard beards, *shaving soap* in a *bowl* is to be recommended. Its lather does not collapse as quickly as that of cream from an aerosol can. It is also more enjoyable to hold a wooden bowl in one's hand instead of a tacky spray can.

❷ Real badger hair is used for the bristles of expensive *shaving brushes* because it is particularly fine and elastic. The back hair of the American badger adds an extra touch of luxury, though it is used only rarely today.

❸ The straight, or cutthroat, razor needs to be sharpened before each shave. The *razor strop* is sometimes a long, rigid strip of leather; and sometimes a flexible hanging strop, which takes up less space.

❹ The *safety razor* makes it possible to enjoy a close wet shave with a reduced risk of injury compared to the open straight razor. However, its replaceable blades have the disadvantage that they are almost too sharp when new, and it is practically impossible not to cut oneself. They lose much of their sharpness, and so scratch the skin, after only a small amount of use.

Shaving at Home

❺ If, no matter how careful one is, one cuts oneself, small nicks and scratches can be closed up with a *styptic pencil* made of aluminum potassium sulfate, which has a mild cauterizing effect, is able to stop bleeding, and acts as an astringent on the injured tissue.

❻ The *shaving mirror* is usually double-sided. One side reflects a mirror image in normal size, the other magnifies it by two or three times. This makes it possible to control the shave precisely.

❼ The real purpose of *aftershave* is to disinfect the skin after shaving, but most men also use it as a fragrance. . Today almost all ranges of toilet accessories include an aftershave with a matching *eau de toilette*, which has a longer-lasting fragrance.

❽ A man who prefers to avoid wet shaving, even though the result is a much closer shave, does not have to wear a beard nowadays. He can always use an *electric shaver*.

❾ Most men are afraid of shaving with a *straight razor*. Associations with film scenes such as the opening of Buñuel's *Un Chien andalou* are only too easily awakened. Nevertheless, straight razors are highly pleasing aesthetically, and mastering the perfect shave with a cutthroat razor lends one an air of manliness. But take care, their use has to be learned and practiced.

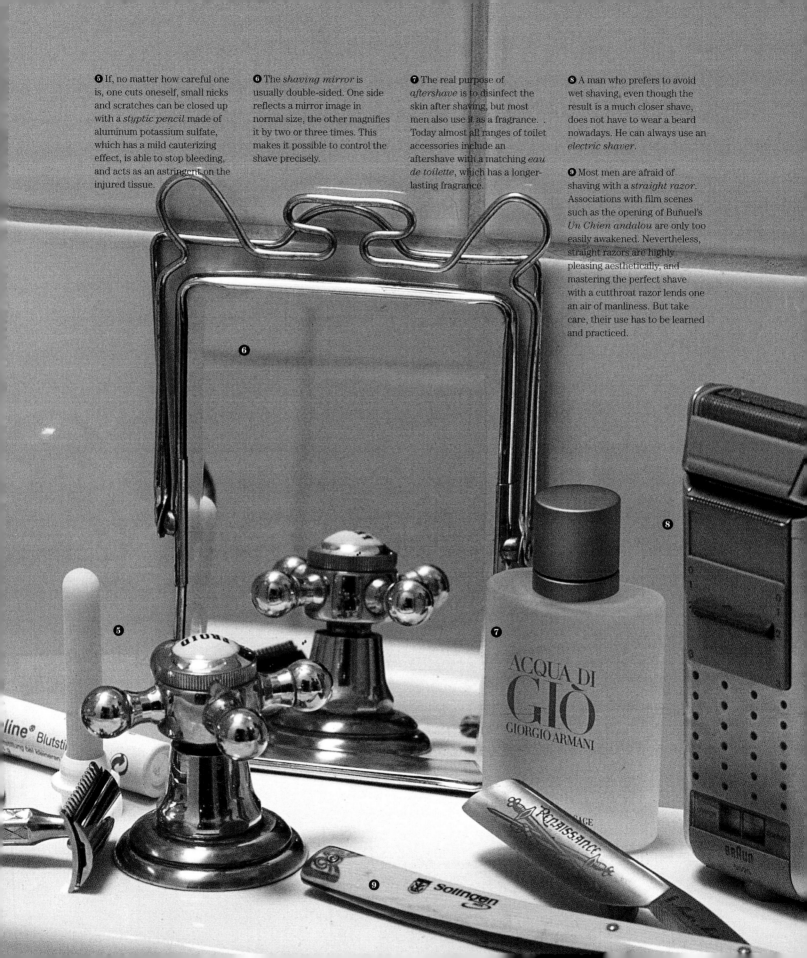

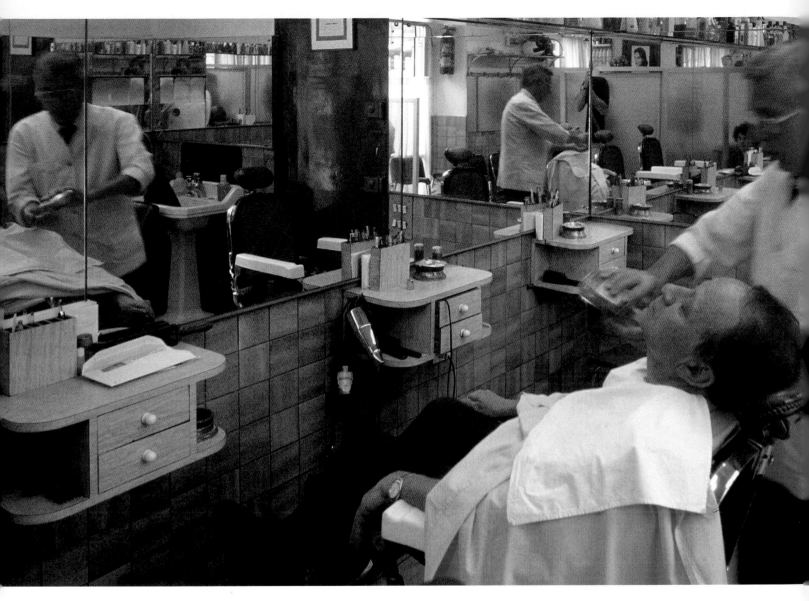

At the Barber's

When Emile Zola spoke of a "ladies' paradise," he was referring to the institution of the enormous department store, that temple of commerce in which fine Parisian ladies abandoned themselves to unrestrained frenzies of buying in the mid-nineteenth century. By contrast, the good old barber's shop is a paradise for men. It is a place where a man can engage in conversations of a particular kind that are only possible with a hairdresser: a little banal, entertaining for the most part, and always highly relaxing. The close physical contact encourages a certain familiarity, which is balanced out by the general nature of the conversation. In contrast to the ladies, a man does not discuss intimate matters with his hairdresser. He is more likely to talk about cars, the weather, recent or upcoming horse races, and what is on television. But, sad to say, the barber's shop is a threatened species, though it has not quite died out completely yet. Fortunately, many European cities still have traditional gentlemen's hairdressers that offer their customers a good shave and a timeless haircut. It is usually men who work in these establishments, true to the old rule that, apart from his wife, a real gentleman does not allow himself to be touched by a woman. His doctor, his tailor, and, indeed, his hairdresser, must be male.

A Good Wet Shave

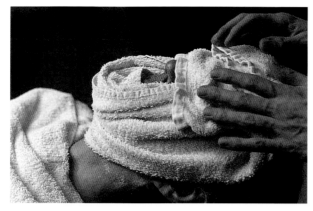

Before the actual shave can commence, the beard is softened with hot towels. This procedure also encourages the blood circulation in the skin of the face.

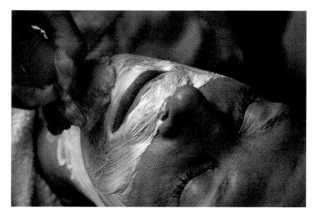

The customer's face is lathered using a real badger-hair brush. The lather softens the stubble and makes it easier to shave.

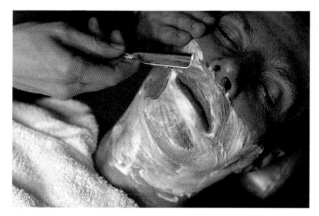

The cheeks are shaved first. The razor is always drawn "with the grain," that is, in the same direction as the hair growth.

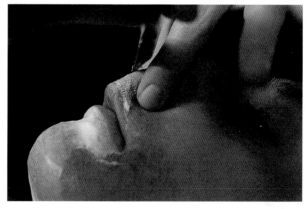

The barber holds the customer gently by the nose so that his upper lip is just tight enough.

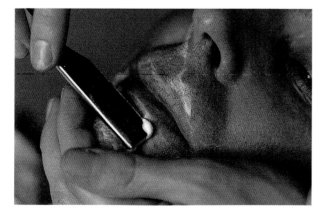

The point of the chin requires particular skill, and no beard should be left underneath the bottom lip. But this is not a problem for a barber who is well versed in his craft.

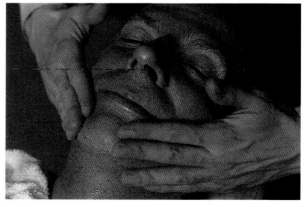

When the shave is finished, the remaining soap is rubbed off, and the skin finally patted dry. This subjects the customer's face to a thorough exfoliation.

The Electric Shaver

Dry or wet? American men were the first to be confronted with this fundamental question about their shaving habits. Approximately 76,000 electric shavers were sold in the USA and Canada in 1934, and in 1937 this figure reached 1.5 million. In Europe it was the Dutch company Philips who were the first to recognize the potential of this new product. At first they considered importing American razors, but soon this plan was rejected and the decision was taken to develop their own model. A certain Lopez Cardoso was dispatched to the USA to purchase the products made by the competition. These were then given a thorough examination at home in Eindhoven. The engineer and inventor Alexandre Horowitz had the idea of replacing the square shaving foil with a round, rotating shaving head. It took him until 1938 to create the prototype: this was a bronze shaving head with three blades rotating 10,000 times a minute inside a cylindrical casing that had 48 slits on its upper side. The device worked so well that the company decided to develop it for mass production. The first electric shaver with a rotating shaving head was ready for public display on March 14,

1939. Six razors, to be precise, were presented alongside radios and lamps at the spring exhibition in Utrecht. Male visitors to the exhibition were invited to come unshaven in order to try out the new "Electrisch Droogscheerapparaat." The crowd pressing round the Philips stand was enormous, and Prince Bernhard of the Netherlands himself watched a demonstration of the new invention. The press were also impressed: *Het Handelsblatt* stressed how many men had indeed appeared unshaven at the fair, while the Utrecht newspaper *Dagblad* noted that beard hair was removed in just five minutes, and the *Eindhovener Presse* was delighted that it had now become impossible to cut oneself while shaving. Initial opinions about the still unfamiliar design of the shaver, which had been christened the "Philishave," diverged widely, but, even though it was compared to the handle on the chain on a toilet cistern, this did nothing to reduce its fascination. As it happened, Philips had built up the know-how for the development and manufacture of electric shavers from their work producing, amongst other things, bicycle dynamos. In this field of activity the company had learned how to produce minute electric motors, which were now used to great effect in their tiny "salt pot" electric shavers.

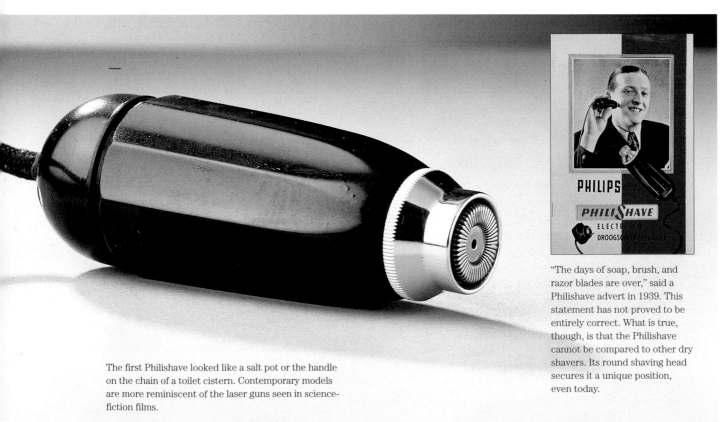

The first Philishave looked like a salt pot or the handle on the chain of a toilet cistern. Contemporary models are more reminiscent of the laser guns seen in science-fiction films.

"The days of soap, brush, and razor blades are over," said a Philishave advert in 1939. This statement has not proved to be entirely correct. What is true, though, is that the Philishave cannot be compared to other dry shavers. Its round shaving head secures it a unique position, even today.

The German company Braun only introduced their first electric shaver onto the market in 1950, 11 years after Philips. Nevertheless, they had the edge over the opposition as far as design was concerned in 1962, when they brought out the *Sixtant* model, because it was the first black shaver to come onto the market for several years.

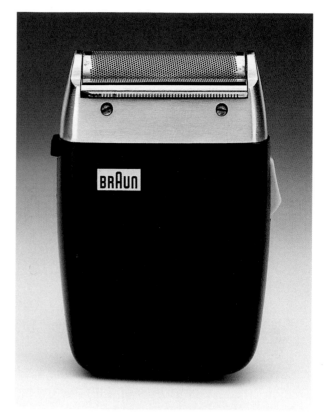

Nor was it by chance that the handle and casing of the first Philishave were made of Bakelite. The housings of Philips radios were made of the same material. The electric shaver thus made a contribution to the more efficient exploitation of the company's Bakelite production. Prior to this, the Philite works had produced doorknobs and even toilet seats. Just as brown Bakelite matched the tastes of the 1930s, the following generations of Philishaves reflected the fashions of their times. In 1948 the Philishave was given a new, streamlined look. No lesser figure than the famous American designer Raymond Loewy was the creator of this design, which remained modern until the late 1950s. This model was also very successful in the United States, particularly the version with two shaving heads. The successor to the legendary egg-shaped razor was a design called "The Pipe," brought out in 1957. When it was presented to the management, though, the new razor was called the "Sir Anthony," an allusion to the name of the company's head of sales, Tony Aaltsz, who was delighted with the new design. The first shaver with three shaving heads appeared in 1966. In 1969 Philips actually developed a prototype model of a special shaver for use in outer space, the Moonshaver, complete with a built-in miniature vacuum cleaner for beard hair and a sparkless motor. It is not certain whether this 12-inch (30 cm) long shaver was actually taken to the moon, but NASA certified it as fully adapted to conditions in space.

In 1975 came the development of the TH range ("TH" stands for "telephone handset"). The design of the Philishave is still based on this concept today. As far as its technology is concerned, it has maintained its unique position because all other electric shavers work with a block made up of a series of blades which vibrate backward and forward under a perforated metal foil. It is a matter of opinion whether better results are attained with this mode of operation, or with the rotating shaving head of the Philishave. Among European manufacturers, though, Philips can point to the greatest experience with electric shavers and, therefore, it might be supposed, have the greatest

competence. For example, the German manufacturers Braun introduced their first electric shaver onto the market only in 1950, 11 years after the first Philishave.

In the end, though, whether or not a man takes to dry shaving is hardly a question of deciding between two different technologies, or the more or less pleasing design. Rather, "wet or dry?" is a matter of principle that men have been discussing since the appearance of the first electric shaver. Those who prefer the traditional method with shaving soap and an open blade treasure it, above all, because it gives such a close shave, but also for its refreshing effect. In fact, wet shaving is like giving one's skin a thorough exfoliation. Not only that, the shave itself is very quick. Indeed, the only arguments against wet shaving are the danger of injury when working too hastily and the fact that water is always needed. Dry shaving is often preferred because it can be done anywhere, provided that an electricity connection or batteries are available, and because it really is very difficult to hurt yourself with an electric shaver. In case of doubt, tradition would probably be on the side of wet shaving, but, after more than 70 years, dry shaving is no longer an alternative that could be described as "modern," although technological advances continue to be made in electric shaving.

Different Men, Different Beards

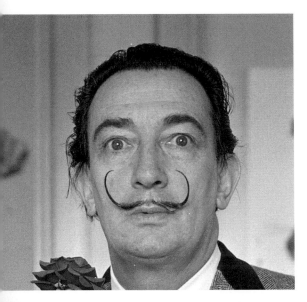

We only mention the gravity-defying twirled mustache for the sake of completeness. It cannot be considered as a serious option. The inimitable Salvador Dalí was himself the only person who could carry it off. Someone who wears a mustache of this kind usually wants to show that, like Dalí, he is an eccentric artist. But a real eccentric will rarely be satisfied with copying someone else's trademark.

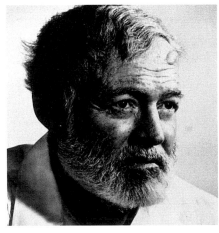

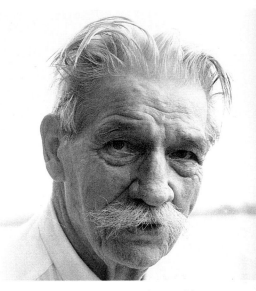

The well-kept full beard, like the one Ernest Hemingway wore, is a timeless classic. Most men try this style once, but very few indeed persevere with it. Most men get rid of their laboriously cultivated full beards because they do not have sufficient hair, the final growth looks too uneven, or the wearer notices that his beard makes him look rather too fierce.

Long, untamed mustaches are rarely met with amongst the style-conscious. They make a man look too wild. It needs the personality of someone like Albert Schweitzer to radiate a friendly aura with this kind of mustache. Few women like this type of mustache because it hides the mouth and is also a great nuisance when kissing.

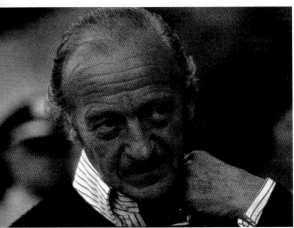

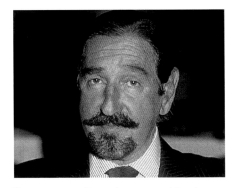

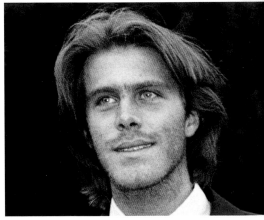

David Niven was one of the most famous men to wear a thin mustache. Someone who decides to wear a mustache like this must always be ready for comparisons with the elegant actor, or at least with the roles he took on. As David Niven usually played gentlemen of the British officer class, this mustache is probably unlikely to suit someone who tends to like dressing in jeans, a polo shirt, and loafers.

The appeal of a thin, clipped mustache derives from the reserved manliness it expresses on account of the quite thick hair growth needed to get a toothbrush mustache to take shape. Someone who wears a mustache of this type is signaling that, although he keeps to form superficially, a volcano is bubbling away underneath the surface.

For many years the goatee was considered unworthy of discussion by those interested in style, until it experienced a renaissance in 1990s youth culture. This beard was seen most seldom on the face of a gentleman. Don Jaime, a famous member of the Spanish Marbella set and the brother of Queen Fabiola (the widow of the Belgian King Baudouin), is a rare exception.

It has taken a long time for designer stubble to become respectable. It is too outrageous a violation of the normal convention that the only alternative to a beard or a mustache is a perfect shave. Even though it is widely found among the creative professions, it is still hard to imagine a London stockbroker or a senior judge with designer stubble. However, since even royal personalities, such as the Italian Prince Emanuele Filiberto of Savoy, are wearing designer stubble, it will possibly gain acceptance at some point.

Caring for Beards and Mustaches

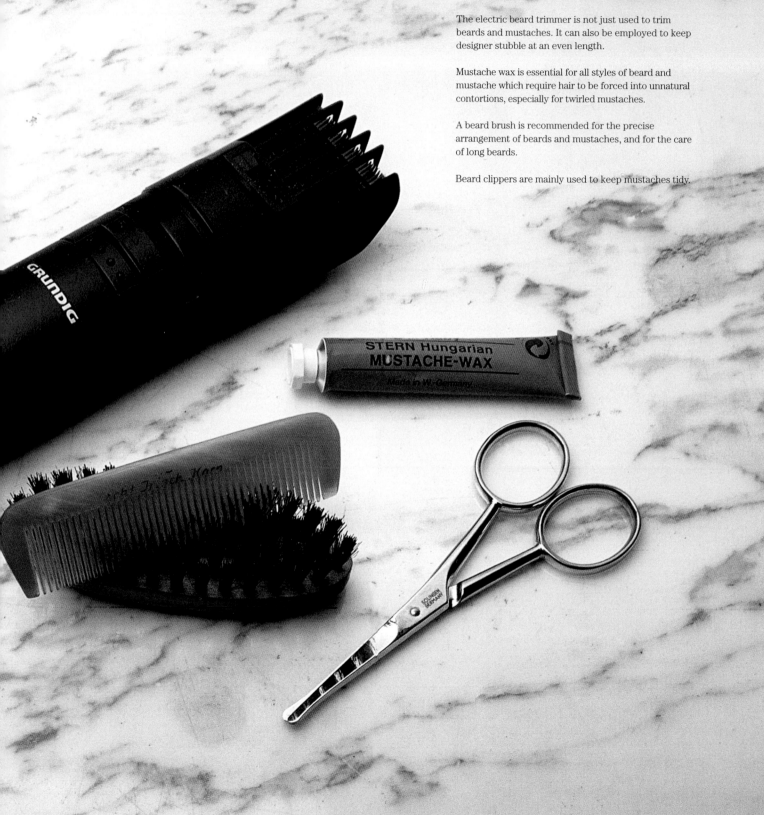

The electric beard trimmer is not just used to trim beards and mustaches. It can also be employed to keep designer stubble at an even length.

Mustache wax is essential for all styles of beard and mustache which require hair to be forced into unnatural contortions, especially for twirled mustaches.

A beard brush is recommended for the precise arrangement of beards and mustaches, and for the care of long beards.

Beard clippers are mainly used to keep mustaches tidy.

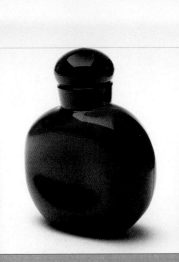

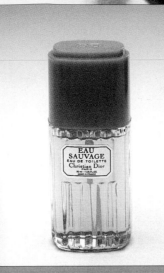

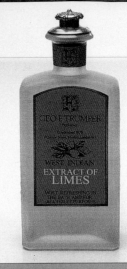

This legendary fragrance from the American designer Halston is still something of a secret outside the United States, probably on account of the fact that Halston has never been as well known in Europe as in his homeland. Halston has gone down in contemporary history, as well as the history of clothing, as the designer of one sensational little hat, Jackie Kennedy's famous pillbox, which she wore on the occasion of her husband's inauguration in 1961. This couturier, who is regarded as the "Yves Saint Laurent of America," has worked for houses as rich in tradition as Bergdorf & Goodman. *Halston Z-14* is a modern fragrance, but not modish. In consequence, it goes well with a wardrobe that places an emphasis on the modern without forcing tried and trusted classics into the background.

Eau Sauvage by Christian Dior is one of the great classic fragrances. If one were to compare this fragrance to a piece of clothing, it would be something like a Hermès necktie. Never controversial or out of place, it is accepted around the world. But, as so often, something that has proved its worth over the years strikes many as dull. Someone who is looking for a scent that will be more expressive of his own individuality is hardly likely to choose this popular veteran.

Someone who is suspicious of the large perfume shops may be most likely to develop a taste for Trumper's *Extract of Limes*. A typical English *eau de toilette*, it is not found on sale in perfumeries, but in old-established gentlemen's outfitters, where this refreshing lime scent is displayed alongside English shirts, neckties, and shoes. It goes best with clothes from the shirt-makers and tailors of Jermyn Street and Savile Row.

Timeless Fragrances

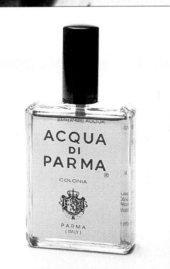

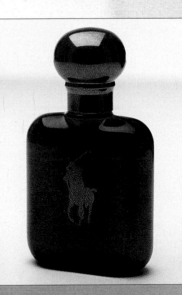

Acqua di Parma would probably have remained an exclusive niche product for ever if top-label designer Diego Della Valle had not adopted the fragrance. Together with Luca di Montezemolo, he bought the brand in 1994, and has helped this fragrance – made from a rose cultivated in Bulgaria, *Rosa damascena*, lavender, and rosemary – to wide popularity, though it caused distress to established customers who found their favorite secret dragged into the light of publicity.

As a fragrance is always sold by means of the design of its bottle and the name of its creator, *Polo* by Ralph Lauren is particularly popular amongst those enthusiastic for this brand. Someone who is not aware of Ralph Lauren will only choose the green bottle with the golden top by chance, but people who value this American designer's style will also appreciate his *eau de toilette*.

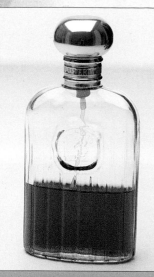

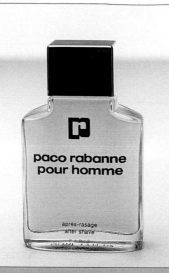

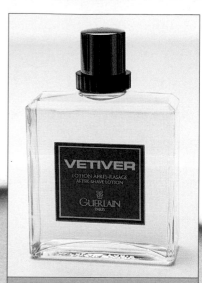

Giorgio of Beverly Hills sounds like a mixture of *La Dolce Vita* and Hollywood. Someone who likes neither the one nor the other will hardly take a liking to this perfume. It really is rather glamorous, and would be just as incongruous with a Citroën 2CV as with a T-shirt, jeans, and boat shoes. At the same time, with its top note of orange and bergamot, it is very refreshing, yet spicy, well suited to a film star's lifestyle.

It is in the Mediterranean countries, above all, that Paco Rabanne's fragrances are well known. They are comparatively rarely worn in central and northern Europe. The name alone seems to clash with a wardrobe of English clothes. With its fresh, spicy top note of bergamot and lavender, *Paco Rabanne pour Homme* really is better suited to the Promenade des Anglais in Nice than to London's Bond Street, though it still sells in England.

Vétiver by Guerlain is one of a large group of fragrances named after an oil extracted from the root of a tropical grass, *Vetiveria zizanioides*. Its sweet, earthy-woody aroma is found in the middle note of this classic perfume from the traditional house of Guerlain. Puig, Roger & Gallet, Lanvin, and Carven also make vetiver products, but the one produced by Guerlain is definitely the best-known example.

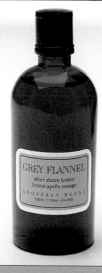

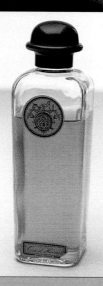

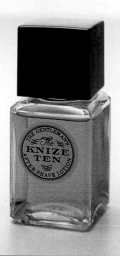

The name *Grey Flannel* would immediately conjure up a quite specific image in the mind of someone scanning the shelves of a perfumery. *Grey Flannel* sounds classical, serious, and refined. A product with a name like this is, one might say, going to be the complete opposite of a fragrance called *Denim*. Fortunately, this classic shows no sign of the fact that it came onto the market in 1976, in the middle of a decade not generally renowned for its timeless style. It goes best with a wardrobe organized along classical lines.

The idea of unisex fragrances is by no means new. In 1951 Edmond Roudnitska created *Eau d'Hermès*, a fresh, flowery scent for ladies and gentlemen. Someone who exudes a hint of *Eau d'Hermès* always scores points amongst perfume connoisseurs. Unlike the modern unisex fragrances of American origin, *Eau d'Hermès* is not for the *hoi polloi*.

Very few people are aware that Knize is, in fact, an illustrious Viennese gentlemen's outfitters, a name renowned throughout the world between the two world wars. Marlene Dietrich, for example, had her famous trousers made by Knize. Someone who uses *Knize Ten* breathes the fragrance of an institution of classic men's clothing, and exudes the scent of real high-class Viennese tailoring.

The Perfumer's ABC

Absolutes
Absolutes are pure, natural oils and extracts of flowers, as well as other vegetable materials. On account of the low yields obtained compared to the amount of raw material used, absolutes are extremely valuable and highly expensive.

Accords
An accord is a mixture of various aromas which produce a harmonious effect. An accord may consist of anything between two and a hundred aromas.

Basic Note
The basic note, or "fond," is the third odiferous element that we perceive in a composed fragrance. After the top note has faded away, we smell the middle note, or "bouquet," which then merges into the basic note. Typical basic notes in gentlemen's fragrances include musk *(Grey Flannel)*, oakmoss oil *(Eau Sauvage)*, ambergris, and vanilla *(Giorgio for Men)*.

Chypre
Chypre is the term for a group of fragrances that combine a fresh top note with a basic note of oakmoss oil, labdanum, and patchouli, to name the main components. Typical chypre fragrances are *Knize Ten*, *Giorgio for Men*, *Polo* by Ralph Lauren, and *Vétiver*

Citrus
Citrus is a fresh top note of bergamot oil, lemon, lime, and mandarin, orange, or bitter orange that is found in many men's fragrances, such as *Eau Sauvage*, *Lacoste*, or *Eau de Sport* by Paco Rabanne.

Eau de Cologne
Eau de Cologne is a solution of 3 to 5 percent perfume oil in a mixture of alcohol and water. *Eau de Cologne* is primarily intended to be refreshing, and consists mainly of citrus oils.

Eau de Parfum
Eau de parfum is a solution of 15 to 18 percent perfume oil in alcohol. It is more expensive than *eau de Cologne* or *eau de toilette* because it contains considerably more perfume oil.

Eau de Toilette
Eau de toilette is a solution of between 4 and 8 percent perfume oil in alcohol.

Fougère
"Fougère" (fern) is the term for a note made up of fresh herbal aromas, such as lavender, on a mossy base. Typical men's fragrances with this note include *Azzaro pour Homme*, *Paco Rabanne pour Homme*, and Dunhill's *Blend 30*.

Leather Notes
Leather notes are typical components of classic men's fragrances. A good example is the leather note in *Knize Ten* that consists of musk, moss, and ambergris.

Light
Fresh, fruity, green, and citrus-based aromas are described as "light." Light aromas are relatively volatile, and are therefore usually found in top notes.

Masculine
Dry notes – such as leather, tobacco, herbs, spices, mosses, and woods – are regarded as masculine. Men's fragrances are generally less floral than ladies' perfumes. In recent years men's fragrances and ladies' perfumes have become ever more similar, a trend that has culminated in unisex scents designed for men and women.

Oriental Notes
Oriental notes are reminiscent of the fragrances of the east. They are sweet, strong, and heavy. Typical men's fragrances with oriental notes include *Ho Hang* by Balenciaga, *KL Homme* by Lagerfeld, and *Open* by Roger & Gallet.

Perfume
The word is a corruption of the Latin *per fumum*, which means "through smoke." In the ancient world fragrant resins were burnt as sacrifices. Today a perfume is defined as a solution of 15 to 30 percent perfume oil in alcohol. Perfume is the most expensive type of scent because it contains the highest concentration of perfume oil.

Spice Notes
Many men's fragrances contain spice notes, such as marjoram, coriander, and pepper. Cinnamon is also popular, as in the middle note of *Santos* by Cartier.

Sweet
Vanilla is one well-known sweet aroma. It is found in the basic note of many men's fragrances, such as *Egoiste* by Chanel, *Men's Cologne* by Cardin, and *Patou pour Homme*.

Tobacco Notes
Tobacco notes are typical of men's fragrances. Apart from substances that mimic the smell of tobacco, use is also made of the aromas of materials employed to perfume tobacco products, such as plum and honey.

Top Note
The top note is the first olfactory impression one gains of a composed fragrance. It must arouse our interest as it is the first thing we perceive when testing. It consists principally of light, volatile aromas, but often contains hints of the middle note and the basic note as well (see entries under these headings).

Wood Notes
Cedarwood, patchouli, sandalwood, and vetiver are typical wood notes. Wood notes are found in many men's fragrances, such as *Davidoff*, *Knize Ten*, and *Halston Z-14*.

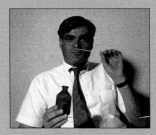

The French call a perfumer *le nez*, "the nose." Someone who wants to pursue this career really does need to have a good sense of smell. But it is even more important to have a feel for aromas: the ability to sense instinctively the associations sparked off by an aroma. This is a matter of "feel" and instinct. But this only places the perfumer in a position to predict, with a certain degree of probability, that a fragrance he composes will have a particular effect. He will never be 100 percent certain in this respect because the human olfactory organ is too idiosyncratic. Although this kind of feel for aromas is, in many ways, a talent, it also has to be trained and cultivated, just like every other talent. Even an experienced perfumer practices daily with a wide variety of aroma samples that he has to recognize and name. Only in this way can he maintain his comprehensive memory of odors, a memory in which he will have stored away up to 2,000 notes. He uses this living memory of smells to create ideas for new compositions, the complex make-up of which he is able to imagine in the same way that a musician can hear not just a melody in his inner ear, but its whole orchestration.

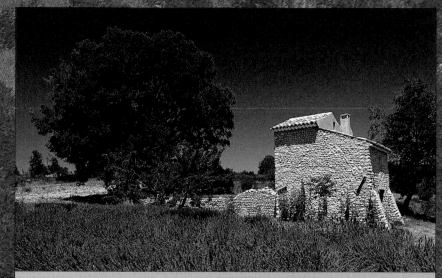

The south of France is generally considered to be the classic region where *Lavandula officinalis* is grown. However, the plant has not always been cultivated for the purpose of making perfumes. The ancient Persians, Greeks, and Romans knew lavender as a medicine, and burned lavender twigs in order to drive illness and malign humors out of sick rooms with smoke. Lavender was also popular as an ingredient in various medicinal drinks, and housewives still use small bundles of lavender flowers to keep moths out of clothes drawers today. Only at the end of the nineteenth century did the common view of lavender change, and its function as a fragrance moved into the foreground. Nevertheless, many people still believe in the various beneficial effects of this typical plant from the Mediterranean region. However, most of us think of lavender above all as an aroma familiar from *eaux de toilette*, perfumes, and soaps.

Provence is the home of many aromas. Here we find the flowers from which the great essences are obtained. The traditional procedure is "enfleurage," which is also known by the less flowery name of the "absorption process." In this process highly volatile and rapidly decomposing odiferous substances are bound in fat. The procedure is simple, but very time consuming. A glass tray is coated with a layer of tallow or lard about ⅛ inch (3 mm) thick, placed into a wooden frame, and covered thickly with heliotrope, hyacinth, jasmine, narcissus, reseda, rose, syringia, tuberose, or violet flowers. When the fat has absorbed all the flowers' odors, the exhausted flowers are replaced with new ones and the procedure is repeated until the fat is completely saturated with aromas. This fragrant pomade is kept for two to three weeks in pure ethyl alcohol, in which the odiferous principles dissolve. The end product is called an extract, or "extrait."

In another procedure linen or cotton sheets are soaked in olive oil, stretched out in wooden frames, and again covered with flowers. After the complete absorption of the odiferous substances, the perfumed oil is pressed out of the cloths. Oil obtained in this way is known as "huile antique."

Today simpler and less expensive extraction methods are more widespread. These involve placing flowers in carbon disulfide or petroleum ether. The final fragrance is obtained, dissolved in alcohol, by means of distillation. This method is more suitable for mass production.

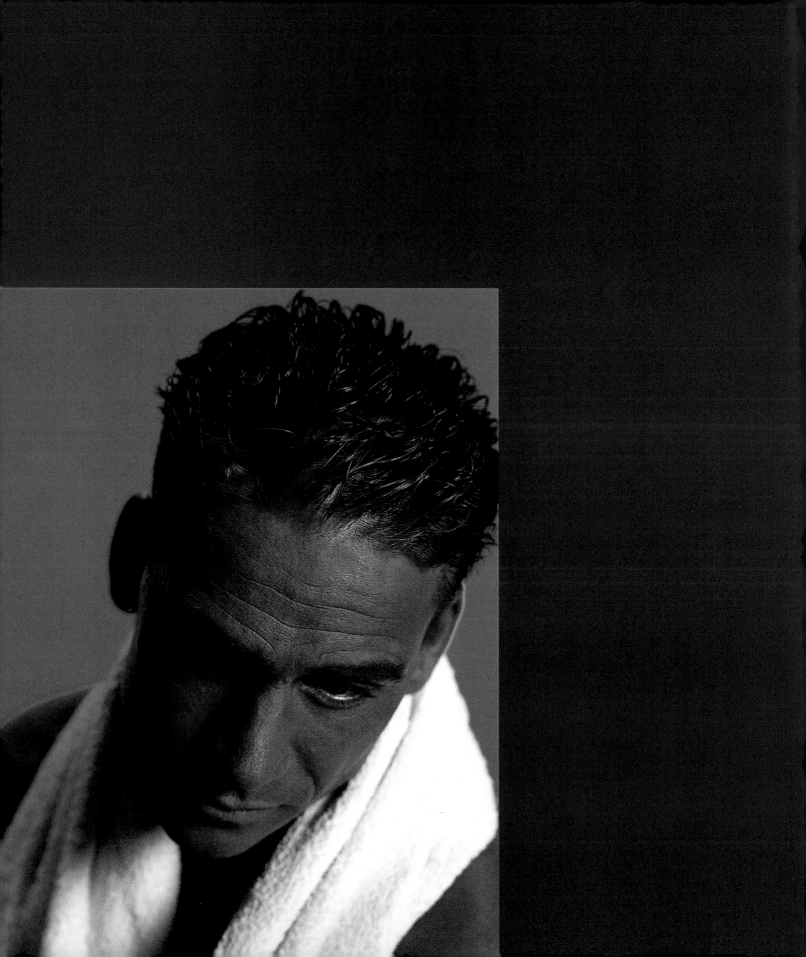

The Hair

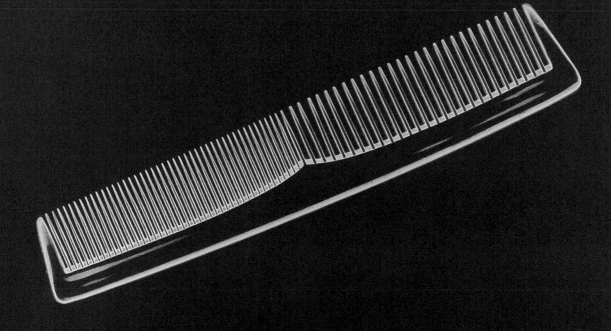

The Joys of Visiting the Hairdresser

The transition into adulthood often begins when a little boy, who is no longer quite so little, is finally allowed to take his place on the "real" chair at the hairdresser's. Somehow or other, as a young child he had always found it embarrassing when he had to sit on a construction that raised him up as he sat, or even a high seat.

Every man has memories like this, unless he is unfortunate enough to be one of those pitiable exceptions whose hair was cut at home by his mother. One can only feel sorry for these men because going to the hairdresser's has a quite particular appeal of its own – as long as it is a real gentlemen's hairdresser's, at any rate. No one forgets easily the unique smell of shaving water and shampoo, the yellowing advertisements for long defunct hair-care products, the hum of the trimmers, or the crackle from the inevitable portable radio.

One day a father takes his son with him for the first time. While his father's hair is cut, Junior takes the opportunity to have a good look at the other customers, who are chatting together, dozing, or reading the paper. He watches with excitement as the hairdresser styles his father's hair with practiced movements, snipping nonchalantly with his scissors. At some point the hairdresser removes the cape with a sweeping movement, and now it is the son's turn.

He feels the hairdresser hold him for the first time. His hair is pulled pretty hard during the preparatory combing, and he has to suppress his initial impulse to run away. Sometimes there are tears if the hairdresser cuts off too much of his hair. His father and the hairdresser stop him weeping by telling him rather ineffectually that his hair really will grow back again. At the end his image in the mirror looks remarkably strange. He runs his hand through his hair to give it its familiar shape and to take possession of it once more.

Despite the alarming nature of this experience, and the worry that the hairdresser might just cut his ear with his clippers, most little boys look forward eagerly to their next visit, probably because the passage of time does not worry us when we are children. For those of us who are older, every visit to the hairdresser tells us all too clearly that, yet again, a few more weeks, or even months, of our life have passed by, gone forever.

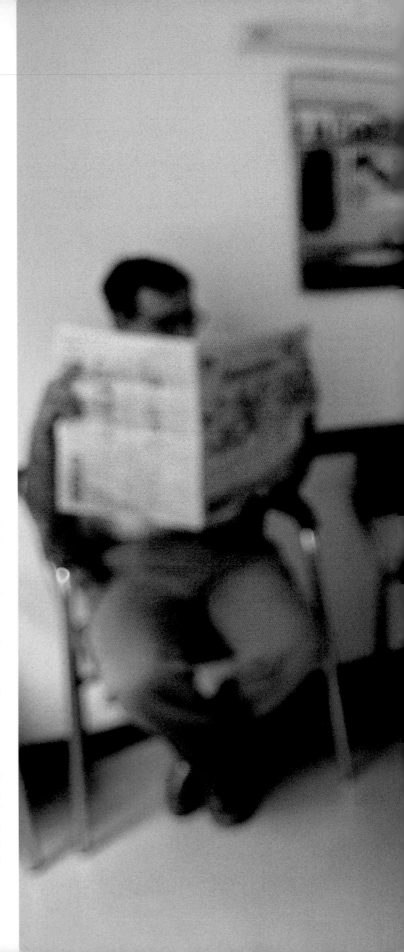

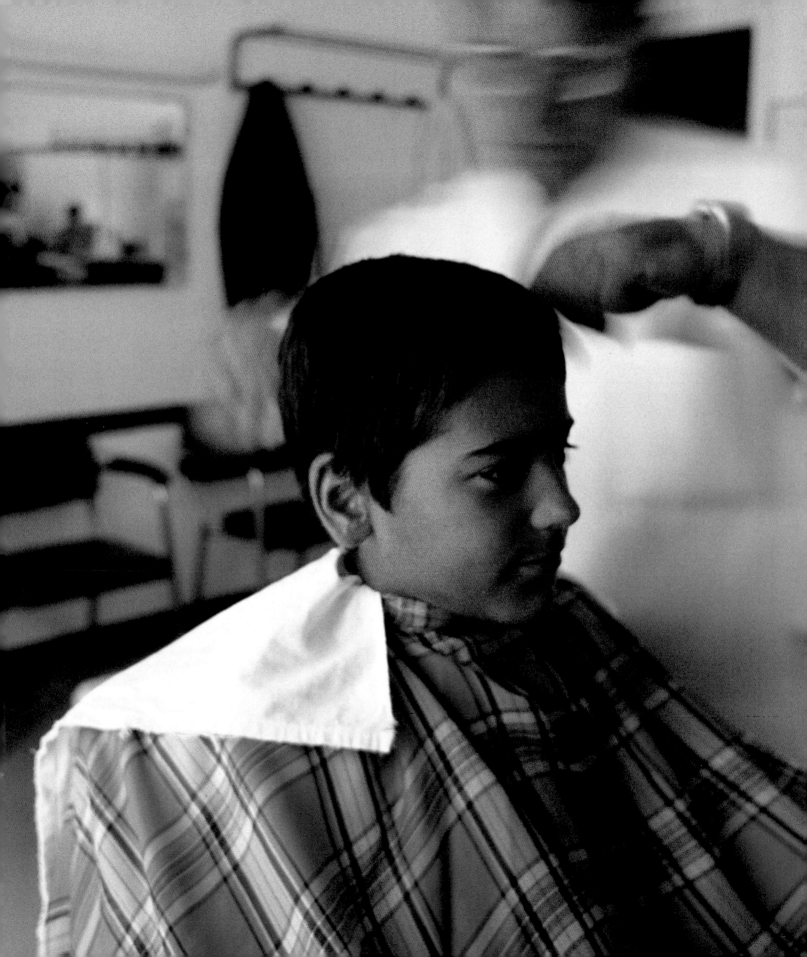

What Should I Put on My Hair?

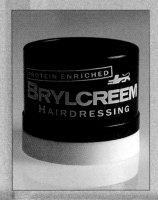

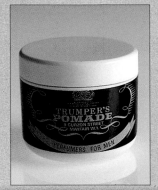

Hair creams, or *pomades*, consist mainly of fat, oil, and wax. Two classic products of this kind are Brylcreem (left), and Trumper's Pomade (right). They can be used to create the shiny Rudolph Valentino look, which is most effective on men with thick, wavy hair. Unlike hair gel, hair creams and pomades do not dry out the hair, though not everyone likes their greasy shine.

Brisk hair cream is just as well known, and trusted, in Germany as Brylcreem is in England and Brill cream in the US. The design of the tube was modernized a couple of years ago, but fortunately nothing was done to alter the perfume formula. As a result, it is not just the shine that gives away hair held in place by Brisk, but also the long-familiar fragrance.

The highly concentrated shampoo pastes made by D. R. Harris of London are truly classic hair-care products. They come in small plastic tubs with screw lids that do not take up too much room in travel luggage and practically never leak.

In consistency, *Brilliantine* is reminiscent of Vaseline. It is recommended for thicker hair and is particularly well suited to the task of taming curls that will not do as they are told. Brilliantine also has beneficial effects on dry scalps.

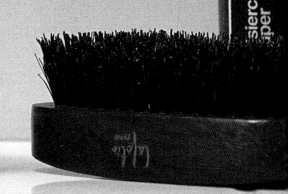

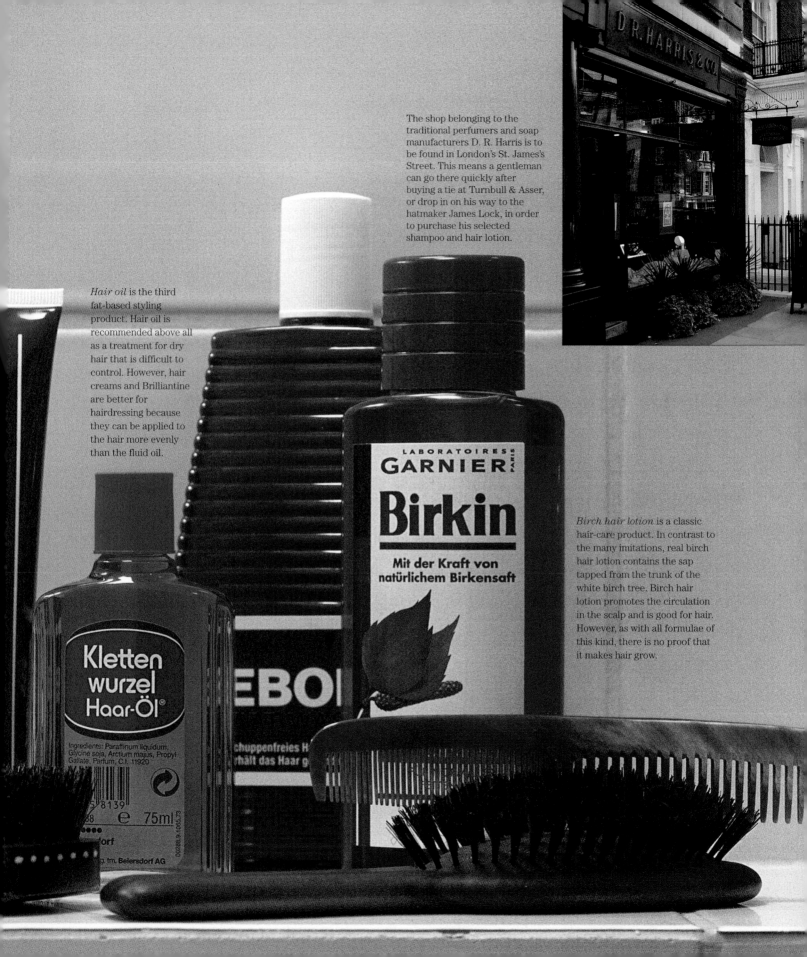

The shop belonging to the traditional perfumers and soap manufacturers D. R. Harris is to be found in London's St. James's Street. This means a gentleman can go there quickly after buying a tie at Turnbull & Asser, or drop in on his way to the hatmaker James Lock, in order to purchase his selected shampoo and hair lotion.

Hair oil is the third fat-based styling product. Hair oil is recommended above all as a treatment for dry hair that is difficult to control. However, hair creams and Brilliantine are better for hairdressing because they can be applied to the hair more evenly than the fluid oil.

Birch hair lotion is a classic hair-care product. In contrast to the many imitations, real birch hair lotion contains the sap tapped from the trunk of the white birch tree. Birch hair lotion promotes the circulation in the scalp and is good for hair. However, as with all formulae of this kind, there is no proof that it makes hair grow.

LABORATOIRES GARNIER PARIS
Birkin
Mit der Kraft von natürlichem Birkensaft

Kletten wurzel Haar-Öl®

Ingredients: Paraffinum liquidum, Glycine soja, Arctium majus, Propyl Gallate, Parfum, C.I. 11920

e 75ml

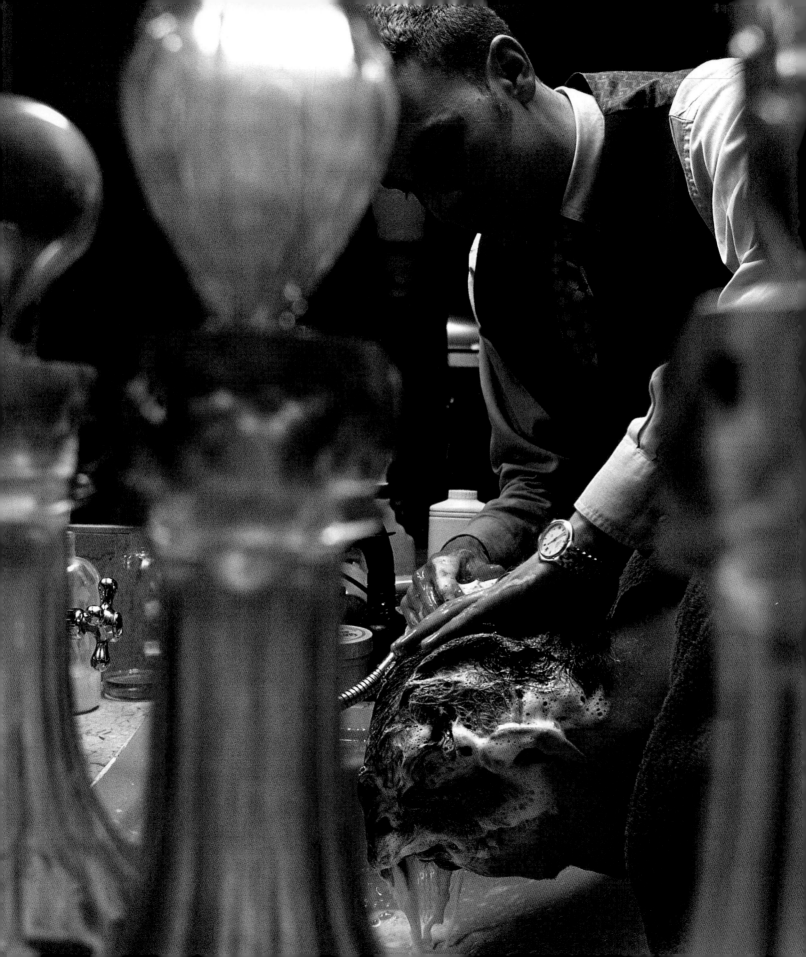

The Right Way to Wash Hair

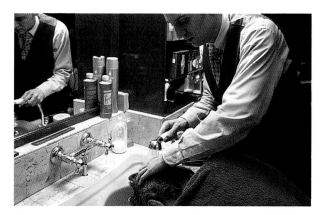

First of all, the hair is wetted thoroughly. Dirt that does not contain grease, such as dust and sand, is carefully rinsed out of the hair at this stage.

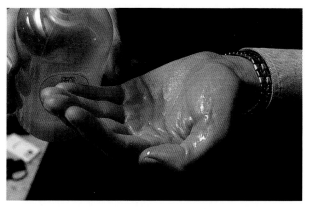

As little shampoo as possible is used. Otherwise, the hair swells up too much. The shampoo is first rubbed onto both palms so that it can be applied evenly.

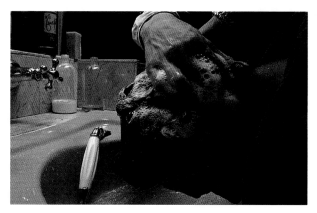

Now the shampoo is carefully massaged in with spread fingers, and not with the flats of the hands. The hair should not be rubbed too roughly when this is done.

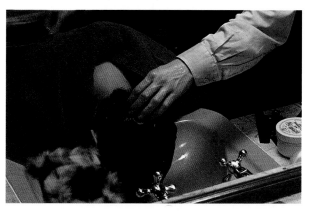

The shampoo must be rinsed out very thoroughly, best of all with lukewarm or cold water. This straightens the hair out. If the hair is particularly dirty or greasy, it may be washed a second time, though one wash is normally enough.

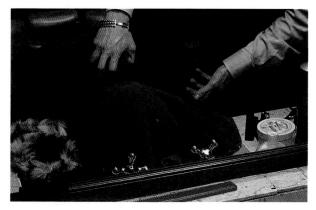

Excess water is pressed carefully out of the hair. Never rub! A hand towel wrapped round the head soaks up more moisture from the hair. If at all possible, the hair should be allowed to dry in the air.

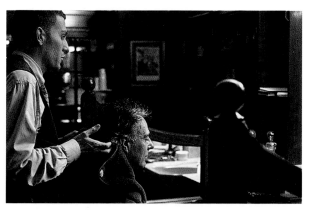

At Trumper's in London a hair wash can be crowned with a head massage. This relaxes the neck muscles, promotes the circulation in the scalp, and has a dangerously sleep-inducing effect.

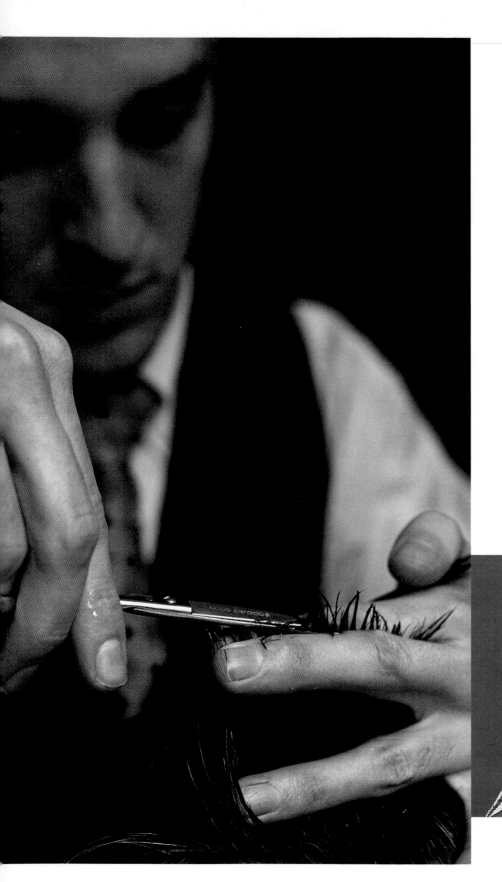

Hairstyles with Character

Until the 1960s the short-back-and-sides was the basic haircut of the twentieth century. The overwhelming majority of men still have their hair cut along these lines. However, men have always worn long hair as well. During the 1960s it was still a sign of protest at, and liberation from, the bourgeois narrow-mindedness of the late 1950s, but by the 1970s long hair had become established as a stylistically acceptable alternative. Nowadays it is regarded throughout the western world as quite normal for men to wear their hair long, even outside the creative professions. This does not mean that the short-back-and-sides has had its day, but it is no longer the only proper haircut for a man, even if it is still the dominant style in conservative circles. Among the young, short hair is once again very fashionable, and it is older men who today tend to have the longer hair.

Short sharp shock: the short-back-and-sides

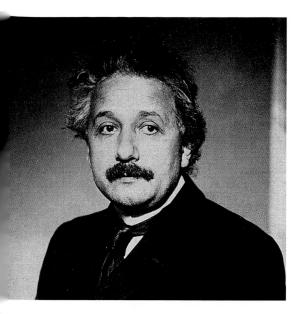

The Genius

Can anyone imagine Albert Einstein with a crew cut, the close crop worn by American GIs? Hardly. The great physicist's tangled, curly hair is the absolutely classic haircut for geniuses, poets, thinkers, and artists, as well as anyone who thinks he belongs in this group. Conductors also love similar manes of hair, which may lie tamely on their heads at the beginning of a concert, but are flying in all directions by the end of the first movement, at the latest.

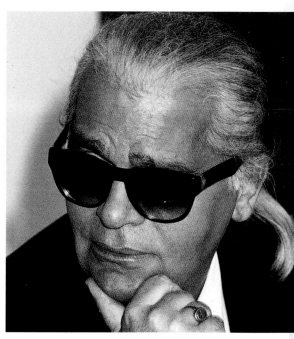

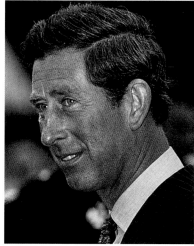

The Aristocrat

This style is the classic among men's haircuts: longer hair on top, no layering, the ears uncovered, and short hair on the nape. Someone who wears his hair this way will always look well groomed, even if no one is going to take him for an art director, architect, or filmmaker. He is more likely to be taken for a lawyer, banker, or stockbroker, which is not really so bad if that is the job one does.

The Dandy

The development of the pony tail has been most interesting. In the 1960s it was still a real rarity, and no one with a pony tail would have dreamed of applying for a job in a bank. Doing so might still be a bit daring nowadays, but it is no longer unthinkable. The men's pony tail, such as the one worn by Karl Lagerfeld, is also remarkable in so far as it is worn by people in spheres that are not just quite different from each other, but quite antagonistic; the athletic doorman of a night club wears a pony tail, but so do the environmentally conscious music student and the pleasure-seeking millionaire's kid. Nevertheless, it is still difficult to imagine a president or a king wearing a pony tail (for the moment, at least).

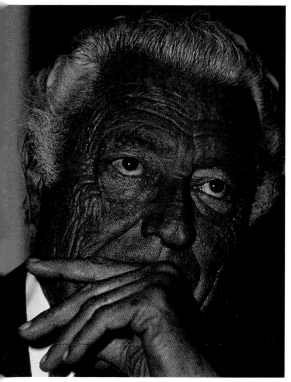

The Italian Look

A man with dark, curly hair can carry off this classic southern European look. It loses none of its attractiveness with increasing age and slowly graying hair, as Fiat boss Gianni Agnelli demonstrates.

The Eternal Youth

His hair is always tousled, falls into his eyes, and is constantly being thrown back with a short movement of the head. This habit just goes with the classic boyish look. Someone who wears a "hairstyle" of this kind has no wish to worry overly much about his hair. Someone like David Hockney, who still looks as if he just arrived home from school, is an example. This haircut looks particularly timeless on men with light hair, since it is just as effective on someone with blond hair as on someone who is graying.

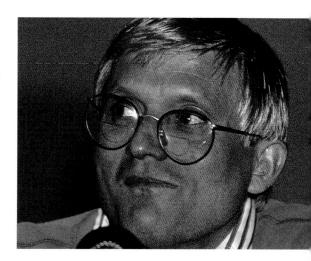

The Toupee: For and Against

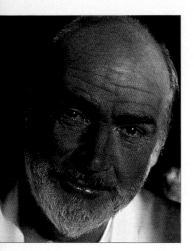

To be bald, or not to be bald? That is the question, for many men. Whether it is nobler in the mind to confess he is thinning on top, or to cover his nakedness with a hairpiece instead, is something that every balding man has to decide for himself. When making this choice, it has to be taken into consideration that not having a full head of hair is a far lesser defect than being badly dressed – and for that matter it is also usually easy to spot a toupee in the kind of situations in which no clothes are worn.

So what is all the fuss about? What most men are interested in are women, and how to impress them. The majority of women may love nice hair, but what is the use of nice hair if the man on whom it grows is a dull, humorless individual? A thick head of hair can never be a replacement for charm. Charm, by contrast, can make up for almost any other defect. Combined with the right wardrobe, charm is completely irresistible.

Someone who counters this by pointing out that even Sean Connery wears a toupee should be reminded that Connery has done this mainly for his film parts. As it happened, Ian Fleming imagined James Bond as a man with hair, so the actor had no choice but to turn up for filming in a toupee. When his roles have permitted it, Sean Connery has appeared bare headed, for example, as the monk William of Baskerville in *The Name of the Rose*. His effect on his female admirers has not been damaged by this in the least.

The only sensible reason for wearing a hairpiece is the protection it offers against the cold. However, a hat or a cap is often a better alternative. It is not for nothing that head coverings are often found on a bald head.

So, instead of pondering over a replacement for our missing hair, we would do better to put our minds to how we can make ourselves more attractive to those around us in different ways. In other words: hair, or the lack of it, is not crucial – no one notices that an interesting, amusing man has no hair. This is true of Sean Connery, just as it is for all of us mere mortals. It is up to us to compensate for this perceived defect by turning on the charm.

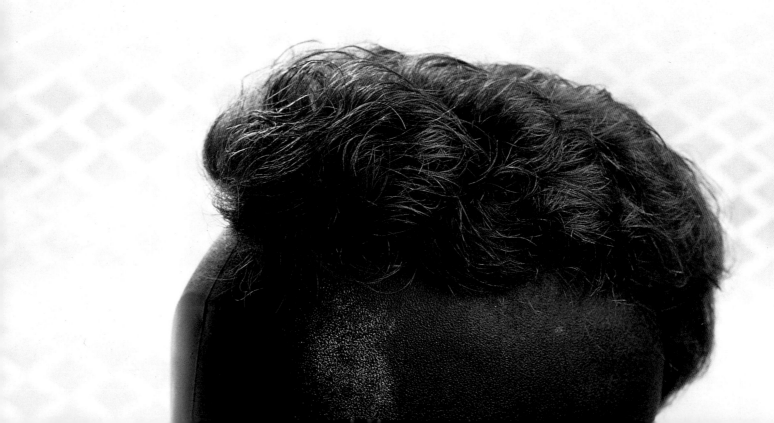

The Fake Hair of the Stars

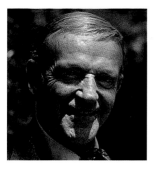

Fred Astaire was only ever seen in his films wearing a toupee. In his private life the dancer often chose to cover his head with a hat or a cap.

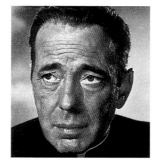

Humphrey Bogart was never once seen in a film without anything on top. In private, though, he showed his bald head without the slightest embarrassment.

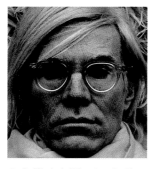

Andy Warhol did not make the least attempt to make his false hair look real. He was not at all worried that his own dark hair could be seen under his silvery-white wig.

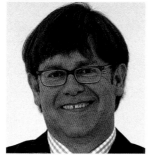

In his early career Elton John distracted attention from his diminishing head of hair with his extravagant glasses. Only his hairdresser can explain why he suddenly has such a lot of it again.

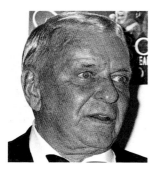

When his hair started to fall out, Frank Sinatra adopted a modest short haircut, from which his next move, to a toupee, was hardly a big step.

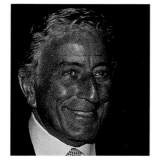

When someone's hair is visibly receding at the temples, but is still conspicuously full on top, as with Tony Bennett, one might almost conclude that he is wearing a toupee.

Chest Hair

Someone who takes care of his appearance often treads a thin line between too much and too little. Some people say that a man should remove his body hair because he also cuts the hair on his head and face, and manicures his nails. Others regard a haircut, shave, and manicure as the normal minimum of body care, but see the removal of body hair as the expression of an excessive desire to

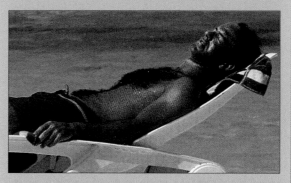

control the way one looks – which, like plastic surgery for purely cosmetic purposes, is to be rejected out of hand.

In Europe there is a tendency to let nature take its course. The traditional English aristocrat would be as unlikely to dream of having his son's flapping ears pinned back as a man from southern Europe to consider doing something to get rid of the vigorously sprouting hair on his chest, back, and legs. It will probably be a while before Italian sun worshippers are able to imagine themselves without their furry chests.

The proponents of body-hair removal mostly come from the United States, where people use ingenious cosmetic methods to modify their appearance and battle against mortality with exercise and diets. However, just the thought of going through the painful process of having their hair removed is disagreeable to many men. In addition, the costs outweigh the benefits, and it is anything but certain that the ladies really do prefer a smooth chest.

Maybe we should simply accept the way we are, instead of wishing for things we do not have. This is true of the hair on our heads, and it should also be true of our chest hair and the other natural hairs on our bodies.

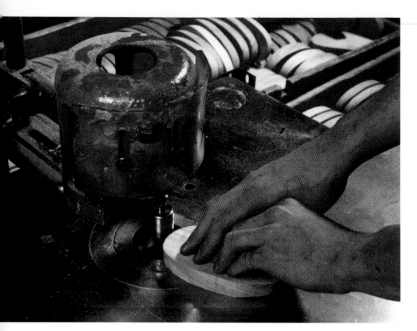

G. B. Kent & Sons still make most of their famous brushes by hand. As a result, the company's products are highly expensive, but also very long lasting.

The Royal Hairbrush

Since 1777 ladies and gentlemen have been able to depend on the brushes made by the company G. B. Kent & Sons when they want to tidy, and look after, their hair. When this company was founded over 220 years ago, no one can have had any idea that Kent would today enjoy a universal reputation as the producer of the best hairbrushes in the world. The company's product range also includes clothes brushes, toothbrushes, combs, and shaving brushes.

Of course, there are also other very good brushmakers, but none of them is as famous as Kent. This is due partly to the Kent brushes' outstanding quality, but also partly to the fact that an English officer and his lady wife would pack Kent brushes in their luggage when they set out to serve the Crown in some distant part of the British Empire. In consequence, Kent brushes began to find their way around the globe long before the company built up a distribution network. Not

only that, Kent products carry the Royal Warrant, the symbol of a company that supplies the British Royal Family and a quality mark that promotes sales in the United Kingdom and elsewhere.

A good hairbrush has three functions. Firstly, it smoothes and untangles the hair gently, thanks to the wild-boar bristles with which it is made. Unlike plastic and metal bristles, wild-boar bristles do not damage human hair because they are themselves hair, a substance related to horn. There are various grades of brush, ranging from soft to hard, for different types of hair. Secondly, brushing the hair cleans it thoroughly of dust, dirt, and dandruff. The third function of the hairbrush is to keep hair looking good by distributing the natural fats that accumulate at the roots all the way along to the hair ends. This natural fat does an excellent job of protecting hair and keeping it healthy. It gives it a good shine and stops the ends from splitting too easily. This aspect is particularly important for men with flowing manes of hair. Since most people now wash their hair every day, the cleansing function is not so important as it once was. Nevertheless every hair on your head will be thankful if it is cared for with a high-quality brush. Not for nothing does the New York doctor and hairdresser Dr. George Michael recommend the purchase of a really good hairbrush in his book *Complete Hair Care for Men*.

The Military Oval is the ideal men's brush: an oval-shaped model without a handle. It is available in various bristle strengths for differing thicknesses of hair. The manufacture of the brushes is very costly, and the classic wild-boar bristle models are still made by hand.

This is done by one of two manufacturing methods. The first is called long-holing. This involves tiny horizontal channels being drilled lengthwise into the back of the brush, and thin wires drawn through them. Next, vertical holes are drilled into the brush from above, and the individual bundles of bristles are inserted and wound around the wires. Brushes produced in this way are very durable and can also be repaired with new bristles.

The second method is facing, in which a horizontal slice, the "face," is cut off the back of the brush. Holes for the bristles are drilled into the face. The bristles are drawn through the holes and wound round tin or silver wires. Finally the face into which the bristles have been inserted is fitted onto the underside of the brush back and fastened firmly.

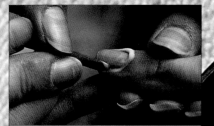

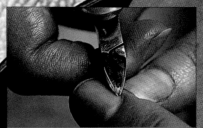

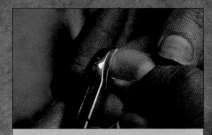

The next stage is to push back the cuticles carefully with a special rosewood stick. The cuticle must never be damaged or removed completely because it protects the nail bed. It is therefore advisable to be particularly careful when doing this.

Any particles of cuticle that remain are removed with special clippers. This also has to be done with great care in order to avoid injuries.

If the nails have become very long, they are first shortened with clippers before the actual manicure is carried out.

The Manicure

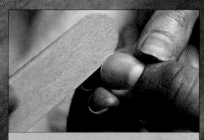

The nails are then filed precisely into shape, first with a coarse file, then a finer one. Men's nails should be semicircular. The customer decides on the length.

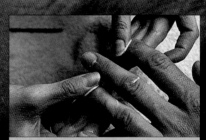

The nails are polished to finish off the manicure. However, this is not compulsory.

The finger tips are immersed in mild soapy water. This makes it easier to clean the nails and also softens the cuticles so that they can be pushed back much more easily.

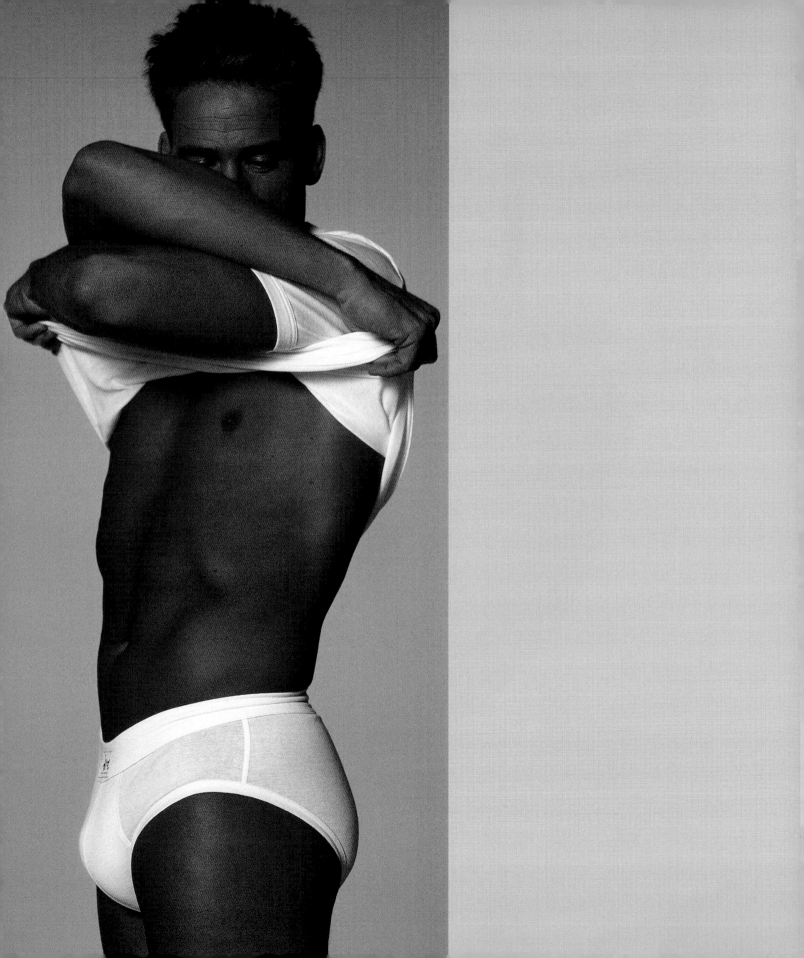

Underwear

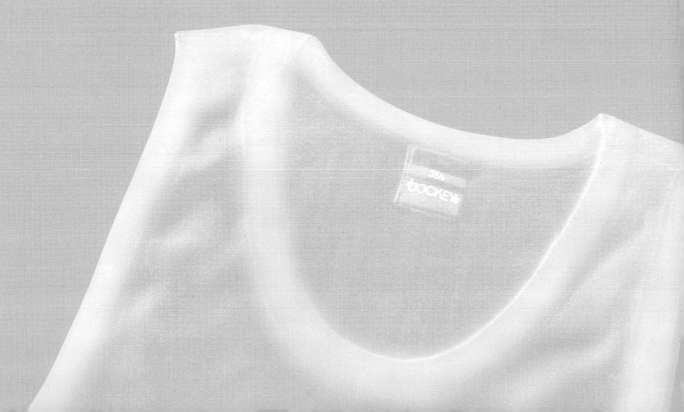

The Most Important Question of All

We begin our discussion of men's clothing with underwear. This is on account of the sequence in which we dress ourselves in the morning, not the chronology of clothing history. It was only in the 1930s that the basic forms of underwear now worn every day finally took shape. It is true that we know about precursors of modern underwear worn in Egypt at the time of the Pharaohs. However, it is difficult to identify these archaeological finds absolutely conclusively as underwear. We may interpret a linen cloth intended to be slung around the hips as an early form of our underpants, but it might also be a piece of outer clothing. It might even be nothing more than a piece of linen. The underpants of the Middle Ages were rather closer to the modern article. These were more or less tightly fitting garments of varying lengths with an opening at the rear, which must certainly have been a practical feature. Only the prosperous could afford the luxury of underclothes of this type. Indeed, underpants for men only became widespread during the third decade of the nineteenth century, when industrial manufacturing first made it possible for the broad masses to afford them. With this development, underclothing finally lost its air of exclusiveness. Style is no longer a matter of whether one wears underwear or not, or the frequency with which it is changed, but is linked to the selection of the right product. This is not difficult since – despite all the variety in this field – only a few designs may be said to enjoy classic status. By "underwear" we mean underpants above all else. The undershirt is becoming less and less significant now that modern men change their shirts once a day, and sometimes more often when necessary. If need be, the undershirt still has a role to play in very hot or very cold climates because, on the one hand, it is warm, and, on the other, it absorbs excess perspiration before it reaches the outer shirt. However, if undershirts do not come to be worn as outer garments – as is the case, for example, with the T-shirt – they will basically become redundant. The same cannot be said of underpants, which men can now buy in the shape of either briefs, with or without a fly, or boxer shorts. The main advantage of briefs is that they give more support and do not ride up, even if you are wearing very light trousers. This is quite likely to happen with boxer shorts if they are worn under extremely light material. Nevertheless, the choice between briefs and boxer shorts is mostly made on the basis of instinct. Even though boxer shorts were very much in fashion during the 1980s, those who are keen on briefs did not allow themselves to be distracted for long. At the same time, someone who enjoys the freedom of boxer shorts will always find the support offered by a pair of briefs restrictive. In actual fact, boxer shorts do have one very real advantage: they can be made to measure. The real joy of custom-made boxer shorts is the opportunity they offer to take one's pick from the whole selection of fabrics held by a well-stocked shirt maker. Stripes, checks, the most various colors and materials, whatever your desire may be, it can be made into boxer shorts, by hand, and guaranteed to fit. However, it is doubtful whether even this would tempt a confirmed briefs wearer to abandon his underwear of choice.

In his book *From A to B & Back Again: The Philosophy of Andy Warhol*, the American artist, who was a dedicated shopper, described in the most elaborate detail how he purchased underpants in the New York department store Macy's: "I quickly found the brand I usually use, Jockey Classic Briefs. They were three for five dollars which didn't seem too inflationary. I read the label on the plastic bag they came in, just to make sure they hadn't changed any of their famous 'Comfort Features' – 'Exclusive Tailoring for Proper Fit to Support a Man's Needs; Contoured Designed Arch Gives Added Comfort No Gaps; Support Waistband is Smoother Fitted Heat Resistant; Stronger Longer Lasting V No Chafe Leg Openings; Soft Rubber at Either Thigh Only; Highly Absorbent 100 Per Cent Highly Combed Cotton.' So far so good, I thought. I checked the 'Washing Instructions' – 'Machine Wash Tumble Dry.' Everything was fine, the same as always. I hate it when you find a product you like that fits a particular need of yours, and then they change it. [...] At least the Jockey Classic Briefs were still Classic." A couple of pages later we learn that Andy Warhol was not always able to afford Jockey briefs: "I used to buy my underwear at Woolworth's so I have a sentimental attachment to it."

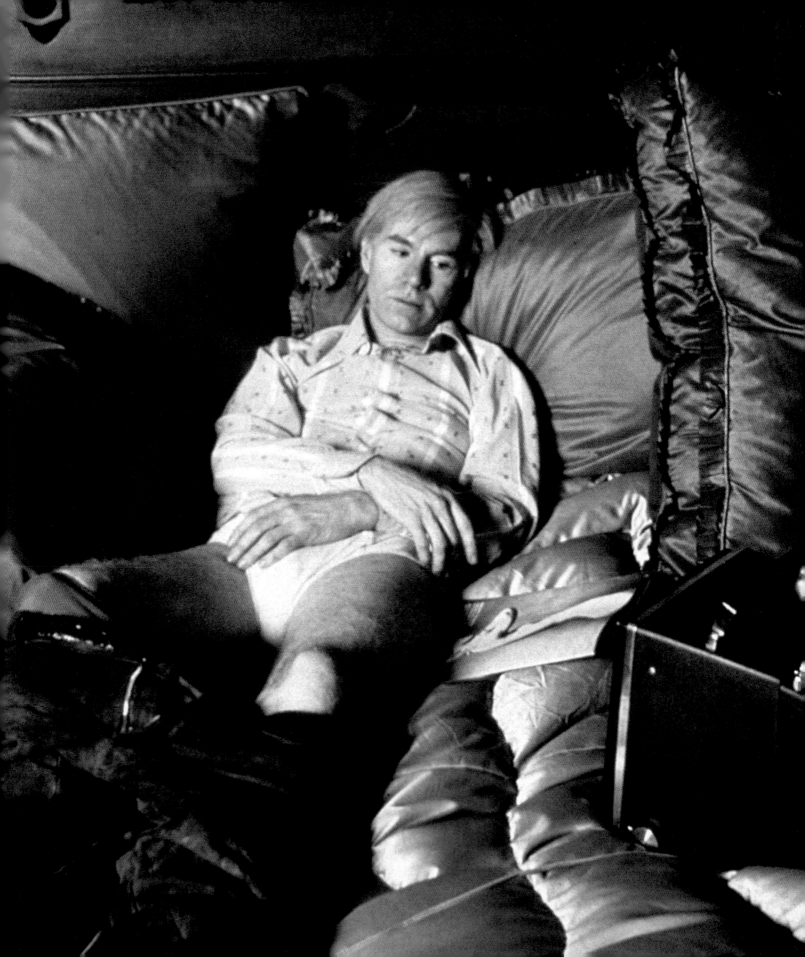

Variations Underneath

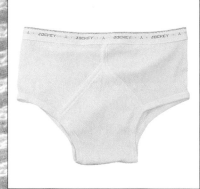

The original Jockey with a Y-shaped front panel. It is available in various grades of material. This model made of 100 percent cotton is a classic design.

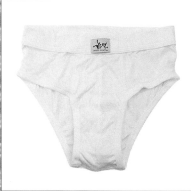

Although Y-fronts offer a superb fit, many men regard the fly as superfluous. For them Jockey make various closed forms, such as Poco Briefs, which give support without the fly.

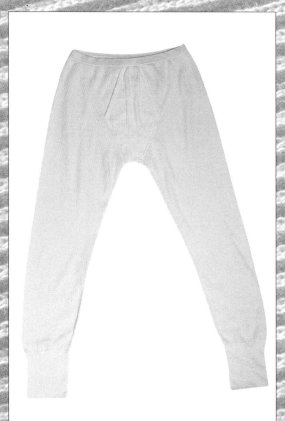

If you spend a lot of time out of doors during the cold part of the year you will certainly appreciate the advantages of long johns, which may not be particularly becoming.

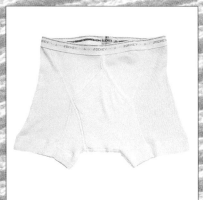

Medium-length underpants are a compromise between boxer shorts and briefs. The advantage of these over boxer shorts is the superior support offered.

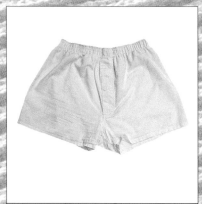

Boxer shorts are the classic alternative to briefs. Only a few men like both types of underpants equally. The supporters of one type of underwear usually have a strong dislike of the other design, and usually make this very clear.

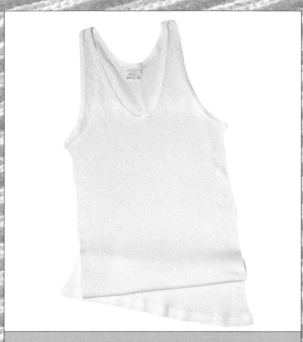

String underwear has the advantage that it is warm in cold weather and cool when it is hot, due to the air chambers that form in the mesh structure of the fabric. The string undershirt is certainly a classic. It was supposedly invented in 1933 by a Norwegian Army commander called Henrik Brun. According to the legend, he sewed himself the first set of string underwear out of old fishermen's nets.

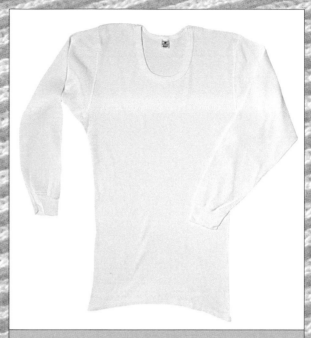

The long-sleeved undershirt serves the same purpose as long johns, that of keeping out the cold. Care should be taken that the sleeves of the undershirt do not protrude from the shirt cuffs in an unsightly manner.

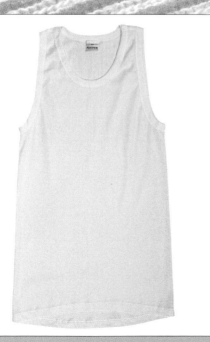

For years the sleeveless undershirt was the very quintessence of unsightly men's underwear. However, in recent years it has seen a revival as streetwear. Whether it will still be worn as an undershirt 50 years from now is doubtful.

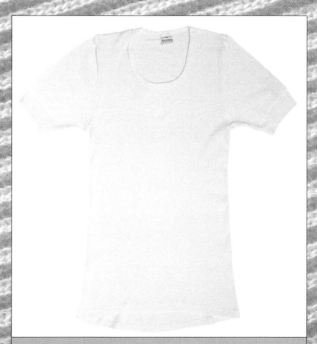

An undershirt with a rather lower, rounded neckline is a good compromise between a sleeveless undershirt and a T-shirt. Its generous cut also means that this undershirt cannot be seen if you wear your collar open.

A Fly-Away Success

The Cooper company was founded in Kenosha (Wisconsin) by a German-American in 1886. In 1934, 48 years later, Cooper introduced a revolutionary new product onto the underwear market under the Jockey brand name. The design was inspired by the short bathing trunks worn on the French Riviera, but what was most innovative about it was the front panel cut in the shape of an upside-down Y. This "Y-front" was extremely comfortable, offering a perfect fit and unprecedented support. The Jockey brand began its unstoppable rise with this patented design. The first licenses were awarded to companies in England, Australia, and Switzerland as early as 1936. Today there are over 120 license holders around the world, and innumerable other manufacturers who try to copy the famous design. This alone does not account for the success of Jockey. It is above all the outstanding quality of the tailoring that puts the original briefs in a class of their own. For example, the elastic band worked into the leg opening only goes round the outside of the upper thigh, which means that it does not restrict the wearer's blood circulation. The massive success of the close-fitting Jockey underpants also has had an influence on our other clothes. The tight fit of the new men's underwear made it possible to cut pants closer in the crotch. Fashionable pants began to cling ever more tightly to anatomies now restrained by Jockey briefs. However, the more spacious waist-pleat trousers were rediscovered when boxer shorts came into fashion again in the 1980s. In any event, with their love of tradition, the tailors of Savile Row have never warmed to men's briefs. They still prefer to cut suit pants with sufficient room for baggy boxer shorts, and their contents.

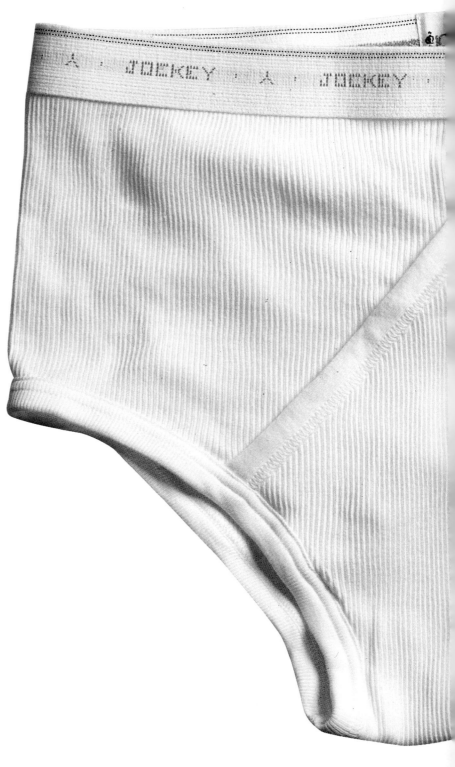

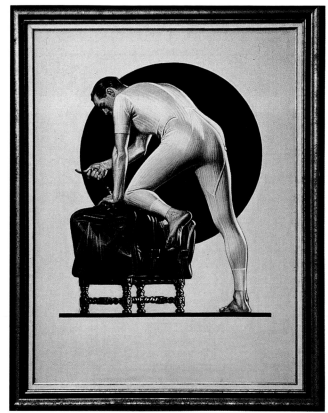

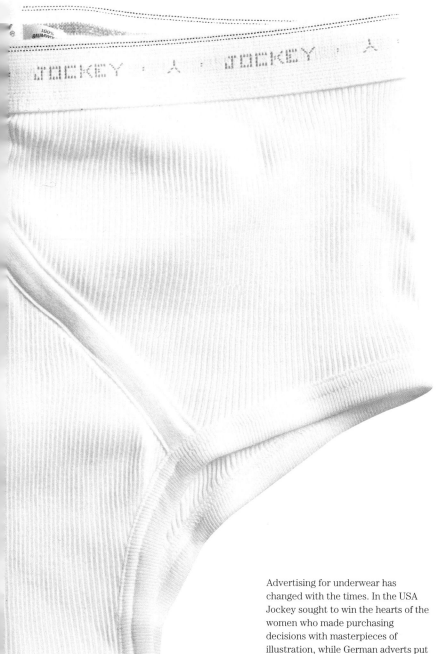

Advertising for underwear has changed with the times. In the USA Jockey sought to win the hearts of the women who made purchasing decisions with masterpieces of illustration, while German adverts put forward purely technical arguments. This lack of emotion in underwear advertising probably explains why German men still spend so little money on these essential garments.

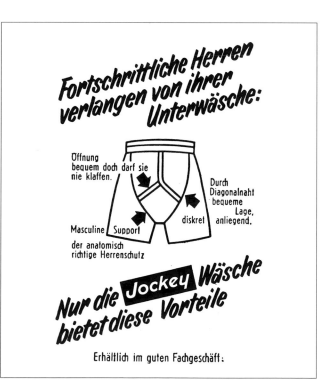

Fortschrittliche Herren verlangen von ihrer Unterwäsche:

Öffnung bequem doch darf sie nie klaffen.

Durch Diagonalnaht bequeme Lage, diskret anliegend.

Masculine Support der anatomisch richtige Herrenschutz

Nur die Jockey Wäsche bietet diese Vorteile

Erhältlich im guten Fachgeschäft:

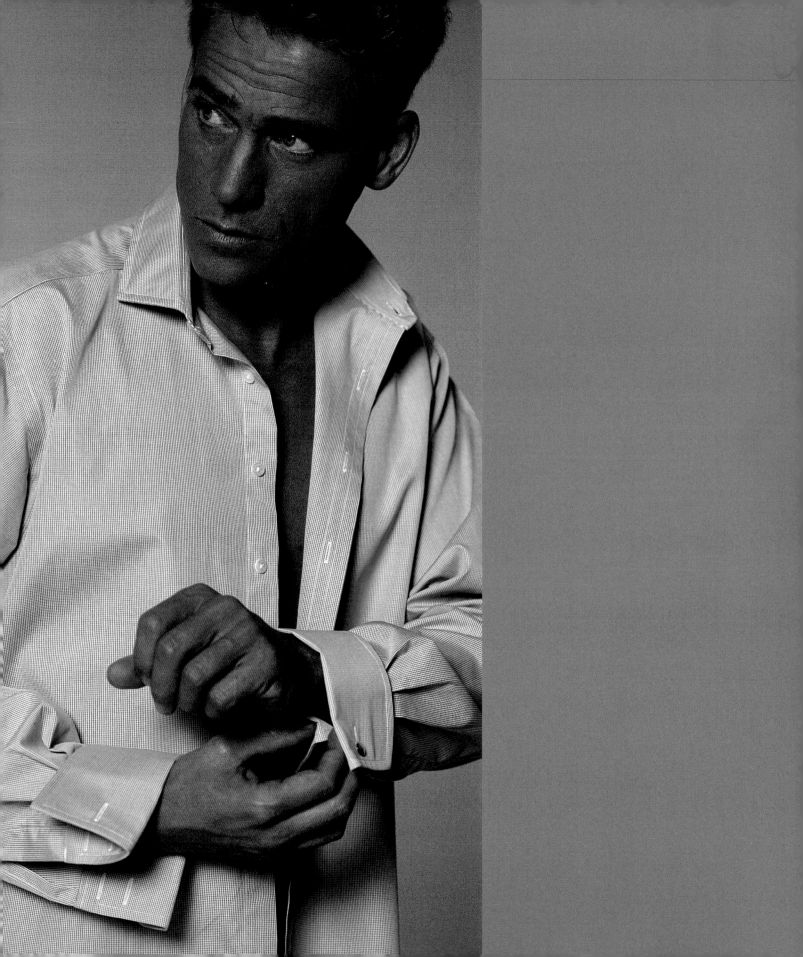

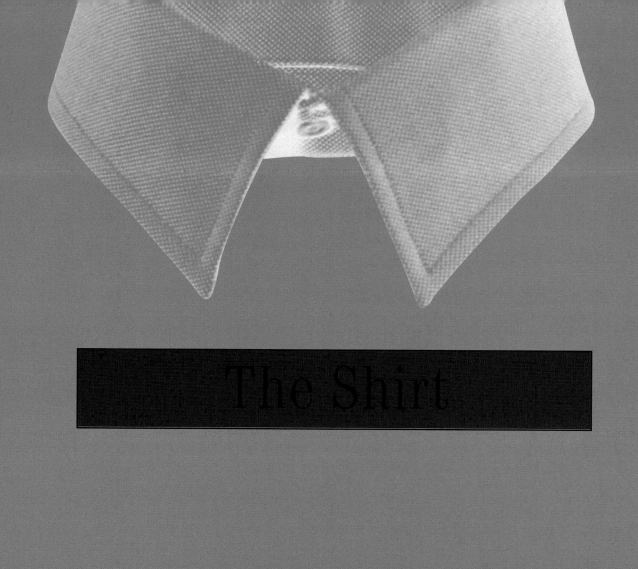

The Shirt

A Gentleman's Shirt

The modern men's shirt has a long history, though its present form began to take shape only at the end of the nineteenth century. In 1871 Brown, Davis & Co. of Aldermanbury registered the first shirt with buttons all the way down the breast. Till then people just pulled shirts on and off over their heads. By this time, though, the shirt had already been established as a piece of outer clothing for a long time. Until the eighteenth century the shirt was worn under the outer garments and was only visible at the collar. As a result, it was originally regarded as underclothing and, to this day, the shirt has not been able to shake off associations with its real roots. Indeed, it is still regarded as a *faux pas* for a man to take off his jacket uninvited, especially in the presence of ladies.

This rule may appear outdated to many people, but if we recall that our modern overshirt was once a piece of underclothing, we will understand how this convention came to exist. It is still as deeply rooted in the collective consciousness as ever, in the western world, at least. An official ceremony at which kings, presidents, and prime ministers appeared in shirt sleeves would be unthinkable.

Until the end of the nineteenth century the white shirt was the epitome of elegance. Only someone with enough money to have his shirts washed frequently, and enough of them to change regularly as well, could afford to wear white shirts. Since the cleanliness of a white shirt would be polluted by any form of work, only a gentleman could wear one – that is to say, a nobleman or wealthy commoner who lived on the fruits of his wealth. Striped shirts only came into fashion towards the end of the nineteenth century, but it was a struggle before they were accepted as part of the city business suit of the time. Patterned shirts always raised the suspicion that they were worn in order to conceal a lack of cleanliness. By way of a compromise, colorful shirts were equipped with white collars and cuffs. These combinations of patterned material with a white collar are still very popular today, though they never have the serious air of a plain white shirt.

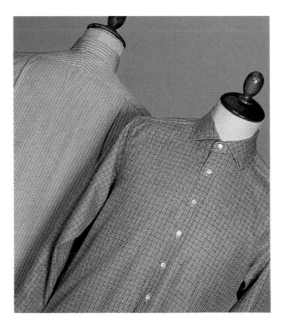

The collar design is one of the essential features defining the style of every shirt. The collars of the early shirts were cut in various ways. The fundamental distinction is that between the stand-up collar and the turndown collar.

Up to the end of the nineteenth century various versions of the stand-up collar held sway, with the size of the necktie determining the width of the collar. The stand-up collar was gradually supplanted by the turndown collar, and since the 1930s the stand-up collar has only been worn with tuxedos and tailcoats. Detachable versions of both the stand-up collar and the turndown collar were also available. They had the advantage that the collar could be washed every day, while the rest of the shirt was spared this treatment. Someone who was in a position to have his shirts washed every day did not need to resort to this expedient, but the detachable collar did offer another advantage in that the shape of the collar could be varied, and this made it possible to suggest that one owned a variety of different shirts without actually having to buy new ones all the time. All the same, the advantages were outweighed by the disadvantages: for example, the laborious task of buttoning on the collar, and the frantic search for the collar button every morning. Isolated eccentrics, such as the American writer Tom Wolfe, whose style of dress is entirely trapped in the taste of the 1930s, still adhere to this fashion. In its current form, the shirt has hardly altered since the end of the First World War. The only feature to have been added is the breast pocket, which was introduced as the three-piece suit with a vest went out of fashion. However, traditional men's shirts still do not have breast pockets, particularly as no one actually has any idea what their function should be.

Good Shirts at a Glance

A good shirt has removable collar bones where required by the shape of the collar. This is particularly the case with turndown and cutaway collars, but collar bones would be out of place in the soft collar of a button-down shirt. Most collar bones are made of plastic, but some gentlemen's outfitters offer brass collar bones as well. Whatever they are made of, they give the collar the right curve and prevent the collar tips turning up. This can be particularly important when the shirt is worn with a necktie.

The origins of the split yoke lie in traditional shirtmaking. As people generally have shoulders of different heights, a split yoke can be used to adjust the fit of a shirt precisely to the customer's stature. On ready-to-wear shirts the split yoke is just a detail which suggests more expensive work; it is a costly detail, though, because every additional seam is a not inconsiderable cost factor when shirts are produced in large numbers. Such details may be unimportant for many, and an unnecessary expense.

Unfortunately, patterns are only matched exactly on very good ready-to-wear shirts, though this is always done on custom-made shirts. For example, stripes or checks should match exactly where the shoulder joins the sleeve. Raised (or "French") seams are used on those parts of the shirt that are subject to particularly hard wear. For a raised seam the two pieces of material are sewn together, turned over, and sewn again. This procedure is expensive, but ensures that the seam will be durable.

The more stitches a seam has, the more durable it will be, with about 20 stitches per inch (8 per cm) on a good shirt. Seams, even parallel double seams, are always sewn with a single needle. The advantages of this are that the seams are more precise, and the material in between them does not go wavy after washing. On less high-quality shirts a machine with two needles is used for double seams. This can sew a parallel seam in half the time.

Material is used generously when good shirts are made, so that they do not slip out of the pants at the back or sides. The back is usually cut somewhat longer than the front to ensure it fits well even when the wearer bends over. The length is right if the front and back parts can be brought together in the crotch. Shorter shirts are best avoided, to save embarrassment.

Traditional buttons made of mother-of-pearl are obligatory features of a good shirt. Mother-of-pearl buttons are so hard that they will break the needle of a sewing machine. The button facing used to be an additional piece of material sewn onto the shirt, but today it is made by folding over the material at the edge of the shirt. A placket front facing is more stable, but can also look a little rustic, so more refined shirts tend to have a single button facing.

A gusset, a triangular piece of material, is usually added for reinforcement in the corner between the breast and the back. You will find this detail on all good shirts. However, there is only one manufacturer that uses this little detail as a marketing tool. The gussets on shirts from Thomas Pink are always pink. This is intended to remind the owner of the shirt of the maker every time he wears it, and would not work for Turnbull & Asser or T. M. Lewin.

On good shirts the cloth of the sleeve is pleated several times where it meets the cuff. In addition there is often a small button above the cuff that prevents the sleeve opening up to reveal the arm in an unflattering way. It can also be unbuttoned to make rolling the sleeve up easier. On very good shirts this buttonhole is horizontal, and not vertical. On the very best shirts it is hand sewn, of course, just like all the other buttonholes.

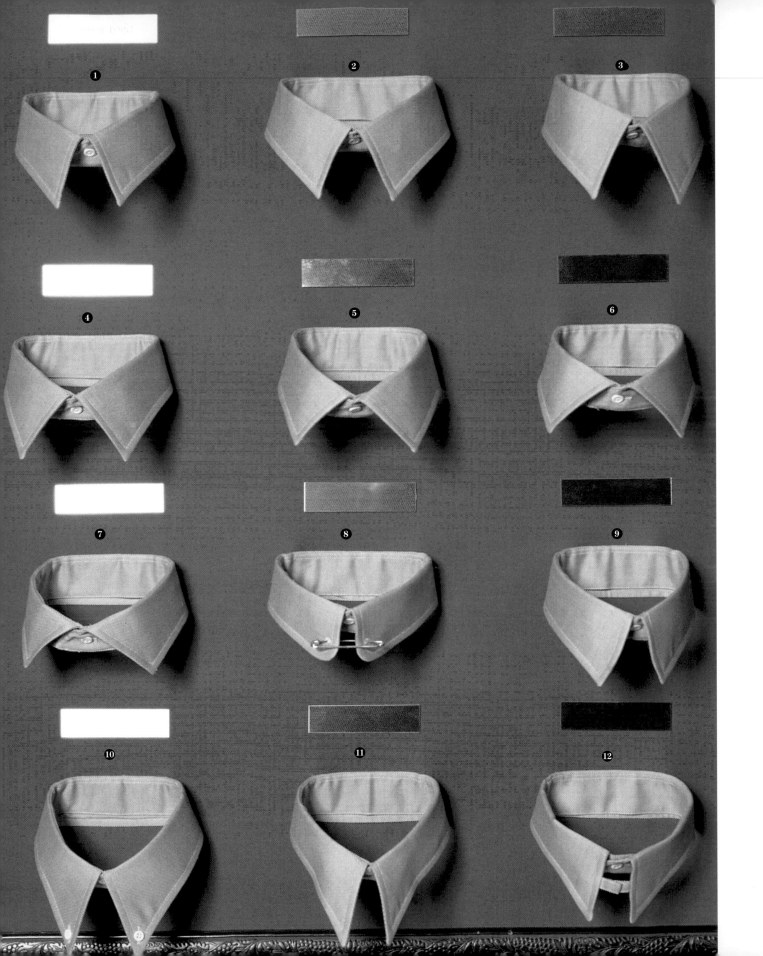

Collar Shapes

❶ The wide turndown collar is the most formal, and at the same time appears the least conspicuous, collar style. The gap between the collar tips may vary.

Thus, examples ❷ ❸ and ❹ are all described as turndown collars, as is ⓫. A broad collar covers more of the neck, making a man who wears it look more "dressed up." In addition, a broad collar allows more room for thick, wide neckties. When a custom-made shirt is made, the width of the collar is adjusted to meet individual requirements. Where necessary, it is possible to make a long neck look shorter by wearing a wide collar, just as a short neck can be made to look longer with a narrow collar. Incidentally, Ronald Reagan admitted to this trick in his memoirs.

❺ This elegant collar shape has many names. Other examples include ❻ and ❼. In English it is called the cutaway, or spread, collar; in German it is the *Kentkragen*, *Haifischkragen*, or *Spreizkragen*. The term "cutaway collar" is internationally accepted. It refers to the typical way in which the collar tips are "cut away" to the sides. In fact, the tips are pulled a long way back on this design and therefore allow a free view of the necktie knot. The cutaway collar always looks more elegant than the extremely classical turndown collar. It is seen a great deal on style-conscious southern Europeans, with or without a necktie. Many people like to wear the cutaway collar with thickly padded, rather wide neckties, which are displayed to full advantage in the large gap between the collar tips.

❽ The pin collar, on which the collar tips are connected with pins of various designs, is also a very American collar style. The pin collar is thus a variety of the tab collar. Although this collar design sometimes looks very elegant, European men mostly find it too affected. In addition, a reflective piece of metal distracts other people's attention from the wearer's face in a disconcerting fashion. As the pin collar can only be worn with collar tips that are relatively close together, it is subject to some of the same disadvantages as the turndown collar.

❾ The great days of the detachable collar are long since past. Only dandies, nostalgics, and the very thrifty still wear it. Nevertheless, it is cheaper to replace a frayed collar than a whole shirt, and many English shirtmakers still offer shirts with detachable collars in their standard ranges. These archaic shirts are somewhat time consuming to put on and take off, but the design exerts a certain fascination over many men. As so often when we meet with apparently anachronistic things, we experience an almost irresistible urge to try them out at least once. This is true of the straight razor, the nightshirt, and suspenders, just as it is for the good old detachable collar.

❿ The real Brooks Brothers soft-roll collar enjoys a special status among collar designs. It looks just as good with a necktie as without. Someone who wears this collar with a necktie will look very "dressed up" as it is quite wide. Nevertheless, the button-down collar looks less formal than other designs. This is a result of its soft finish and the casual look of the buttoned collar tips. However, only American manufacturers make a good job of this collar. On European versions the collar is usually too narrow, the collar tips are at the wrong angle to each other, and the collar never rolls quite as it does on a real Brooks Brothers shirt.

⓬ With the tab collar we are leaving the certain fields of tradition. It was supposedly first worn by the Prince of Wales, later Edward VIII, on a journey to the USA. Americans adopted the style with enthusiasm, and to this day the tab collar is more popular in the United States than in Europe, though the small strap emphasizes the knot of the necktie very elegantly. However, this collar cannot be worn without a necktie, which may be a disadvantage for a business traveler who wants to drink an aperitif with his shirt open after his work is done. It may also be that many men find handling the tab collar simply too fussy.

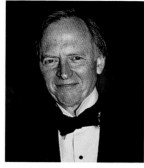

The American author Tom Wolfe is regarded in the United States as a great dandy. He is known to favor old-fashioned, stiff detachable collars. He could hardly have chosen another detail of men's clothing with which to express more clearly his distance from an unbuttoned American society, in which everything is designed for comfort.

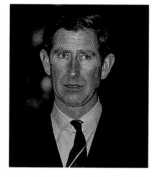

Prince Charles has been wearing shirts with more or less widely spread cutaway collars since his early youth. Either he chose the right collar design instinctively, or his shirtmakers – Turnbull & Asser – advised him well. What is true is that this collar always looks much more friendly, and at the same time more refined, than a turndown collar with its collar tips pointing more directly downward. What they say of the corners of the mouth is also true in this respect: the higher they are, the nicer they look.

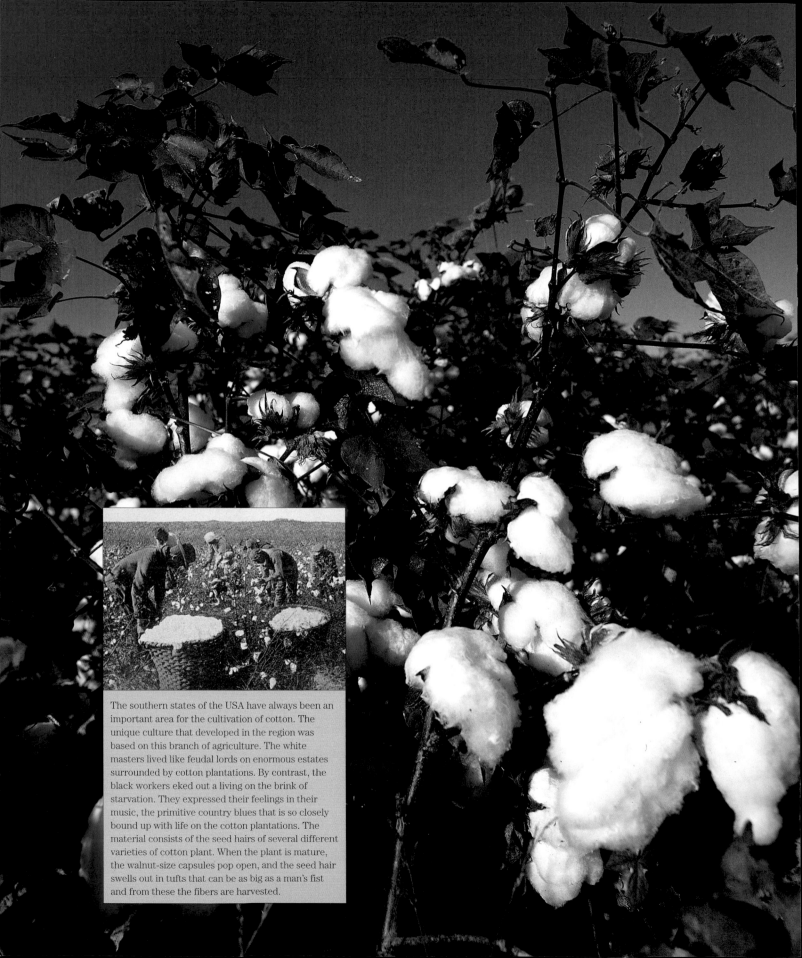

The southern states of the USA have always been an important area for the cultivation of cotton. The unique culture that developed in the region was based on this branch of agriculture. The white masters lived like feudal lords on enormous estates surrounded by cotton plantations. By contrast, the black workers eked out a living on the brink of starvation. They expressed their feelings in their music, the primitive country blues that is so closely bound up with life on the cotton plantations. The material consists of the seed hairs of several different varieties of cotton plant. When the plant is mature, the walnut-size capsules pop open, and the seed hair swells out in tufts that can be as big as a man's fist and from these the fibers are harvested.

Cotton

Cotton was already being cultivated in India over 5,000 years ago. From there, it spread to China in the eleventh century. The Incas were cultivating cotton in Central America during the same period. In the Old World the Arabs found cotton in Persia and introduced it to North Africa, Sicily, and southern Spain.

For a period of 300 years Venice was the leading market for cotton from the Levant. In the seventeenth century the Netherlands became the main trading center for this valuable raw commodity. Cotton processing on a large scale began in Great Britain and Switzerland in the eighteenth century. The invention of the spinning machine and the mechanical loom made it possible to process even greater quantities of the material, which was now grown mainly in the southern states of the USA from where much of the world's cotton still originates today.

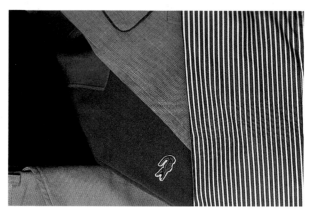

Cotton is still ahead of real wool as the most important textile commodity. Indeed, there would be enormous gaps in our wardrobe if it were not for cotton. Shirts, jeans, chinos, trenchcoats, underclothing, pajamas, socks, summer suits, light pullovers, and sweatshirts – all of them are made of cotton.

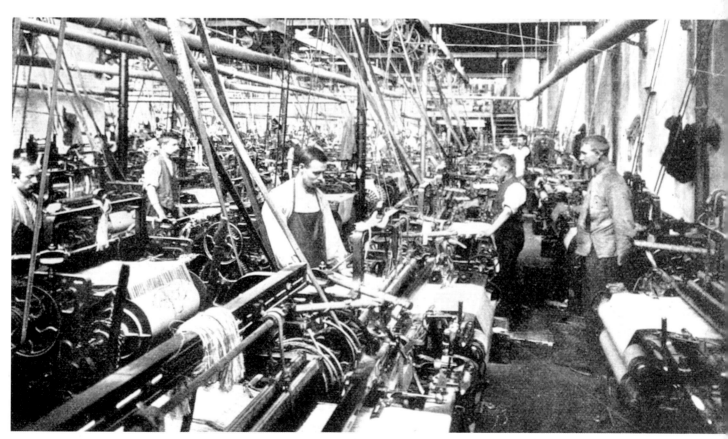

The longer the fibers that are harvested, the higher the quality of the cotton. The fibers are sorted, or "stapled," by length; long and short-fiber cottons are therefore described as either long staple or short staple. The longer fibers measure about an eighth of an inch (about 3–3.6 mm). Apart from the length of the fibers, their fineness, strength, softness, color, and luster are also important. Colorless cottons with a silky luster are regarded as particularly valuable. The best varieties are Sea Island Cotton from the USA and Egyptian Mako.

The Stuff that Shirts are Made of

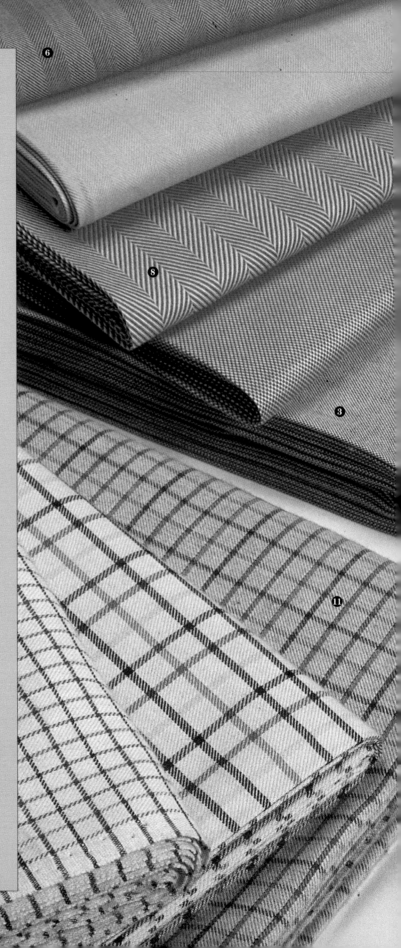

❶ Cotton batiste is a light plain weave of fine, high-quality yarns. Batiste made of Egyptian Mako cotton is also described as Swiss batiste.

❷ Poplin is the term for a fabric made using fine warp yarn and a thick filling. The filling gives this material its character.

❸ Oxford is a coarser kind of weave in which dyed and undyed threads are combined together. It makes soft, but hard-wearing, shirts. There are many different varieties of Oxford weave, but they always look somewhat less refined and formal than those made from batiste or poplin.

❹ Royal Oxford is a somewhat more refined version of the otherwise rather homely Oxford weave. Like conventional Oxford, it is made by weaving together dyed and undyed threads, but the yarns used are much finer. This means that a shirt made of Royal Oxford feels silkier and much softer to the touch than does a normal Oxford shirt.

❺ Sea Island is always the most expensive cotton. It is woven from a greater number of threads than poplin, which gives this material a silky feel. While poplin weave has about 100 threads to the inch (2.54 cm), in Sea Island there are 140 threads to the inch. Stripes or checks in this material therefore have clearer definition and deeper, stronger colors. This is why Sea Island is particularly well suited for conspicuous patterns. The material is so fine that it is sometimes mistaken for silk.

❻ Ribbed twill has a characteristic diagonal structure like that familiar from the material used in chinos. The typical, lightly shimmering look of ribbed twill gives plain shirts an interesting accent.

❼ Pinpoint is a combination of cotton poplin and Oxford. It is woven of long-staple cotton, and, as in Oxford, only the warp yarn is dyed.

❽ Herringbone twill is a close relative of ribbed twill. In both kinds of material the threads are woven to form a diagonal structure. In order to achieve the typical herringbone effect the direction of the diagonals is changed at intervals of a fifth of an inch (5 mm), which creates a zigzag pattern.

❾ Although silk shirts are to be purchased on every corner nowadays, really high-quality shirts made of this material are still very expensive. Many business travelers have their English custom-made shirts copied in silk by Chinese tailors in Hong Kong.

❿ Brushed cotton is used for soft leisure shirts. It is produced in plain colors, various checks, and Scottish tartans. In Europe brushed cotton is particularly familiar and popular in the style of the famous Tattersall check.

⓫ Another leisurewear classic is Viyella, a mixed weave that combines the warmth of wool with the comfort of cotton. Viyella is used mainly for the production of Tattersall check shirts. Tattersall is named after Richard Tattersall, an English horseman who used the pattern for horse blankets.

Folding Your Shirt

When you have finished ironing your shirt, you should let it cool off for half an hour on a clothes hanger. Then button it up carefully and lay it with the front side down on the ironing board.

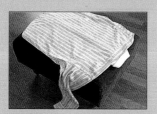

Fold over one half as shown in the picture. Depending on the size you wish the folded shirt to be, fold it over about halfway along the shoulder.

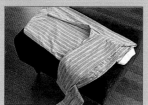

Next fold the sleeve downward. If the shirt has double cuffs, turn the cuff flat on its side.

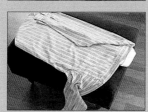

Now fold the other half over. Make sure that the fold runs down from the shoulder at right angles to it.

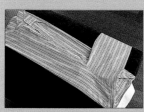

Fold the second sleeve in. The shirt should now be a long rectangle. It should not get narrower toward the bottom.

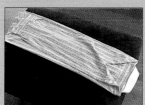

Turn the lower part of the shirt over the cuffs. Fold the shirt so that the bottom hem of the shirt touches the collar.

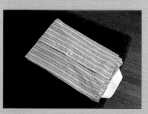

Turn the shirt over and store it in a cupboard or a chest of drawers. If you have the space, it is better not to fold up your shirts, but to keep them on hangers.

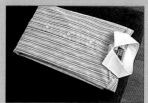

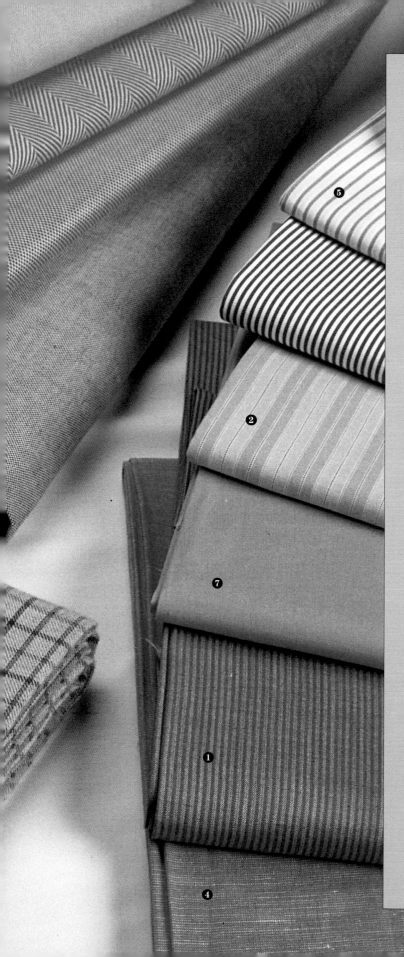

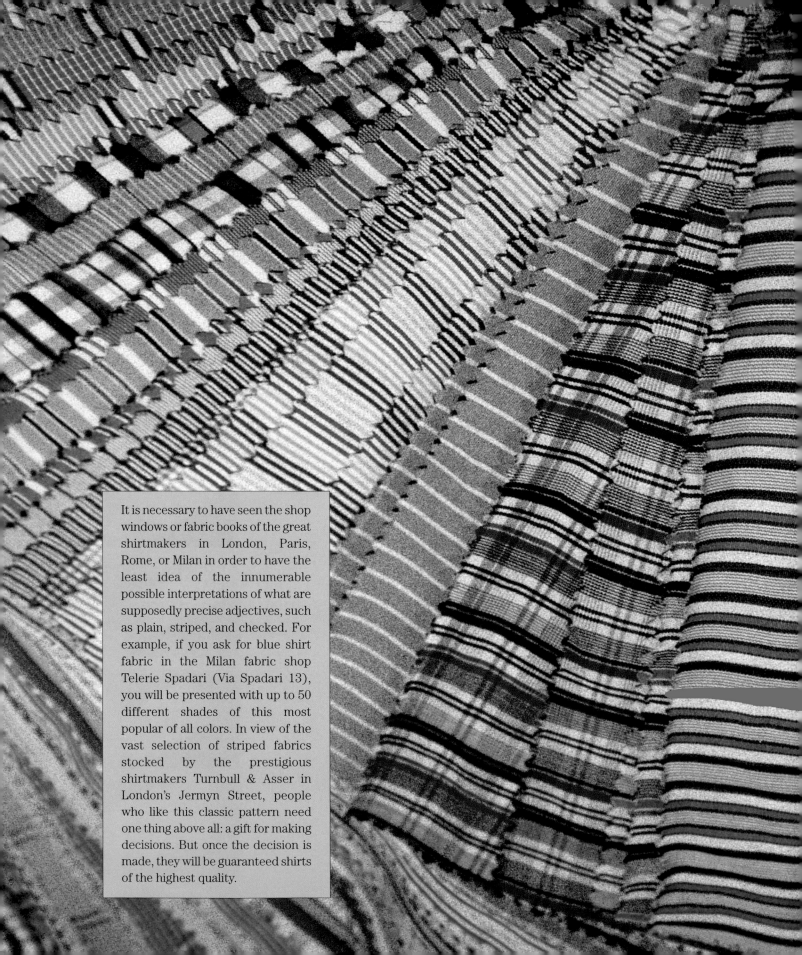

It is necessary to have seen the shop windows or fabric books of the great shirtmakers in London, Paris, Rome, or Milan in order to have the least idea of the innumerable possible interpretations of what are supposedly precise adjectives, such as plain, striped, and checked. For example, if you ask for blue shirt fabric in the Milan fabric shop Telerie Spadari (Via Spadari 13), you will be presented with up to 50 different shades of this most popular of all colors. In view of the vast selection of striped fabrics stocked by the prestigious shirtmakers Turnbull & Asser in London's Jermyn Street, people who like this classic pattern need one thing above all: a gift for making decisions. But once the decision is made, they will be guaranteed shirts of the highest quality.

Jermyn Street

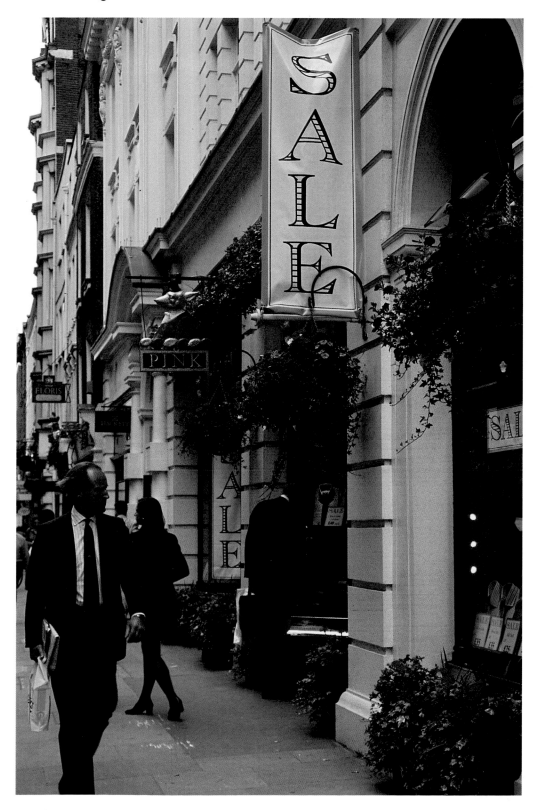

Jermyn Street is a mecca for people who love classic English shirts. There you will find nearly everything your heart could desire: not just shirts and neckties, but also exclusive toilet accessories, pajamas, and underclothes. The area may not have enjoyed exactly the highest of reputations when the tailors started settling there, but that meant that the shops could be rented at reasonable charges. Today, however, Jermyn Street is an address renowned around the world, and the rents are absolutely astronomical.

The Best English Shirtmakers

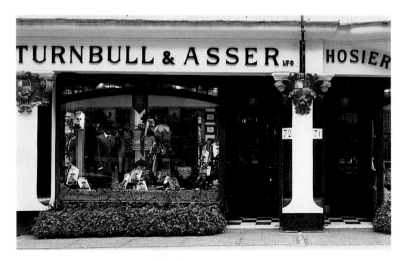

No. 71 is the most famous address on Jermyn Street. An unbelievable selection of materials for custom-made shirts, ready-to-wear shirts, and neckties has been on sale here since 1904. The minimum order for custom-made shirts is six garments, and the delivery time is twelve weeks. However, the wait is worth it for the quality of the finished product, as well as the prestige that attaches to shirts from Turnbull & Asser.

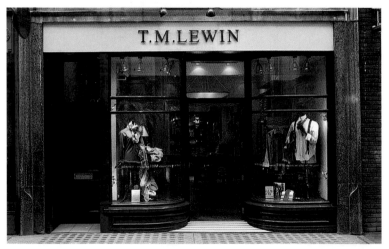

At No. 106 we find T. M. Lewin, a company founded in 1898 by Thomas Mayes Lewin. The Lewin shirt is cut relatively close to the body with a somewhat broadly spread and relatively narrow turndown collar. T. M. Lewin's superb shirts have no rivals as far as quality is concerned, though their designs might be described as rather modern by Jermyn Street standards. Lewin are famous for their enormous choice of club, school, and regimental ties, and also have an efficient mail-order service.

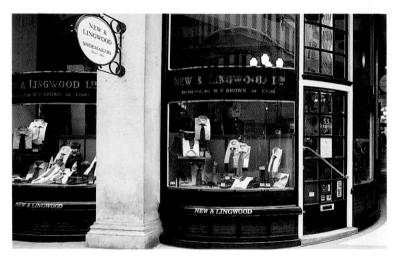

New & Lingwood at No. 53 Jermyn Street are one of the famous names among London shirtmakers. Their shirts are typical of Jermyn Street, and will appeal to anyone who likes wearing loud striped shirts with his dark business suits. New & Lingwood also offer an excellent range of shoes.

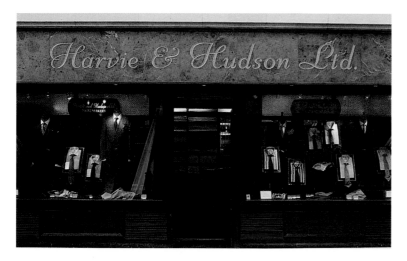

Harvie & Hudson are to be found at No. 77. Apart from typical Jermyn Street shirts, they also offer suits, jackets, and trousers. Striped silk shirts with matching neckties are a specialty of the house. The atmosphere in the shop is somewhat stiff, though this probably constitutes a great deal of its appeal. However, the spoilt continental shopper will find the ambiance very "understated." In truth, Harvie & Hudson's legendary reputation rests solely on their shirts.

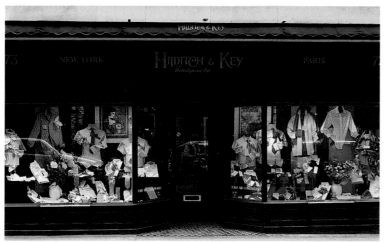

At No. 37 and No. 73 we find Hilditch & Key, another Jermyn Street legend. There is no need to travel to London to purchase Hilditch & Key shirts because they are also on sale outside England – in Paris, for example, at Rue de Rivoli 252. Hilditch & Key's end-of-season sales are famous. It is even possible to take advantage of them by mail, thanks to a service known as "Sale by Mail."

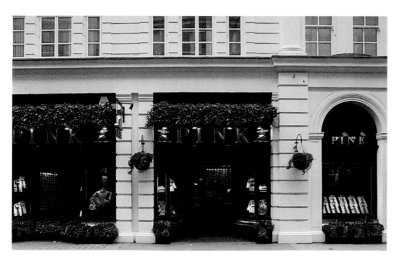

At their spacious premises Thomas Pink offer meticulously tailored shirts in a large selection of designs and cottons. Thomas Pink have always tried to attract younger customers, and there is no doubt that they succeed in doing this at their shop in Jermyn Street. The sales staff are helpful and provide customers with test shirts in various sizes on request so that you do not have to buy a pig in a poke. The Pink shirt has a relatively stiff semi-cutaway collar and a moderately spread collar that is best worn with a necktie. Thomas Pink also run an excellent mail-order service that delivers anywhere in the world.

How a Custom-Made Shirt is Created

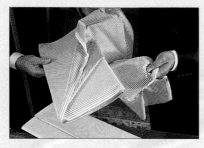

The Düsseldorf custom tailor and shirt-maker Heinz-Josef Radermacher stocks a huge range of materials. The word "striped" alone is inadequate to describe the variety on offer. He also offers plain materials in all shades, various checks, and more unusual patterns, such as herringbone.

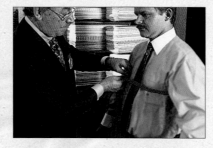

Measuring up is a fascinating moment, an almost holy ritual in all kinds of custom tailoring. First, the tape measure is passed under the armpits and around the chest. Whether the shirt is to be tight here or not will only be decided later when the paper pattern is drawn up for cutting out.

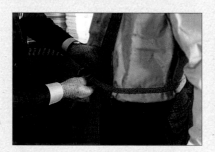

Next the waist measurement is taken. If the customer was being measured for a suit, measurements would have to be taken above the waistband of the pants and the vest.

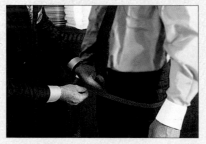

Now the hips are measured. When this is done the customer should make sure his pockets are empty and stand with his legs together, to ensure accuracy.

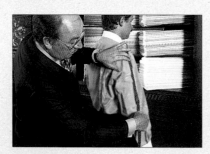

Both arms are measured separately. Most people have arms of different lengths, so this is important.

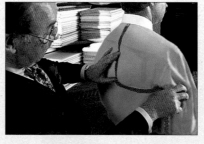

The width of the back is an additional measurement that is used to check the chest measurement that has been taken.

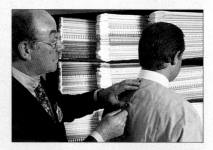

The back measurement determines the total length of the shirt. The collar is not included when this is taken.

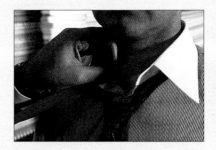

The neck must be measured exactly. Enough room must be allowed to ensure that the collar does not become too tight later due to washing. When this is done, the customer should say how narrow or wide he wants the collar.

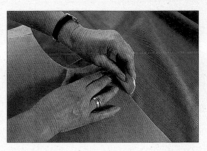

After the measurements have been taken, the pattern is drawn up on paper, cut out, and traced onto the cloth. When working with patterned fabrics, the cutter must take account of the pattern sequence so that all the lines run together perfectly on the finished shirt. Traditionally, the material is cut out with large shears.

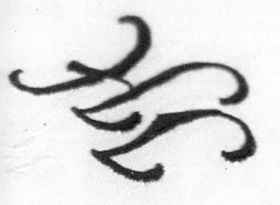

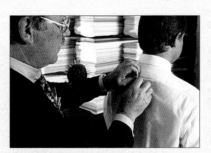

The fitting is used to ensure that the garment fits perfectly. Shoulders of different heights are compensated for at this stage by adjustments to the yoke.

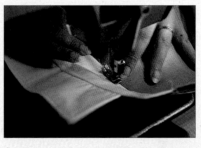

Even the most traditional shirtmakers now use sewing machines wherever possible. However, much is still sewn by hand.

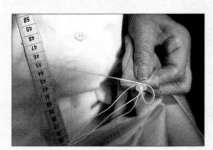

As a general rule, buttons are always sewn on by hand. However, the buttonholes are only sewn by hand at the express request of the customer.

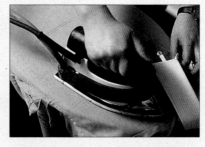

All that remains to do is iron the finished, sewn shirt to a professional standard before it is wrapped in plastic for handing over to the customer.

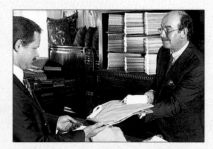

The finished shirt can be picked up a couple of days or weeks after the fitting. It can also be mailed to the customer on request.

Checks for the Weekend

In the 1980s there was a series on television based on the memoirs of the English country vet known as James Herriot. It was not only worth watching for the stories, but also for the costumes. Each character was dressed with total authenticity, and every last detail was correct. The viewer could identify the class and profession of every character in the series at a glance. However, what united the vet with the lord and the farmer was a shirt that is just as much a part of English rural life as the Barbour jacket and Hunter "wellies." In color, it is usually a creamy white, but is also available in light shades of beige. However, its most important feature is a mesh check of dark brown, green, burgundy, blue, or black stripes known as Tattersall check. It is said that this pattern is named after the horse market run by a man called Richard Tattersall where the horse blankets were decorated with exactly this type of check.

Today Tattersall check is more than a symbol of English rural life. For many years it has been regarded as an essential component of the classic weekend outfit, especially in fall and winter, when it is combined with a lambswool or cashmere pullover, a tweed jacket, or a blazer. The Americans have adopted this typical English check as a favorite pattern for the button-down shirt, and conservative New Yorkers wear it with chinos or corduroy pants when they drive down to their houses in New Jersey at the weekend. The comfortable check also has another significant group of customers in Europe and the USA. It is often found on the shirts worn by academics at Oxford, Cambridge, and the Ivy League universities, a fact of which the costume designers of Hollywood are well aware. Whenever a professor appears in a film, you can be sure that he is wearing a tweed jacket and a Tattersall check shirt. Tattersall checks also appear again and again in the collections of the great shirtmakers, but the best still come from the traditional English manufacturers. The American Tattersall check shirt with a button-down collar is also a real classic, and should definitely be on your shopping list for your next trip to New York. You will also find it in European stores and outlets that sell clothes by Ralph Lauren, who include it in their collection almost every year. The Tattersall check thus combines the features of classic and casual, traditional and fashionable, ensuring its continuing popularity.

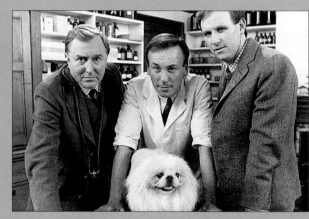

The Brooks Brothers Shirt

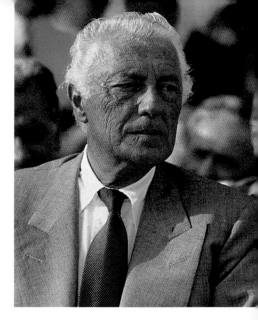

Gianni Agnelli is one of the best-known men to wear a Brooks Brothers shirt with a soft-roll collar. The fact that he wears this shirt is the highest accolade for American fashion. A man like the seriously rich "avvocato" could also buy from the best Italian and English shirtmakers. The fact that, even so, he wears a shirt off the rack really does testify to the quality of the product.

The Brooks Brothers shirt rose to its current triumphant position in the 1980s. When out-and-out Yuppies from Europe traveled to New York, they always returned home with a real button-down shirt in light blue, white, pink, yellow, mint, stripes, checks, or tartan. People who did not go to New York themselves would ask someone else to purchase one for them, together with genuine dark-blue Levi's 501s, and cordovan shoes from Alden, or penny loafers from Bass. At the time the button-down shirt was a hot new discovery for the youthful readers of the men's fashion magazines, but it had been known to insiders for a very long time. It was certainly well known in the United States because, at least according to the company's official history, the button-down shirt had been sold by Brooks Brothers in Madison Avenue since 1900.

It is claimed that John Brooks, the president of the high-class American gentlemen's outfitters, noticed at a polo match in England that the tips of the polo-shirt collars were fastened to the breast with tiny buttons that stopped them from fluttering into the players' faces. Inspired by this, he had the button-down shirt made, and from then on it became an indispensable part of the Brooks Brothers range. It does not matter whether the story is true or not, it is still a nice story. In all likelihood, this version of the origins of the American button-down shirt was deliberately put into circulation by the English in order to put down the American's brilliant invention as a copy. Some of the evidence tends to support this: neither the modern polo shirt nor the shirts worn by real polo players display even the most distant similarity to the button-down shirt.

Whatever the truth of the matter, the button-down shirt is one of the few American contributions to classic men's fashion. Its eccentric charm even allows it to take its place alongside the finest English and Italian products, but only if it really does come from Brooks Brothers. Strangely enough, no one has ever succeeded in copying the cut of the Brooks Brothers soft-roll collar in a satisfactory way – one more reason to seek out the shop at 346 Madison Avenue, at the corner of 44th Street, next time you are staying in New York. When you are there you will need to ask specifically for the soft-roll collar in the shop because a European-style version has also been put on sale recently in the birthplace of the classic button-down shirt.

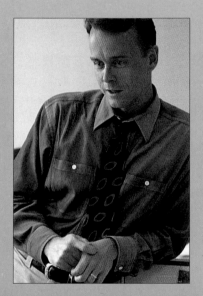

Contrary to European prejudices, strict dress codes are followed in the USA, particularly on the east coast, and apply above all to business life. If you have your "wing tips" given a deep shine by one of the many bootblacks in Manhattan in the morning, you will be surrounded by men all wearing suits. In summer the suit can be beige, olive, or light blue, just as long as it is a suit. The sole relaxation of this rule ever to have been introduced is "casual dress Friday." Friday is regarded as a day when one can appear, if not in jeans and a polo shirt, at least in a sports jacket, chinos, and a somewhat lighter shirt, the "Friday shirt." The Brooks Brothers mail-order catalogue regularly devotes a whole page of its own to the Friday shirt, and there we find all the popular materials, such as fine-yarn chambrays, the somewhat coarser Oxfords, and, of course, the various typical patterns, such as "mini-plaids," candy stripes, and "mini-Tattersalls" that put us in the right mood for the weekend with a dash of color.

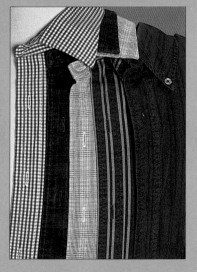

The Right Shirt – the Right Fit

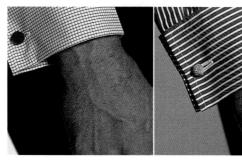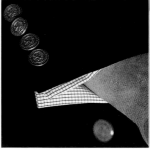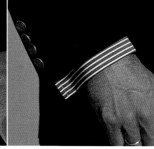

Wrong

Many men buy shirts with sleeves that are too short. Others may pay attention to the length of the sleeves, but forget that shirts only shrink to their final size after being washed four or five times. In consequence, a shirt should neither have the final sleeve length nor the final neck measurements when it is bought. As a matter of course a good shirtmaker will add just enough material to ensure that the shirt fits perfectly after it has been washed several times.

Right

When the sleeves are the right length the cuff covers the wrist and reaches just to the root of the thumb. The sleeve must be long enough to fit well even when the arm is bent, and not just when the hand is hanging down vertically. Otherwise the shirt sleeve is pulled into the sleeve of the jacket when you sit down and lift your arms. The cuff should be tight enough to stop it from slipping too far down the hand, though this is only a danger when the sleeves are too long.

Wrong

Most men buy shirts with sleeves that are too short, and jackets with sleeves that are too long. As a result, their shirt cuffs are hidden by their jacket sleeves, creating the impression that they are wearing short-sleeved shirts. Moreover, an otherwise well-fitting jacket automatically looks too large if the sleeves are too long.

Right

If the shirt and jacket have sleeves of the correct lengths, at least a half inch (1 cm) of the shirt cuff will show, and some men prefer even more. In extreme cases the jacket sleeves appear to be too short in relation to the length of the jacket, but as the jacket is never worn without a shirt this is not conspicuous and can even look good. A length of shirt cuff extending from the jacket sleeve makes your arms look longer, provided the sleeves of the shirt are the correct length. Someone who has short arms can certainly make use of this.

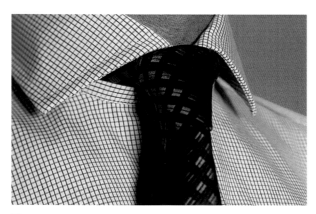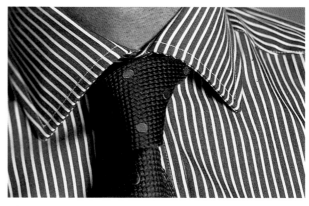

Wrong

The shirt collar must be of such a size that the necktie knot does not lift the tips of the collar away from the shirt breast. The collar tips must stay on the breast of the shirt, even when you turn your head. Of course, the collar tips may also be lifted up if the knot of the necktie is too large. It is best to use the knot that you prefer to wear as a standard. It is therefore worth taking along your favorite necktie when you buy a shirt in order to test the shirt out in the shop with it.

Right

The tips of a well-cut collar touch the breast of the shirt and will not lift up when you move your head. They are forced into this position by the necktie knot itself, though the collar must be of a certain size for this to happen. The collars of really good shirts are always cut large enough to fit well, regardless of whether fashion dictates wide or narrow collars. Someone who insists on buying small, narrow collars should not wear heavy Jacquard neckties.

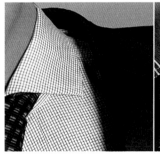 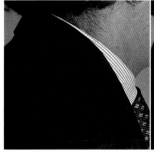 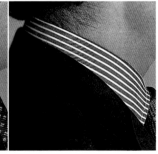

Wrong

If the outer edge of the shirt collar is not covered by the lapel, the collar is usually not cut perfectly. The harmonious relationship between the shirt collar, the necktie, and the jacket is disturbed if the material of the shirt breast shows between the shirt collar and the lapel. Obviously, this problem occurs very rarely with double-breasted jackets, and never with a well-cut suit.

Right

The outer edge of the collar and its tips should just be covered by the lapel of the jacket. Only in this way is perfect harmony created between the lines of the shirt collar, the necktie, and the lapel which encloses them. A shirt collar with tips pointing sharply downward is most unlikely to be covered by the lapel unless the jacket is very tight and high cut. The cutaway collar generally looks elegant because its outer edge is always covered by the lapel, even if the jacket is less well cut.

Wrong

The shirt collar is too narrow if it is covered at the back of the neck by a well-cut jacket collar. Unfortunately, many manufacturers follow fashion blindly when it comes to the width of the shirt collar. However, traditional shirtmakers in England and Italy know how very important the width of the collar is and that this feature, of all things, must never be subjected to the vicissitudes of fashion. This is particularly important because the necktie can often be seen at the back of the neck if the collar is too narrow, something that is definitely to be avoided.

Right

The shirt collar will not be covered by the jacket at the back of the neck if it is the right width, provided the jacket is well cut. In this connection, it should be mentioned that jacket collars are cut to suit well-fitting shirt collars. The fit of the jacket collar is therefore judged by its relationship to the shirt collar. As a result, the shirt collar should definitely be a perfect fit before you buy a jacket or have yourself measured at a tailor's.

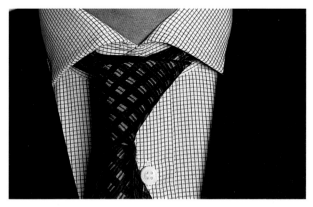 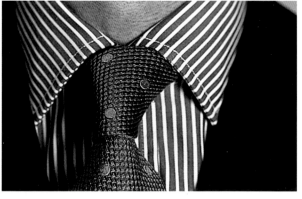

Wrong

The shirt collar must be cut so that the knot sits exactly in the middle of the upper part of the triangle and does not slip down. In this illustration the knot of the necktie does not fill out the two sides of the collar up to the topmost corner. If this is not due to an incorrectly knotted necktie, you should not buy a shirt with which this happens. It is impossible to create complete harmony between the necktie and a shirt with a collar like this.

Right

The knot of the necktie must sit exactly in the triangle between the two sides of the collar and stay there, regardless of whether the top button of the shirt is done up or not. Many men have a habit of not only leaving this button open, but of not even pulling the necktie tight. This is an ugly half-measure: someone who does not like neckties should not wear them, and should instead simply leave his collar open.

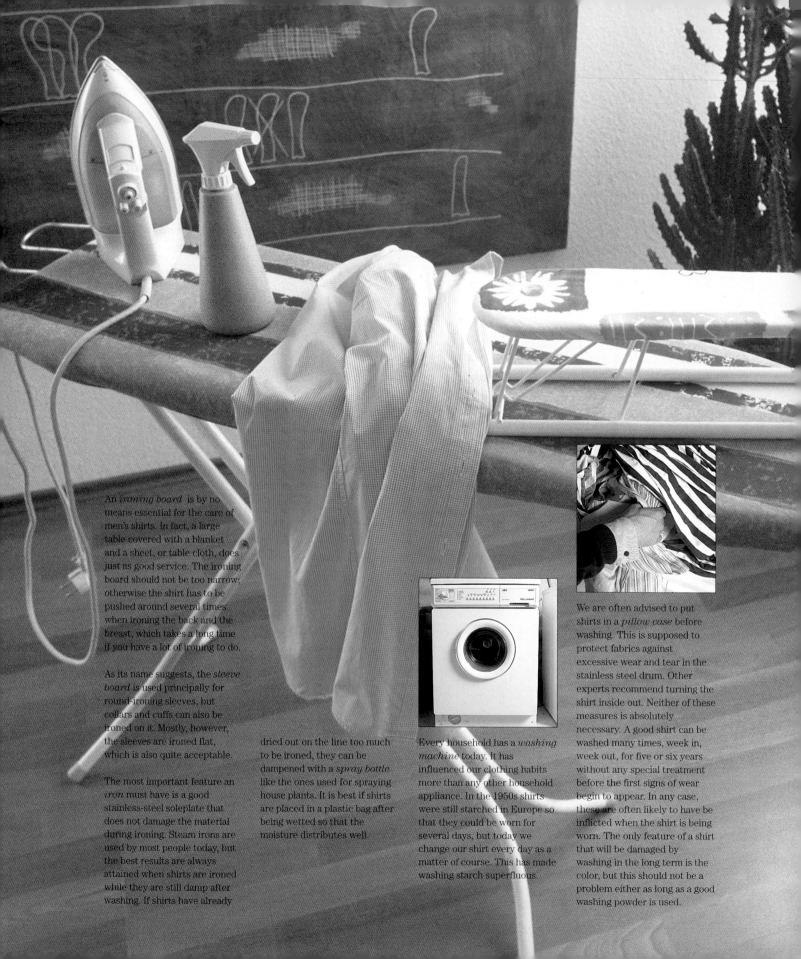

An *ironing board* is by no means essential for the care of men's shirts. In fact, a large table covered with a blanket and a sheet, or table cloth, does just as good service. The ironing board should not be too narrow; otherwise the shirt has to be pushed around several times when ironing the back and the breast, which takes a long time if you have a lot of ironing to do.

As its name suggests, the *sleeve board* is used principally for round-ironing sleeves, but collars and cuffs can also be ironed on it. Mostly, however, the sleeves are ironed flat, which is also quite acceptable.

The most important feature an *iron* must have is a good stainless-steel soleplate that does not damage the material during ironing. Steam irons are used by most people today, but the best results are always attained when shirts are ironed while they are still damp after washing. If shirts have already dried out on the line too much to be ironed, they can be dampened with a *spray bottle* like the ones used for spraying house plants. It is best if shirts are placed in a plastic bag after being wetted so that the moisture distributes well.

Every household has a *washing machine* today. It has influenced our clothing habits more than any other household appliance. In the 1950s shirts were still starched in Europe so that they could be worn for several days, but today we change our shirt every day as a matter of course. This has made washing starch superfluous.

We are often advised to put shirts in a *pillow case* before washing. This is supposed to protect fabrics against excessive wear and tear in the stainless steel drum. Other experts recommend turning the shirt inside out. Neither of these measures is absolutely necessary. A good shirt can be washed many times, week in, week out, for five or six years without any special treatment before the first signs of wear begin to appear. In any case, these are often likely to have been inflicted when the shirt is being worn. The only feature of a shirt that will be damaged by washing in the long term is the color, but this should not be a problem either as long as a good washing powder is used.

Washing and Ironing – the Fundamentals of Shirt Care

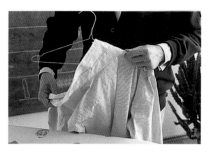

It is best to take the shirt from the line while it is still damp. Then it can be ironed with a minimum of effort.

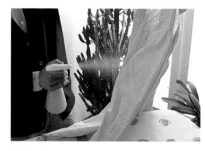

If the shirt is still too dry, you must dampen it thoroughly with water. A spray bottle is used to do this.

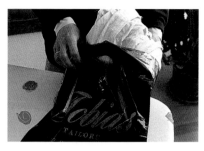

Keep the dampened shirt for half an hour in a plastic bag. This ensures that the moisture distributes evenly through the cloth.

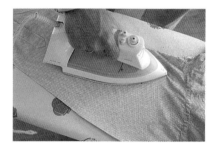

Begin with one of the sleeves. Stroke it smooth and begin ironing in the middle of the sleeve. Iron from the center outward, otherwise light creases will be pressed into the material. Only iron the folds at the end. If you are using a sleeve board, pull the sleeve over it and iron it even and smooth. Round-ironed shirts are supposed to be stored hanging up.

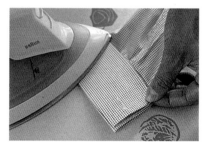

Iron a single-button cuff with the buttons facing upward. A double cuff has to be treated differently. Unfold the cuff and iron it completely smooth. Then fold it to the desired shape and iron in the folds. Fold the cuff once in the middle and iron the fold in so that the buttonholes lie flat on top of each other.

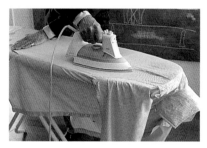

Place the back of the shirt with the inside down on the ironing board. Pull the shirt tight and iron it smooth. When you do this take care with the back pleat. It must be ironed evenly. Place the back pleat on the edge of the ironing board so that it runs parallel to one side. Hold the shirt tight while you iron in the pleat. Repeat the whole procedure from the other side.

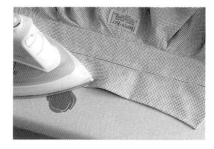

Iron the collar from the tips in so that no creases in the material are left on the outside. This is particularly important with soft button-down collars. Turn the collar over and iron it on the inside. Now insert the collar stiffeners into the collar and turn it over. It is not necessary to iron in the fold of the collar.

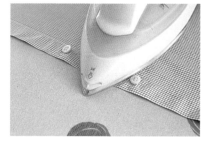

Now iron the breast of the shirt. First lay one half on the ironing board with the outside up and iron it smooth. If it is the right side with the buttons, then iron carefully around the buttons. Repeat the process for the other side.

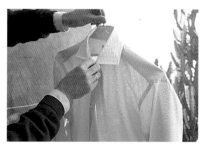

It is best to keep shirts hanging up. Or you can always iron your shirts one by one as and when you need them and then put them on straight after they have cooled. If you want to leave your ironed shirts stored flat, use the instructions for folding given on page 57.

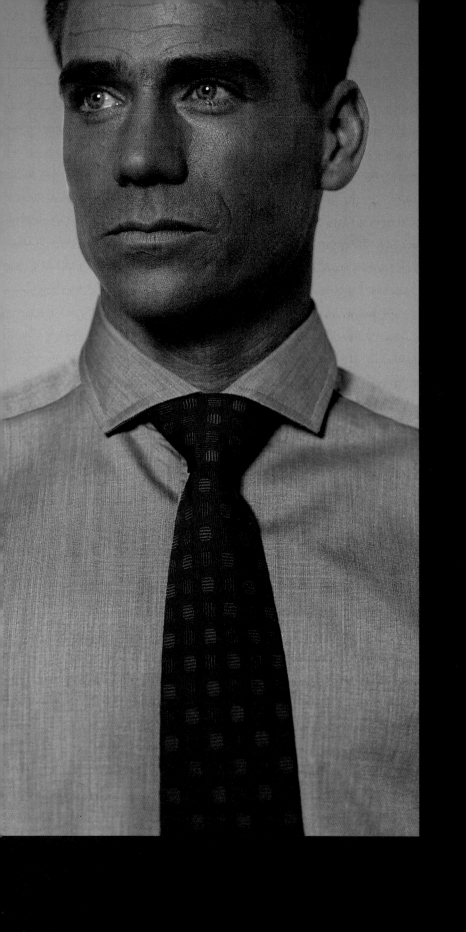

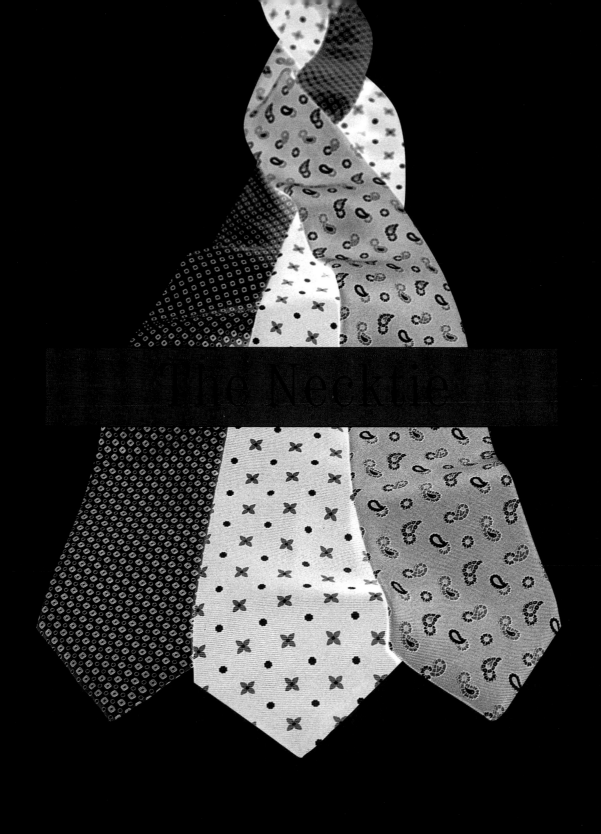

The Necktie

From Neckcloth to Ornamental Neckwear

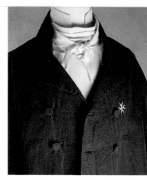

Many works discussing the origins of the necktie mention Trajan's Column in Rome as the earliest recorded evidence for the predecessor of this item of ornamental neckwear. However, the cloth worn by Roman legionaries around their necks at the beginning of the second century AD bears only a very distant resemblance to today's necktie, being just a piece of fabric wrapped around the throat. The real predecessors of the necktie are the neckcloths or cravats that were part of men's clothing from the middle of the seventeenth century. Even the most expensive handmade necktie of our time is cheap compared to the lace cravat worn by King Charles II of England in the year 1660. It cost 20 pounds 12 shillings – and that at a time when a couple of pounds sterling was a good annual salary.

The first real prototype of the modern necktie is to be found in eighteenth-century America. It was called the "bandanna" and was a large patterned cloth wrapped several times around the neck and tied with a bow. Bandannas were popularized by the American boxer James Belcher. In early nineteenth-century England an entirely new mode was introduced by George Brian Brummell. A legendary dandy and style-setter, he condemned all exaggerated fashions and pronounced that a gentleman's clothing should never be conspicuous or overelaborate. He created a look consisting of a blue tailcoat, beige vest and trousers, black boots, and a dazzlingly white cravat. "Beau Brummell," as he was

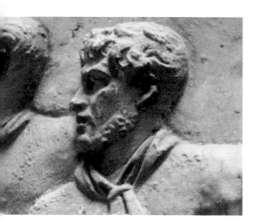

Trajan's column, in Rome, shows men wearing the *focale*, a neckcloth or kerchief worn as protection from the cold.

known, always had a large quantity of starched white linen cravats ready to hand. If he was not pleased with the knot he had just tied, he would take a fresh cravat and repeat the process, continuing until he was satisfied. It could take a long time – and his stocks of linen cravats, like his laundry bills, were enormous. The modern necktie does not call for this kind of thing.

The immediate forerunners of today's necktie were the first school and club ties. In 1880 the members of Exeter College, Oxford, tied the bands of their straw hats around their necks with a simple knot, thus inventing the first club tie. On 25 June of the same year they ordered neckties in the appropriate colors from their tailor, setting an entirely new fashion that was enthusiastically copied by other English clubs, schools, and colleges. The precursor of the patterned necktie was the "Macclesfield tie," so called after the town in northwest England where raw silk from India and China was woven. Around the year 1900 Macclesfield was producing an unprecedented variety of neckties for members of the expanding middle class, who wanted to announce to the world, through their neckwear, that they had succeeded in life.

The modern necktie has existed in its present form since 1924, although neckties that look quite modern are featured in photographs predating the First World War. Before 1924, however, they were usually cut in the direction of the weave of the fabric and then lined with a different material. Made by this method they soon wore out, and the knot left unattractive creases. Jesse Langsdorf of New York found the solution when he cut cloth for neckties on the bias at an angle of 45 degrees to the weave. He also cut the silk not in a single piece but in three sections that were then sewn together. He patented this innovation, and later on sold his invention all over the world. Most good neckties are still made in the same way today.

The modern necktie is usually regarded as formal wear, but that does not mean it cannot be fashionable. Television presenters and other men in the public eye often set the scene for what is regarded as fashionable in necktie wear. Politicians, however, tend to be more conservative in their choices of necktie, the better to suit the seriousness of their offices.

Stars of the Stripes

A man wearing a necktie in the colors of a regiment, college, school, or club is telling the world that he belongs to that particular institution – and moreover that he belongs to a certain social class, at least in England, where neckties of this kind first developed. Men who are not United Kingdom citizens sometimes buy such neckties for stylistic or aesthetic reasons, and there is nothing wrong with that. Problems arise only when a foreigner doing business with an Englishman happens to be wearing, for instance, the necktie of a famous rowing club to which of course he does not belong – while the Englishman does. The chances of committing this social *faux pas* in England are relatively high, on account of the existence in the country of a huge number of color combinations that mean something. Here are some of the best known.

The Staffordshire Regiment

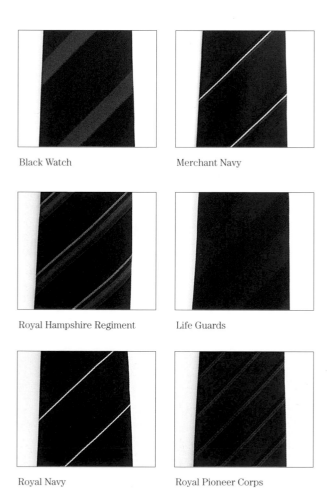

Black Watch

Merchant Navy

Royal Hampshire Regiment

Life Guards

Royal Navy

Royal Pioneer Corps

A Good Necktie

The most important quality of a good necktie, unfortunately, cannot be pictorially illustrated: it must feel good, so you should pick up a necktie and feel it before you buy. It is often suggested that you should crumple the silk to see if it creases. However, if you do try this experiment, do it carefully. Other methods of testing a tie, such as pulling at certain threads, are not necessarily a good idea either, and anyway the results are not always conclusive. Your instant tactile impression is the best guide. If you like what you feel, you are probably right to go ahead and buy the necktie.

A good necktie is usually cut in three parts. If you look closely you will see the seams between the separate sections. Even in neckties of high quality, these seams are machine sewn. The seam holding the necktie together on the inside, however, should be sewn by hand if the necktie is sold as "handfinished" or "handmade."
English manufacturers whose neckties legitimately carry that description include Drake's, Charles Hill, and Holliday & Brown. They supply neckties to Gieves & Hawkes, Turnbull & Asser, Hilditch & Key, and many other famous firms.

In the United Kingdom, Tobias Tailors of Savile Row also produce remarkable handmade neckties. They are not manufactured in a factory but made individually by seamstresses specializing in neckties. This method guarantees that the customer will not find his necktie on sale under three different labels. In France, the most famous handmade neckties come from Charvet, whose boutique in the Place Vendôme offers the largest range of woven silk neckties to be found anywhere in the world. Each item is a masterpiece of the textile manufacturer's art.

The loop where the narrow end begins can be sewn to the underside of the necktie, and in the neckties produced by many manufacturers both ends of the loop disappear into the central seam. However, while this detail is an indication of the time devoted to making the necktie, it says nothing about the quality of the silk or the fabric of the interlining and the lining. Charvet neckties, for instance, which are indisputably of the finest quality, have only a simple label sewn on.

Characteristic of Italian neckties is the feature called "self-tipping," meaning that the tips of both ends are lined with the fabric of the necktie itself. But self-tipping too is simply a stylistic touch rather than proof of the quality of the silk, so, as we suggested above, your best course of action is to feel the necktie before going into the technical details.

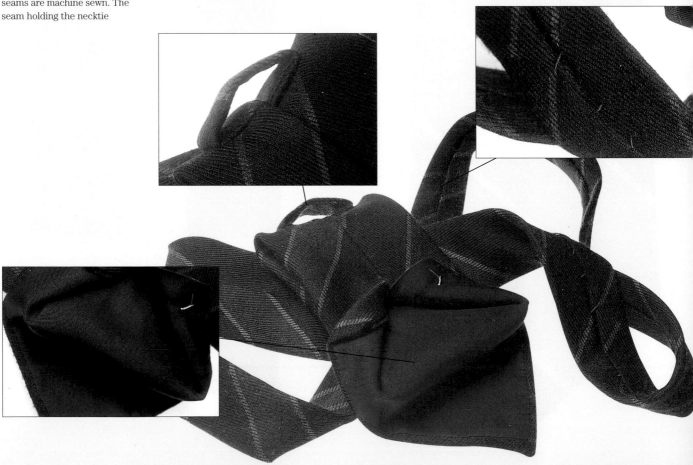

Woolen Neckties

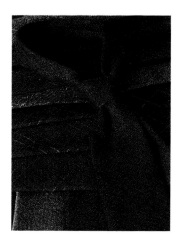

Knitted and woolen neckties do not form part of the English gentleman's city wardrobe. He may wear a woolen necktie in the country, but he is more likely to leave the knitted variety to artists, academics, writers, editors, and journalists. Similar unwritten rules hold good outside the United Kingdom. All over the world, a woven silk necktie is the kind for formal wear. None the less, knitted and woolen neckties can be worn with a business suit or even in the evening if you go about it the right way.

The formal version of the knitted necktie is black or dark blue. It is the same width as an ordinary woven necktie, looks good with light shirts, and is perfectly correct worn with a dark gray suit. Knitted neckties in single colors also go well with patterned shirts. However, if you are not quite sure of yourself in questions of style, it is better to avoid a knitted necktie, since its very simplicity calls for a sure hand in combining it with the right shirt.

There are almost as many different patterns and colors for woolen neckties as for their silk counterparts. In England wool is correct for weekends and the country, so the neckties of famous colleges, regiments, and clubs are often available not just in silk but in woolen versions that can be worn with a tweed suit. As mentioned above in the chapter on the shirt, the Tattersall check shirt is very popular in academic circles. The same is true of the woolen necktie, which is often seen around the necks of professors and lecturers who like to dress as if they were off for a country weekend, perhaps to demonstrate that they have nothing to do with the city and the ordinary world of moneymaking. Like the knitted necktie, the woolen necktie is usually in a single color, so it can easily be combined with a check shirt. However, there are also

woolen neckties in stripes and all the classic patterns, such as paisley and foulard. Many patterns have rural motifs such as ducks, pheasants, or horses. Italy produces some very elegant woolen neckties; those made by Nicky of Milan are particularly exquisite. Indeed, it is true that woolen neckties are worn almost as much as silk ones in Italy.

Woolen neckties are usually made of pure wool or cashmere, but there are also mixtures of wool and cashmere, wool and silk, or silk and cashmere. But whatever the material of which a woolen necktie is made, it is warmer than its silk counterpart, so it is particularly in fall and winter that a woolen necktie makes a comfortable, elegant alternative to one made of silk.

Perhaps a woolen necktie can never acheive the crisp formality of silk, but it nonetheless has its place in the gentleman's wardrobe.

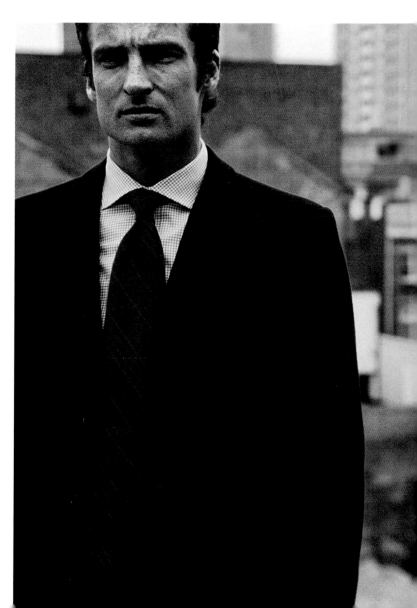

Some of the finest cashmere neckties in the world are designed by the English designer Michael Drake. Not surprisingly, his assistant Robert Godley is pictured wearing one here.

The Best of the Best

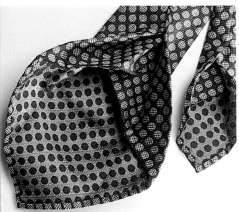

The best neckties are made of pure silk or wool, but the information "All silk" or "100% cashmere" on the label does not tell the whole truth about the necktie. Strictly speaking, the label ought to say "Shell fabric all silk," or "Shell made of 100% cashmere," since in even the best handmade neckties the interlining is not made of silk or cashmere. The fabric of this interlining is not usually mentioned, and makes no difference to the final product. However, there are some neckties made entirely of silk, containing no interlining of any other material. These rare masterpieces of the necktie maker's art are of course rather expensive, and are described as "seven-fold ties." The name explains the method of manufacture, which uses a great deal of material; a square piece of silk is folded seven times into the shape of a necktie which owes its volume not to any additional interlining but simply to the folded silk, so that it really is 100 percent silk. The "seven-fold tie" is the *non plus ultra* of tiemaking, and the ultimate in understatement.

The Mecca of all aficionados of expensive Hermès leather goods, silk scarves, neckties, and accessories is 24 Faubourg St. Honoré. Every year, thousands of customers from all over the world visit the Paris boutique.

A Great Success from the Grande Nation

The Hermès necktie is one of a small number of exclusive products regarded as symbols of good taste all over the world. Neckties in an even more sophisticated style certainly do exist, and more unusual and much more expensive ones are also available. But no other necktie is so far above criticism and changes in taste and fashion as the Hermès tie. If you take a couple of Hermès neckties on a business trip and combine them skillfully with your shirt and suit, you will never risk being incorrectly dressed anywhere you go.

It is difficult to say just what is so special about the Hermès necktie. Perhaps its inimitable style, or perhaps the power of the Hermès brand name, synonymous with luxury for many decades. When the Hermès necktie first came on the market in 1953, no one could have guessed that over six million would have been sold 34 years later. Yet at that time the firm of Hermès could already look back on 116 years of existence. Thierry Hermès laid the foundations of the firm's present success in 1837. Under his son Emile-Charles, it moved to its now famous address in the Faubourg St. Honoré. The first branch was opened in New York in 1929. This was the beginning of the worldwide success of Hermès, which now sells not just leather goods, silk scarves, and neckties, but also clothing, fine perfumes, and accessories of all kinds.

If the fancy takes you, you can be dressed from head to foot by Hermès, and you can furnish your home almost entirely with products sold under the same brand name. Anyone can be part of the Hermès legend simply by purchasing a necktie with the prestigious logo. Some men apparently buy at least 40 a year; there are two new collections annually, each consisting of 20 designs, and in addition 10 collections of reissues of older patterns. Most of the designs are available in four to five colors. Serious collectors of these neckties often hope to fill gaps in their collections at airport boutiques, where with luck they may find a design long since sold out in the local Hermès boutique. It may seem remarkable that Hermès can continually come up with new designs for neckties, but there are apparently infinite variations on patterns possible. The firm will no doubt keep on producing new ones for many years to come. In spite of the great variety of patterns, customers have a clear favorite, the *chaîne d'ancre* pattern, which sells 6,000 neckties in every collection. Perhaps there is one hanging in your own wardrobe?

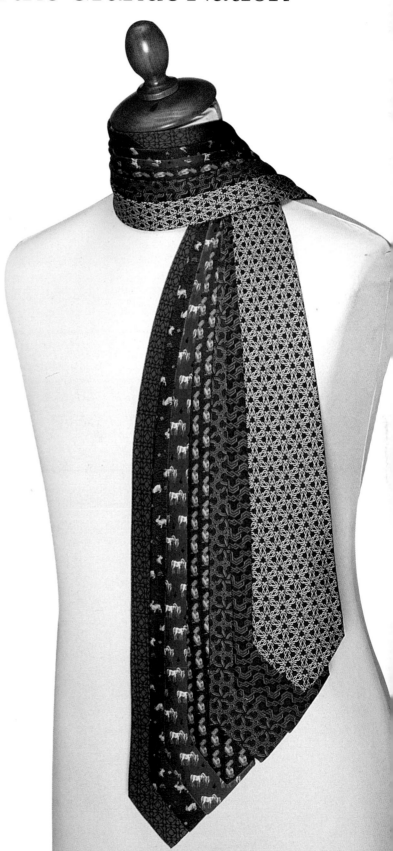

The Origins of Silk

Ever since its discovery, silk has been considered the finest and most beautiful of all woven textiles. For centuries it was reserved for the rich and powerful, who wore the shimmering fabric as a sign of their prosperity. It comes from the silk moth, whose caterpillars (known as silkworms) wrap themselves in a cocoon of silk threads before pupating. The best known of the silk moths is *Bombyx mori*, which eats mulberry leaves.

Rearing silkworms has always been the first step in manufacturing silk. There are records of silkworm rearing (sericulture) dating back to the third century BC. The Chinese were the first to master the art, and they guarded their knowledge jealously for a long time, since silk brought to the courts of Europe along the Silk Roads was a major part of their export trade. However, China eventually had to face competition when sericulture spread to Korea and Japan, and later to India and Persia. Byzantine monks were the first to introduce silkworm rearing into Europe. Today, France and Italy have joined India, China, Japan, and Korea as silk-producing countries. The process is both very time- and labor-intensive. First the silkworms have to spin their cocoons; then the pupae are killed with either hot vapor or hot air.

The sericulturist's part in the process is over at this point, and the threads of the cocoon are unwound in a special factory. The cocoons are first soaked in water to remove the sticky substance gluing together the threads, which can then be unwound with the aid of special brushes. Of the 3,300 yards [3,000m] of threads in a single cocoon, only about 300 to 900 yards [300–800m] will be suitable for making high-grade raw silk. The silk is refined further by boiling in a soap solution to remove any remnants of the silk gum; this process is called "boiling off." Then the silk threads are spun and woven.

The complexity of the process of producing silk makes it relatively expensive. It is also regarded as a high-quality material, hence its use in neckties and other garments.

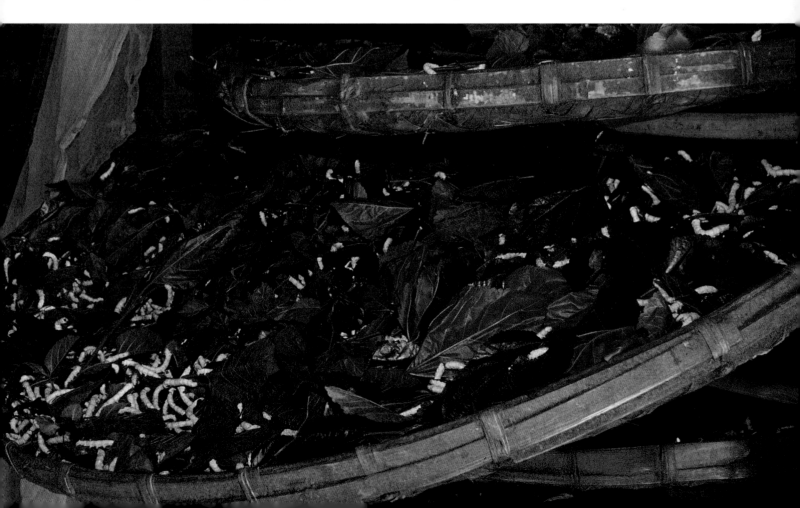

Making a Necktie

The workshop of the English manufacturer John Comfort, founded in 1908, has a long tradition behind it. It is in Leyton, a suburb in northeast London. However, very few customers have ever seen the workshop with its relaxed and friendly family atmosphere. Most customers visit the showroom in New Bond Street for their neckties.

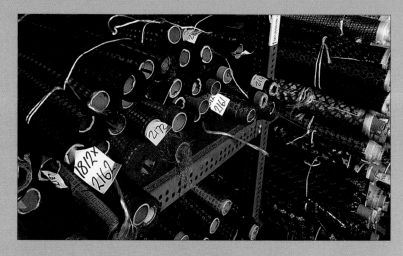

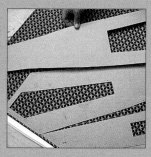

A modern necktie usually consists of three parts. At John Comfort, the fabric is not individually cut by hand with scissors. However, even for machine cutting it must be carefully adjusted by hand, and an accurate eye is necessary.

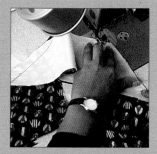

The three parts of the necktie are sewn together by machine. This is usually the case even with manufacturers who describe their neckties as handfinished. Only a very few firms can still truthfully say that every seam is genuinely sewn by hand.

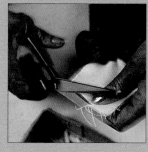

The necktie has a cotton interlining which gives the tie the correct volume, and in wear it affects the size of the knot.

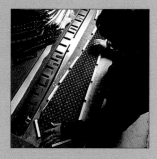

Technically speaking, the mark of a handmade necktie is that the central seam inside the tie is sewn by hand. At John Comfort this is done by a machine which imitates the slight irregularities of hand sewing very closely.

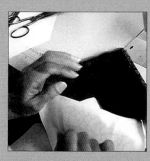

Both ends of the tie have a colored lining into which the interlining is tucked, as if into a pocket. This lining is sewn in separately by machine.

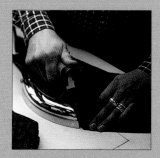

Pressing is another step distinguishing the handmade necktie from the factory-made item. If the necktie is "handfinished" or actually "handmade" it is pressed by hand. At John Comfort the pressing is done by machine.

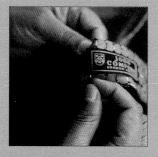

The John Comfort label, or the label of the firm under whose name the necktie will be sold, is now sewn on. Since John Comfort neckties are often marketed under different brand names, many men do not know they are wearing a product of this old family firm.

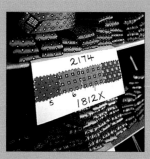

John Comfort always has thousands of finished neckties, bow ties, and cravats in stock so that the firm can fill orders at short notice. Customers do not usually visit the firm itself.

The Master of the Custom-Made Necktie

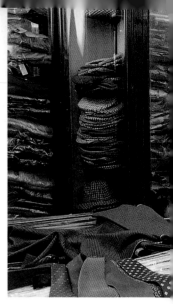

Nothing has changed since Eugenio Marinella opened his store in 1914. Maurizio Marinella is the grandson of the founder of the firm. He stands behind the counter himself from morning to evening, unless he is away on business; at least once a month he goes to Rome or Milan with fabric samples to take orders from regular customers.

What did Mikhail Gorbachev, George Bush, François Mitterand, Oscar Luigi Scalfaro, and Helmut Kohl have in common? You might say it was the mark they all made on the political landscape of their countries – unless you knew that these five statesmen all patronized the same maker of neckties: Marinella of Naples. The store opened in the Piazza Vittoria in 1914, supplying first Neapolitans and then customers from all over the world with the finest of neckties. Its products can be custom-made if required, so a customer can choose a dozen neckties for his new sports jacket and have them cut to exactly the length and width he likes best. He can also decide on the thickness of the interlining, which will affect the thickness of the knot. The customer really is king here, with the power to determine all the crucial details of a necktie. Anyone who thinks that a small store like Marinella could never justify the expense of paying so much attention to detail would be wrong; more neckties are sold here in an incredibly small space of only 24 square yards (20 sq m) than in many gentlemen's outfitters with premises on several floors. The firm makes a profit not by charging an exorbitant price per item, but from the custom of a great many fashion-conscious men from Italy and all over the world.

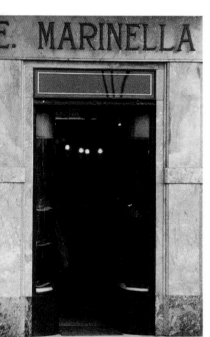

The real shrines of classic gentleman's wear are often to be found behind unassuming façades – like that of the necktie business of E. Marinella in Naples.

However, it is no coincidence that this place of pilgrimage for necktie enthusiasts is to be found on the map of Italy. The men of no other nation attach such importance to their clothing, as is shown by the obviously secure future of this small specialist necktie firm. In England, the superior quality of your shirt is traditionally thought more important, and the choice of neckties is rather limited, since for decades the design of a man's necktie was determined by the colors of his school, college, club, or regiment. As a result, even individually custom-made neckties are less stylistically significant in the United Kingdom. France is the only other country that could be the home of a firm like Marinella, for like the Italians the French appreciate tradition, quality, and above all style. Charvet in the Place Vendôme in Paris, for instance, is another place where you can have your neckties made individually to measure.

Marinella's fame is due not just to the method of handmaking neckties but also to the incomparable range and quality of the fabrics it keeps in stock. Three times a year Maurizio Marinella visits England to buy fabric, using the business contacts built up by first his grandfather and then his father in over 80 years. Marinella sells off the rack neckties as well as individually made items, and Maurizio Marinella has the former made for him in England. He entrusts his custom only to the top specialists; Drake's, for instance, supplies both fabrics and ready-made neckties. Drake's fabrics for Marinella are exclusively designed and manufactured for the Neapolitans. Marinella proves that even today small family firms can survive and prosper if they offer really high quality and individual service. In addition, the firm's tradition shows that a customer who is confident of his style and understands fashion still knows best what suits him, and why would he be satisfied with a gentleman's outfitter providing a choice of a few dozen neckties at most throughout the season, when Marinella can offer over 3,500 different fabrics and patterns in all?

Marinella's range of styles may seem to undermine its ability to appear exclusive. How does one identify the Marinella style, when there are so many? The answer is in the quality of the garment, and it is this that primarily attracts high-profile customers.

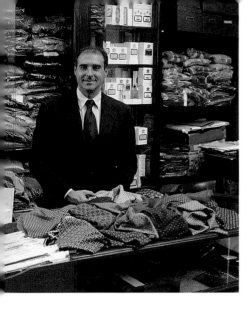

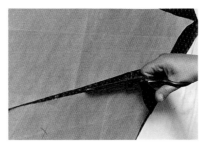

At Marinella the cutting is done by hand, using shears, in the good old way. There is a paper pattern, like a tailor's, which can be adjusted to the customer's own requirements for the length, width, and volume of his necktie.

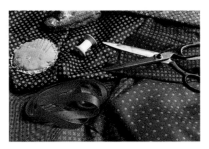

"Self-tipping" is typical of Marinella neckties; the outer lining is made of the same material as the necktie itself. The lining is measured so that none of the interlining will show when the necktie is a finished garment.

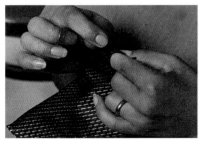

The separate sections of a Marinella necktie are sewn entirely by hand. This method gives the necktie its superior durability and elasticity.

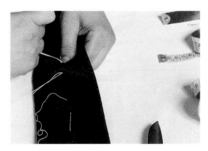

As with a custom-made suit, the Marinella necktie is first basted together with white cotton thread and afterward folded into its final shape.

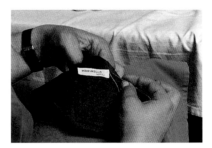

When the necktie has been pressed by hand the Marinella label is added, a discreet statement that it is one of the best ties in the world.

The Business Necktie

Classic business patterns are anything but original; that is not supposed to be their point. Only the smallest of details should indicate whether this is an ordinary necktie or a first-class item. Understatement does not work unless an unobtrusive exterior conceals really top quality, as in the neckties made by Marinella of Naples. People who have read that Marinella provides the best neckties in the world and will make them to measure may be disappointed to see how plain the firm's designs are, but in fact their excellence resides in that plain quality. The saying that "less is more" is perfectly true of ties. For businessmen, as well as politicians, Marinella's reputation for quality is of prime importance, and hence the firm's large number of business customers.

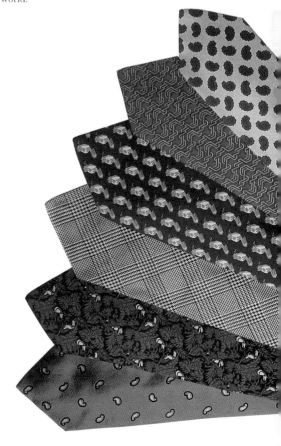

The Four-in-Hand

One of the modern leaders of men's fashion appears in British history books and the annals of international style under three titles: first as the Prince of Wales, second as King Edward VIII, and finally as the Duke of Windsor. Each title covers one phase in the life of a man who was born in 1894 and died in 1972. His period as king was the shortest, and for the sake of convenience we will call him simply the Duke of Windsor here, although he also introduced or popularized major innovations in fashion while he was Prince of Wales. His main connection with the subject of this chapter is the Windsor knot, which was named after him, although photographs tend to suggest that he did not actually wear it himself, and that the voluminous knots of his neckties were probably the result of a thick lining rather than the double Windsor knot. Suzy Menkes, who mentions this fact in her book *The Windsor Style*, adds that the Duke of Windsor had his neckties made by Hawes & Curtis – always with a particularly thick lining, another reason why he personally may not have worn the Windsor knot, which becomes far too bulky when the lining of the necktie is thick. Try it for yourself with ties made of different materials with different thicknesses of lining. The four-in-hand knot, when tied in a rather thick tie, produces exactly the same look as the knot worn by the Duke of Windsor in many photographs. This is perhaps an example of myth being taken as reality, as has happened in many different cases throughout history.

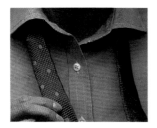

Place the necktie around your neck with the broader end on your right. It must hang lower down than the narrower end.

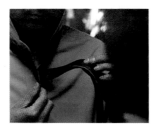

Take the broad end in your right hand and move it left and across the narrow end, holding the narrow end in your left hand. Now pass the broad end around the narrow end.

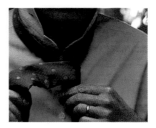

Pass the broad end on around the narrow end so that it is lying on the left again. The shape of the knot is beginning to materialize.

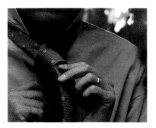

Now pass the broad end underneath the half-formed knot, raising the knot slightly as you do so.

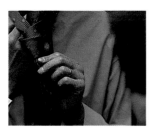

With your left hand, pass the broad end over the half knot from underneath, and pull the whole of the broad end through to the front.

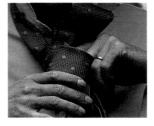

With your right hand, pass the broad end of the necktie between the layer of the knot which is now on top and the layer directly underneath it, and pull the broad end through.

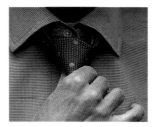

Hold the narrow end of the tie firmly and slowly tighten the knot. Do not forget to do up your shirt button.

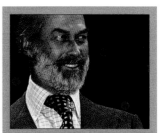

Prince Michael of Kent has two stylistic peculiarities which have earned him the reputation of being a near eccentric. He is the only notable member of the Royal Family to wear a beard, and he has a liking for "kipper ties," broad neckties in the style of the 1960s. His ties are notable not just for their breadth but for their designs and materials.

How to Tie a Necktie

1. The simple four-in-hand knot is the most stylistically attractive and versatile knot to wear. It is stylistically attractive because the long shape of the knot lengthens the look of the throat area, and its slightly diagonal line gives an interestingly asymmetric effect between the two ends of the necktie; versatile because however thick or thin the necktie, it will give a good result.

2. The Windsor knot is symmetric, but perhaps for that very reason rather boring. It is often wider than it is high, so the optical effect is to shorten the throat area in a less pleasing manner than that of the four-in-hand. It really produces satisfactory results only with very thin neckties, but then its triangular shape looks odd in contrast to the otherwise rather long and slender general effect of the necktie.

3. The knot of your tie should suit your shirt collar. The four-in-hand knot looks good with any shape of collar. The "cutaway collar" (see pages 52–53) is the only one that really combines well with the Windsor knot, but even then the four-in-hand usually looks more elegant if the necktie is the right thickness and width.

4. You should not exert force in tying a necktie. A knot pulled too tight and squeezed in at the sides will not look very elegant.

5. Try out neckties made by different manufacturers until you find a brand you really like. A very slender, straight four-in-hand knot can be tied in Hermès neckties. If you like a thicker knot, try Drake's of England's ties. It is also well worth considering custom-made neckties.

The Windsor Knot

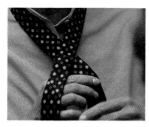

To tie a Windsor knot, start with the broader end hanging much further down on the right. Take the broader end in your right hand and pass it to the left over the narrower end, which you are holding in your left hand.

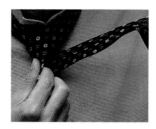

Pass the broader end from left to right under and around the narrow end. Then pull it over the knot and down toward your body through the loop that has been formed.

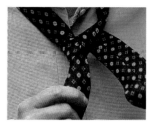

The broader end is now hanging down on the right, wrong side facing up.

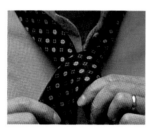

Now take the broader end and pass it left around the half knot.

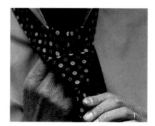

Next, with the thick end of the necktie in your left hand, pass it up from below and behind the knot and through the loop around your neck.

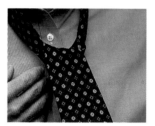

Pull the broader end forward over the half-completed knot and let it hang down.

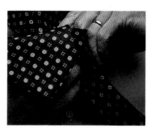

Next, put the tip of the broad end underneath the outer layer of the knot.

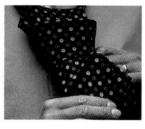

Pull the broad end right through and carefully adjust the knot, holding it gently and pulling the narrower end.

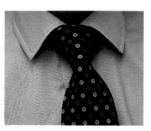

The broader end of the necktie should now hang down further than the narrow end. If not, tie another knot or tuck the narrow end into your waistband.

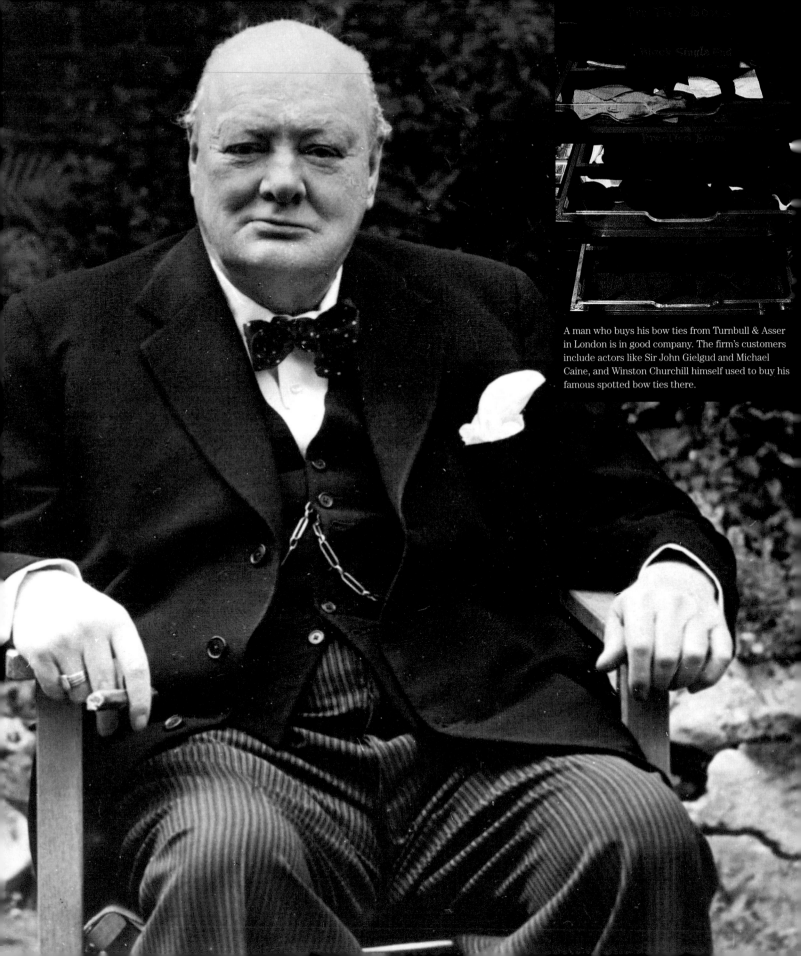

A man who buys his bow ties from Turnbull & Asser in London is in good company. The firm's customers include actors like Sir John Gielgud and Michael Caine, and Winston Churchill himself used to buy his famous spotted bow ties there.

The Bow Tie

The bow tie is closely related to the ordinary necktie, but unlike the necktie its bow still shows that it is descended from the neckcloth, its predecessor. Until the nineteenth century neckwear for men consisted of square cloths folded once into a triangle and then knotted in various ways or tied with a bow. The smaller and narrower those neckcloths became, the more they resembled our present bow tie. Its shape has hardly changed since around 1870. However, over the course of time the bow tie has ceased to be an equally acceptable alternative to other forms of necktie (the standard long necktie or the ascot tie), and is now a product for a special niche market. There is one principal reason for its decline: most men do not know how to tie it – and anyone with the faintest idea about style knows that ready-made bow ties are beyond the pale. But a bow tie is still worn with a tuxedo or with tails, and on those occasions a man usually gets his wife or a friend to tie it. The bow tie is one of those things that every man tends to try and then abandon at some point in his life, like smoking a pipe or growing a beard. Some men really like bow ties and wear them almost all the time, but they are increasingly in the minority, whether because there always seems to be something slightly comic about the bow tie, or because a shirt front seems naked without a standard necktie, or because bow ties seem rather effeminate. In any case, they have become so unusual today that anyone with a bow tie immediately attracts attention. Some men in the public eye have made bow ties their "trademark". You will attract plenty of comments on the first day you wear one, a disadvantage that anyone rather shy or reserved will anticipate, and it will probably put him off the whole idea. There is something to be said for the bow tie, all the same. You cannot drop your food on it, and it is the only alternative for a man who dislikes wearing a standard necktie but still wants to be correctly dressed.

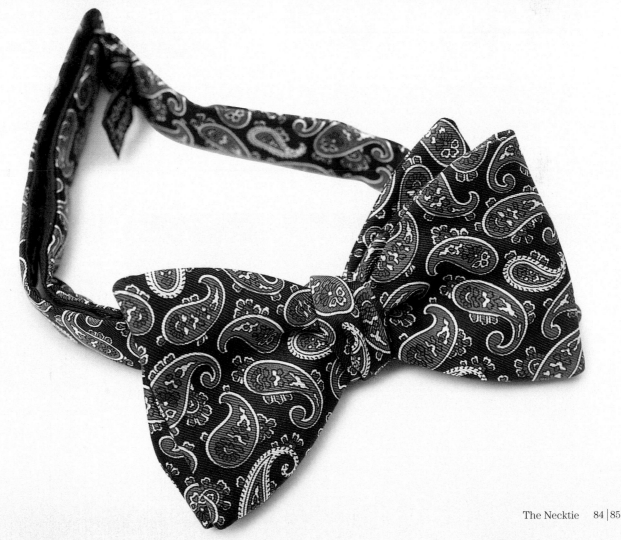

Tying a Bow Tie

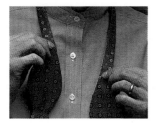

Adjust the bow tie to the right size before putting it around your neck. Unlike standard long neckties, bow ties need to fit the width of the neck exactly.

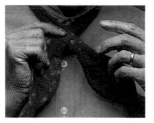

Put the end on the left over the end on the right so that both ends cross at the narrow area behind the oval curve.

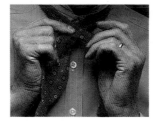

Take the left end through the loop now surrounding your neck, and pull both ends to make a loose, simple knot.

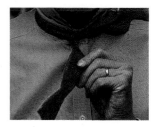

Take the end now on the left in both hands and fold it to the right in the middle of the oval.

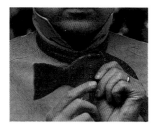

Hold the folded end in the thumb and forefinger of your left hand.

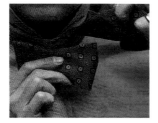

Take the right end and place it exactly in the middle of the left end, which is held in your left hand, so that the right end hangs down over the knot. Hold both ends with the thumb and forefinger of your left hand.

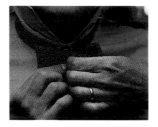

Now pass the right end of the bow under and around the folded left end of the bow. You now have a loop.

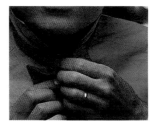

Take the right end around the folded left end again and pass it to the left through the loop you have made – preferably folding the part of the bow on the right first. Press the part on the right with your thumb and fold it at the same time.

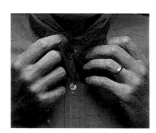

Push the folded right end far enough through to stay in place. Now let go with both hands, and you will see the final form of the bow materializing.

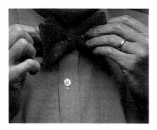

Hold the part of the bow on the right firmly in your right hand, and using your left hand take the end of the bow that is already halfway through by the fold in it and pull carefully. Now you will see the reason for the curved shape of the bow tie in its untied state.

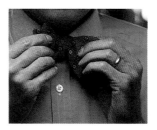

To adjust the bow, take the ends lying opposite each other – the two open ends and the two folded ends – and pull carefully until the bow is firmly tied.

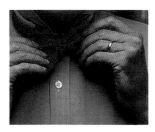

The finished bow will look slightly different every time, but at least the fact that it may not be perfect shows everyone that you tied it yourself. But always make sure that in the first step you place the left end over the right end, or the operation will not work.

The Cravat

Whenever a film script calls for a playboy to appear, the character is regularly shown wearing a cravat, usually with a navy blazer or a shawl-collared knitted jacket. One imagines authors of popular novels wearing them, also film directors and millionaires, and perhaps now and then an officer of Her Majesty's forces, but only at the weekend. These typical associations of the cravat do not really do it justice, since it is an attractive way of lending the casual weekend look that touch of formality and elegance you sometimes want between Friday evening and Sunday evening. A plain outfit of Tattersall check shirt, jeans, a bottle-green V-neck pullover, and burgundy Weejun loafers from Bass is both elegant and casual when worn with a paisley cravat. Similarly, a combination of gray herringbone tweed jacket, dark gray flannels, a white shirt, and black brogues looks more casual if you exchange your magenta and green striped club necktie for a cravat. A cravat emphasizes the sporting look, or lends a light touch to a more formal outfit. However, some men do not like this kind of nuance, and prefer a clear distinction between the formal and the casual to the in-between stage represented by the cravat. If you would rather look formal even at the weekend, they say, why not stick to your guns and wear necktie, shirt, and jacket, instead of going in for half-hearted measures like the cravat? But other men do not care to wear an open-necked shirt, which they feel is just a bit too casual, exposing too much throat, and for them the cravat is highly recommended; it helps them to demonstrate, even at weekends and off duty, that they like to observe a certain code of dress.

The word "cravat" has an unexpected etymology. It comes from the Serbo-Croat word *Hrvat*, meaning "Croat," or native of Croatia. Croat soldiers in the French army during the Thirty Years' War wore the familiar garment, and it became referred to in French as a *cravate*. Similar use of "cravats" can be seen in some military uniforms today, although they are neither silk nor patterned like the ones shown below.

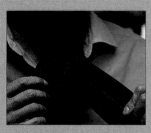

First place the cravat loosely around your neck.

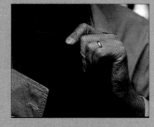

Then take hold of the right end and place it over the left end.

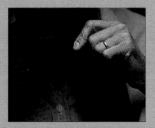

Pass the right end over and around the left end, put it through the loop thus formed from underneath, and pull it through and up.

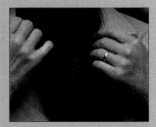

Place what started out as the right end of the cravat precisely over what started out as the left end and is now underneath it, and adjust both ends.

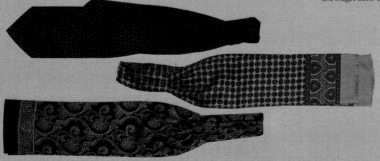

The cravat is always made of pure silk. It can be bought in a vast selection of different patterns and in all qualities, depending on what necktie-maker you buy from. Unlike standard neckties or bow ties, cravats are never in one solid color or striped. Classic designs are paisley or foulard prints, or similar patterns.

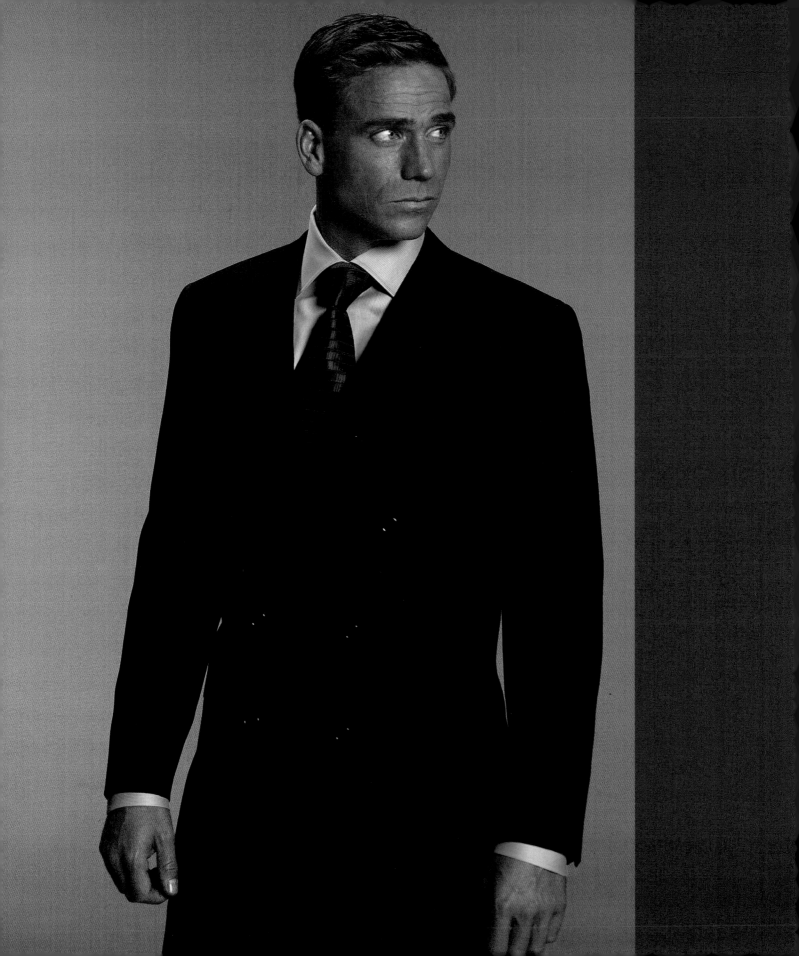

The Suit

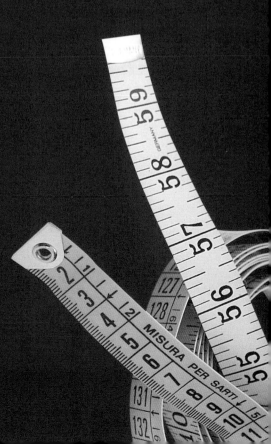

Style in the Suit

The suit is still the most elegant item of clothing a man can wear so long as its cut, color, and fabric are correct – meaning that they suit the occasion, the time of day, the season of the year, and the climate. There are good reasons for listing cut, color and fabric in that order, since cut is really the most important factor. If you are in any doubt, then it is better to buy a well-cut suit in a fabric that may not be of the very top quality than a poorly cut suit in a better fabric – although the suit above all is not an area where compromises should be made. By a good cut we mean the basic pattern that has been used again and again since the 1930s, irrespective of fashions and trends, and is now regarded as the international standard by all good tailors and manufacturers of ready-made clothing. The cut of a good suit should look "natural," that is to say, it should bring out the best in its wearer, resorting to corrective measures only with real problem figures. This is an especially important feature in relation to the shoulders of the suit. A rather thin, small-boned man will look best in a suit with a narrow cut and little or no shoulder padding, narrow lapels, and close-fitting trouser legs. An athletic, broad-shouldered man will not need shoulder padding either, and again, the suit can be cut to suit his natural measurements. If the wearer has a corpulent figure, it is even more advisable to avoid anything in the cut of the suit that would make him look even larger.

The traditional colors regarded as correct for a suit are dark blue, dark to very light gray, and black. It should certainly be in one of those colors if it is to be worn for business in such fields as finance, the law, commerce, or politics. A brown or green suit will do only at the weekend or for sporting occasions – but more about that later.

Today's suits are made in fabrics of much lighter weight than in the past, when offices were either heated by coal fires or not at all. However, there are still considerable differences in the weight and thickness of the materials used, and you should start by thinking exactly where you will be wearing your suit: will it be in the chilly north or in a mild Mediterranean climate? Will

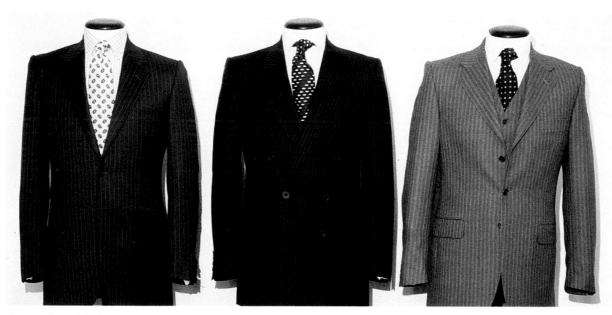

The two-piece suit is the most usual model today. It has two buttons and two side vents, and trousers with or without cuffs. There are variations on this basic model. It is possible to have either three buttons and a center vent at the back of the jacket, or three buttons and two side vents.

The double-breasted suit always has two side vents, never a vent at the back of the jacket. In continental Europe it may have no vents at all, but that is not *comme il faut*. A jacket without any vents will hang well only when you are standing and if you do not put your hands in your trouser pockets. However, as this habit is regarded as bad manners in Germany, many German suit jackets accordingly have no vents.

It used to be quite difficult to buy a well-cut suit with a vest off the rack. Luckily for men who appreciate this classic type of suit, some traditional gentlemen's outfitters such as Gieves & Hawkes have begun offering them again.

you be driving to a stuffy office from your comfortable home in a heated car, without feeling any great change of temperature, or will you reach it after a long journey commuting to work through drafty subway stations and cold streets? One way or another, the best suiting fabric has always been (and still is) pure wool, even in summer, for no other natural material drapes so elegantly – or is so crease resistant. If you do find creases in a pure wool suit after you have been sitting for a long time, they will hang out again quite soon. In fact it does not matter if a perfectly cut suit looks a little crumpled; it is still more elegant than a suit without a single crease in it, but of poor or even just average cut.

Since we have used the word "suit" so often already, it is about time to provide a brief definition; a suit is a set of clothing consisting of trousers and jacket made from the same fabric. That may sound obvious, but it is worth mentioning, since until the end of the nineteenth century a gentleman used to wear a tailcoat, frock coat, or morning coat with a vest of a different fabric, and trousers in yet another material. At first the combination of matching jacket, vest, and trousers – a suit – was worn on informal occasions. It was not until the end of the 1930s that the suit became the accepted uniform of all office workers. But although the suit is now formal wear par excellence, a style-conscious gentleman – in particular one with a sense of tradition – still wears the old combination of morning coat, vest, and striped trousers for weddings, funerals, and grand formal occasions.

At first, then, the suit came in three parts: jacket, trousers, and vest. Today it is more usual to have a two-piece suit consisting of jacket and trousers. The vest is dying out, although since it has been doing so ever since the Second World War, perhaps we may conclude that it is not going to become extinct just yet. However, it is no longer part of the traditional custom-made suit, since offices today are usually too warm for anyone to need an additional layer of clothing under his jacket. Unless you feel the cold very badly, you are almost obliged to do without a vest – but perhaps you work in an office where it is not felt incorrect to take off your jacket and go about in vest and shirt sleeves.

This introduction to the subject of the suit would not be complete without a little geographical information. England is the land of origin of the suit, and indeed of modern gentlemen's fashions in general. The basic pattern of suit now accepted, copied, and varied all over the world was developed in the United Kingdom at the beginning of the twentieth century, and until the

Button Undone

At first sight it looks as if a button is missing, but look more closely and you will see that it is simply undone. Purely by chance, of course. Perhaps the wearer of this suit recently

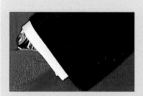

pushed up the sleeves of his shirt and jacket to wash his hands, and then forgot to do up the last button. Or is that really the reason? No, of course not. After all, no one would forget to button up his shirt or overcoat. A man who leaves a button on his sleeve undone is making a statement along the lines of: "Look, I can undo the buttons on my sleeve, and only the sleeve buttons of really good suits can be undone. My suit is a good one – and expensive." Sleeve buttons that really undo are far from being the most important or even the most expensive mark of a good suit – but they are its most striking feature. Hence the undone button.

Second World War London was the undisputed capital of fashionable menswear. Thanks to the tailors of Italy, however, England no longer has a monopoly on style, even if it can still offer the very best of tailoring. However, English tailoring by no means shares the Italian concept of elegance that chooses the fabric, color, and cut of a suit by esthetic criteria and makes it on the same principles, instead of simply observing the strict rules of dress imposed by a social upper class. In fact the Italians are better than the English at making suits from lightweight fabrics, since they live in a hot country, or at least those in the south of Italy do. Today, then, we can choose the best suits from various different sources according to our tastes and our requirements: a pinstriped suit from London, a summer suit from Rome, or alternatively an English suit made in Italian silk or an Italian suit made from Scottish tweed. But England and Italy alike offer the cut and quality that make a really good suit.

Tailors in other countries naturally aspire to the positions of quality maintained by those in Italy and England, and the Italian diaspora in the USA certainly provides fertile ground for producing good tailors. Nevertheless, it is these two countries that retain a reputation for excellence that seems unassailable.

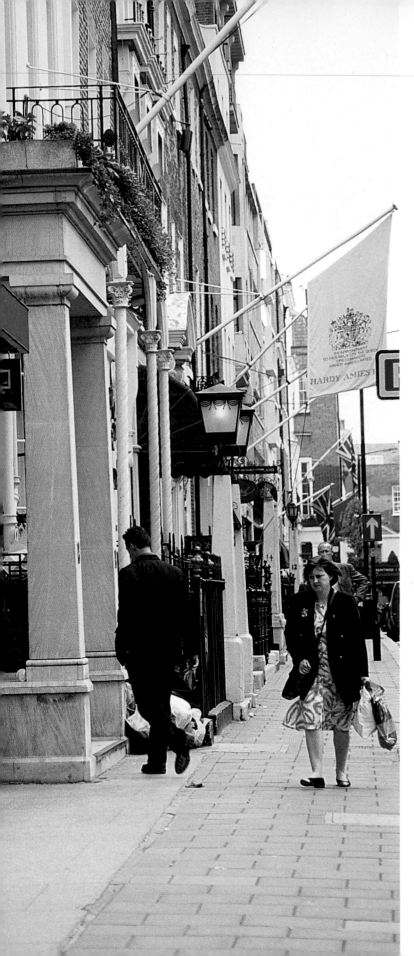

The Mecca of the Custom-made Suit

In the modern world, where people think more of the designer than the craftsman, Savile Row is one of the last outposts where designing a garment is the province of the craftsman who makes it, in this case the tailor. However, let us not forget that there is a division of labor even in Savile Row. The cutter could be called the architect of the suit; he designs its cut and then cuts out the pieces. The tailor is the man who really puts the suit together. To continue our analogy, he is the construction worker. Tailors usually specialize in jackets, vests, or trousers – the English terms are "coat maker," "waistcoat maker," and "trouser maker." The cutter adjusts the suit when the customer tries it on, in a procedure known as fitting. Then the suit goes back to the specialist tailor with the cutter's adjustments marked. Theoretically, the cutter could make the suit from start to finish, since by the time a tailor has risen to the responsible position of cutter he will know his trade inside out. This knowledge of the actual methods of tailoring is what distinguishes the cutter from the designer, who needs to know the craft of tailoring only well enough to make marketable items – more particularly for manufacturing on a large scale. The true craft of tailoring is an old-fashioned cottage industry, well appreciated by the real gentlemen who consume its fine products.

SAVILE ROW W1
CITY OF WESTMINSTER

Savile Row is the Mecca of all aficionados of custom tailoring. In fact the style of a particular tailor here may not be especially English. From the end of the nineteenth century onward many excellent Jewish tailors emigrated to London from Poland, Russia, Hungary, and Germany. They combined the elegance learned in their native lands in continental Europe with the English style, thus making a notable contribution to the fame of Savile Row.

Custom tailoring is no longer the only way to get a suit that fits well, and it is often far from the best way. Sad to say, the art of tailoring has sunk to a lamentably low level in most countries of central and northern Europe, and a custom-made suit will be only as good as the tailor who cuts and makes it. However, if his customers cannot tell the difference between a really good piece of work and one that is only average, the tailor will have no incentive to excel. And how are his customers to recognize the best if they have never seen anything but off-the-rack suits made for what is supposed to be the average figure? England and Italy are the only countries where there is still a constant influx of new customers who genuinely understand the tailor's craft.

By comparison with the golden years of the past, of course, even English and Italian tailors are less important than they used to be, at least in terms of output. However, there is still sufficient demand in London, Rome, Milan, and Naples to maintain many good tailoring establishments. Their customers still know the subtle difference between custom tailoring (or, to use the British term, "bespoke" tailoring) and "made to measure." The accepted definition of bespoke or custom tailoring is: "a garment cut by an individual, for an individual, by an individual." An individual cut is devised for each customer, depending on his measurements and his requirements, and it will be precisely adjusted to his figure and his character. "Made to measure" tailoring means that a standard cut is adjusted as far as possible to the customer's measurements and personality. Even if "made to measure" tailoring is entirely done by hand to all the rules of the tailor's craft, it will naturally lack the individuality of a custom-made or bespoke suit, and that individuality is not found anywhere else on earth in more concentrated form than in Savile Row and the neighboring streets. There were still hundreds of tailors working in this "golden mile" up to the 1960s. At the end of the 1980s there were only about 50 firms left, most of them one-man businesses whose proprietors acted as cutters, usually commissioning outside workers to do the actual tailoring. In spite of this reduction in quantity, many of the tailors in business today still offer really top quality – both small firms and large, well-known names. A famous name over the door does not necessarily guarantee you the best suit, or ensure that the customer will really get what he hoped for. He may find "his" tailor in a smaller, less conspicuous firm, since the really important point is for the cutter to understand the customer's personal wishes and tastes almost intuitively, which is essential for translating them perfectly into the suit.

Another consideration is the noticeable difference between Savile Row prices. This difference is the result of overheads: the costs incurred in addition to the price of the fabric and the labor. In a firm like Huntsman, where every piece of clothing is made on the premises, these overheads are of course higher than for a single cutter who sends the pieces of fabric out to specialist coat makers, waistcoat makers, and trouser makers. Both methods of work have a long tradition behind them, and neither necessarily guarantees the desired result. A newcomer to the world of custom tailoring should either rely on personal recommendation, or choose a tailor whose "house style" he already knows and likes – or go in search of one himself. But be wary of any firm promising to supply a suit in 24 hours or even less. The total time it takes to make a genuine custom-made or "bespoke" suit is about 40 hours, so the 24-hour suit is an impossibility. A minimum of several days from measuring to the first fitting is the rule, if the tailor's time allows. It will then usually be another six to eight weeks before the suit is finally ready, and if you go to a very large, well-known firm you may have to wait some months for the great moment when you can set eyes on the suit you ordered and wear it for the first time.

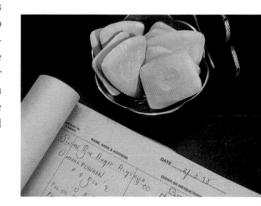

The tailor's chalk is ready to hand – fitting can begin.

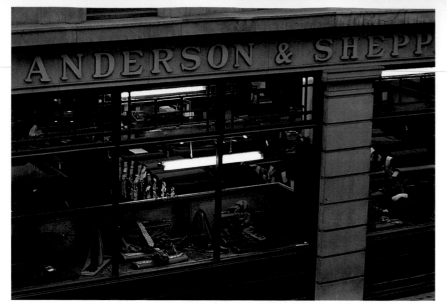

Anderson & Sheppard has been one of the most successful of Savile Row tailors for many years, and is an established institution. The firm's many American customers have contributed a great deal to its reputation; they particularly like the "soft look" of the house. Anderson & Sheppard understands the usual discretion exercised by tailors as a strict vow of silence toward the press. However, it is common knowledge that Prince Charles is among their customers. His double-breasted suits are a good example of the firm's style. For many years, Anderson & Sheppard has also been the only Savile Row tailor to make sleeves with buttons which cannot be undone.

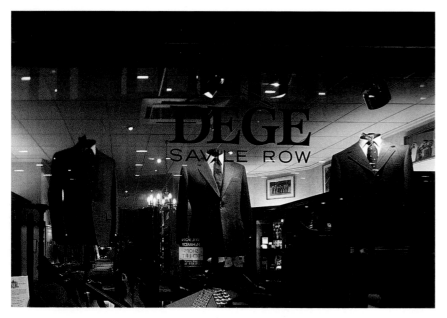

The famous traditional name of J. Dege & Sons at 10 Savile Row accommodates a number of tailors, some of them firms with their own long tradition behind them. They include Wilkinson & Sons, founded in 1662; Rogers & Co., founded in 1774; and John Jones, founded in 1827. Customers will naturally get a suit in the style of whichever particular firm under this roof they patronize. J. Dege & Sons itself makes menswear of a sporting and military cut that appeals to many customers from those fields. The firm regularly visits military bases to take orders. If a customer has no particular wishes, Dege will supply a suit of typically English cut with a long, waisted jacket and sloping shoulders.

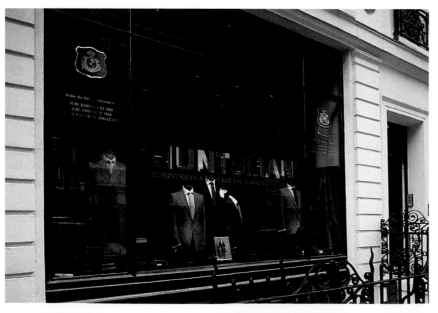

H. Huntsman & Sons was founded in Bond Street, and has been in its Savile Row premises since 1919. Wear for hunting and riding used to be the specialty of this tailor and marked the house style. Jackets are close fitting and have high shoulders and a well-emphasized waist. Huntsman is regarded as the most expensive of Savile Row tailors, but even here prices are no higher than those charged by a good tailor on the continent of Europe. Huntsman prides itself on the craftsmanlike quality of its tailoring, although it is not in fact above the generally high level of the other firms mentioned here.

"*L'Etat c'est moi*," said King Louis XIV of France – and you might say, "Savile Row is Poole." At the beginning of the nineteenth century this firm, founded in 1806, employed over 300 tailors and was the largest enterprise of its kind anywhere in the world. Poole's list of customers reads like a cross section through the history of the nineteenth and twentieth centuries. Even today, its international customers still include many members of the aristocracy. Despite the firm's glorious history, the atmosphere at Poole's is very easy going today, not just as regards the friendly relationships between the staff but in the advice given to customers. No one has a particular style forced on him, and this attitude has certainly contributed to the firm's lasting success. Customers also like the slightly shabby charm of the salesroom; the present head of the firm, Angus Cundey, has stood out for years against the introduction of air conditioning.

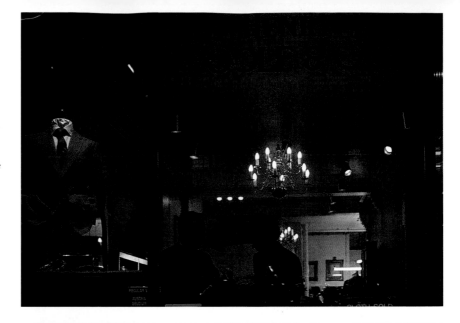

At Tobias Tailors in No. 32, the cutter John Coggin and tailor John Davis still help to fill each order themselves. At Huntsman or at Poole, the customer must rely on the cutter to mark up all the alterations made in fitting clearly enough with his chalk for the tailor in the workshop to follow them. At Tobias Tailors, however, John Davis is present at all stages up to the final fitting, and notes the customer's mental and physical characteristics for himself. If possible, the cutter John Coggin also helps with the making of the suit, so that it is very much all of a piece in craftsmanship and style. Since both men know their craft inside out, the first fitting can take place quite soon, long before the fabric, once cut, would have reached the tailor in an order given to most large tailoring firms. Customers new to Savile Row and connoisseurs alike are welcomed at Tobias Tailors, where receptive ideas of style go hand in hand with traditional concepts of Savile Row quality – and all this at a comparatively modest price.

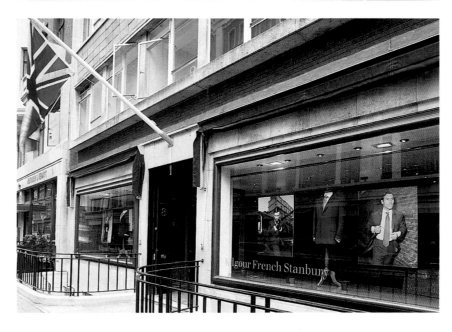

Kilgour, French & Stanbury at No. 8 in the famous street is one of the great old names of Savile Row, although you might easily forget that on entering the recently refurbished and air-conditioned premises. They suggest a background for the up-to-date products of the house, which likes to attract customers aware of the latest trends. But do not be deceived: the cutters and tailors at Kilgour, French & Stanbury still make some of the best suits in Savile Row.
Keeping up with the times, it is now on the Internet, where you can find the tailor's homepage, with information and the latest offers. For instance, there is a special discount for young executives (under 25).
Bernard Weatherill, the leading specialist in hunting and riding wear, operates under the same roof. The cutter George Roden is the last man working in his craft who still makes riding breeches to measure.

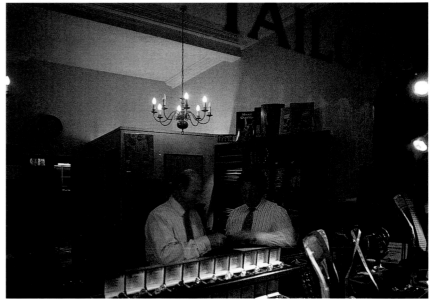

The English Suit

On the underside of the left lapel, below the buttonhole, there is a horizontal *loop* to hold the stem of a flower worn in the buttonhole. This detail is typical of custom-made suits, although it would be no problem to add such a loop to ready-to-wear suits. But presumably only Savile Row customers wear flowers in their buttonholes.

In a traditional English suit like the one worn here by Robert Gieve the *shoulders* have very little if any padding. Instead, they usually slope slightly. However, different tailors have different ideas on the details of shoulder shape.

Anyone with a little expertise in menswear will know that the *sleeve buttons* of a good suit can be undone. This is a feature you will see on the jackets of expensive suits made in Italy. In Savile Row of course the sleeve buttons are also made to undo – although only the two lower buttons of the three or four that actually appear on the sleeve. This means that the sleeves can be turned up when the wearer washes his hands. If necessary the tailor can also shorten the sleeve. The buttonholes of all the sleeve buttons will be cut open and stitched only at the customer's special request.

The waist of the jacket is high and its coat tails fall softly over the hips. This *hourglass cut*, which is also found in many uniform jackets, looks best on slim men. It is typical of the tailors who used to specialize in officers' uniforms and riding clothes.

The *trousers* are cut to rest high on the hips and sit relatively close to the leg. Cuffs are not as common as on the continent of Europe – even the trousers of a double-breasted English suit seldom have cuffs. Traditionally they are held up by suspenders (or in British English "braces"). Some tailors claim it is impossible to keep trousers in place properly without suspenders, others consider them the favorite method because they make it easier to fit the trousers. Another method of holding trousers up without using a belt is a waistband that can be adjusted by buckles or elastication. Any way of avoiding a belt is advisable if the wearer of the suit is short, since a belt divides his figure in half and will make him look even shorter. Suspenders, on the other hand, have an elongating effect, and another advantage is that the trousers will hang properly in any position. Some people even claim that wearing suspenders helps a man walk more confidently. The old recipe for a good carriage – "Stomach in, chest out" – still holds good, and it is easier to follow that advice if you are sure your trousers will stay up.

The classic English suit has two long *side vents*. They enable the wearer to put his hands in his pockets comfortably – a habit that is not regarded as bad manners in England, as it is in Germany. The three-buttoned jacket, often a feature of a tweed suit, traditionally has a back vent instead of side vents. Jackets without vents are very unusual and immediately attract attention. The Queen's husband Prince Philip, for instance, often wears suits without vents in the jacket. His tailor used to be Teddy Watson of Hawes & Curtis, who then entrusted the Duke of Edinburgh to his cutter of many years' standing, John Kent.

Patterns & Fabrics

White pinstripes on a blue background are the undisputed classic. In London this pattern still remains the uniform of most stockbrokers, bankers, lawyers, and politicians, and the fabric also frequently appears on the runway in designer collections.

Gray pinstripe consists of narrow stripes on a gray background, and is the most popular alternative to blue pinstripe. This fabric has sometimes given Englishmen a reputation for dressing like "gray mice."

Dark gray, almost black pinstriped fabric is the ultra-conservative city variant for those of a more discreet nature.

Nailhead is another classic pattern, and comes in shades of gray and blue gray. It is less conspicuous than striped cloth.

Plain worsted fabrics are available in all weights and colors, depending on the use for which the suit will be worn. You would choose a medium weight for a suit that will be worn all the year round, preferably in dark blue or (for the city) shades of gray.

A chalk-striped pattern on a gray background is a classic for double-breasted suits. Edward VIII, then Prince of Wales, popularized this look back in the 1930s.

Strictly speaking, Prince of Wales check or Glen check (as it is known in some continental European countries) is a colored check superimposed on a Glen Urquhart check. Patterns of this kind were designed for the English landed gentry who had settled in Scotland but did not have their own clan tartan. Since they still wanted to dress their employees in a recognizable pattern, the latter wore specially designed "district checks." The Glen Urquhart check was that of the estates of the Countess of Seafield. In England, Prince of Wales check is not worn to the office but is kept for casual suits worn at the weekend, although it is accepted business wear in the rest of Europe and in America. It is thus not surprising that European and Americans conventions on business wear often seem unacceptably showy in conservative England.

GIEVES
&
HAWKES
No.1 Savile Row

A Suit from Gieves and Hawkes

The shop front of Gieves & Hawkes is unusually showy for Savile Row. You often find the best tailors on quite small premises, sometimes even working in basements. Not so at Gieves & Hawkes at 1 Savile Row, where the firm has premises that once served as the headquarters of the Royal Geographical Society.

A new customer of Gieves & Hawkes is first escorted to the Adam Room on the upper floor where, in a relaxed atmosphere, the foundations are laid for a relationship of trust between customer and cutter that may last for decades. While the customer talks about himself and his habits and expresses his preferences for the cut and fabric of his suit, the cutter forms a picture of the customer from what he sees and hears, and working on that basis develops the contours of the suit the customer wants.

Experienced cutters usually know what a customer wants after a few minutes, even if he has not yet made his mind up himself. The cutter is aware more of the customer's needs and can advise him accordingly.

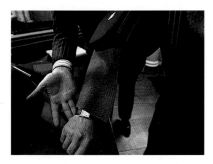

When they have agreed on the cut of the suit and all its details, customer and cutter choose a fabric together. The cutter will tactfully guide a new customer in what he thinks is the right direction, and the customer would be wise to listen to what is usually very good advice.

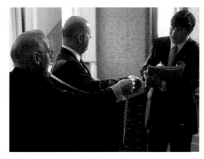

When taking measurements Peter Smith also notes down any physical peculiarities, using a discreet code. DRS means "dropped right shoulder"; FS stands for "forward stomach"; and BL 1, 2, or 3 means "bow legs to the first, second, or third degree."

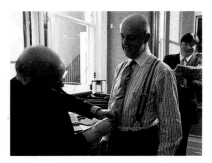

The customer who visits a custom tailor for the first time, after unhappy experiences of ready-made suits, will find that he need not apologize for his physical imperfections or be penalized for them by clothes that hang badly. Even if he has a round stomach or flat buttocks, his trousers will fit perfectly.

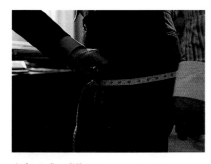

At least five different measurements are taken for the trousers. In what can be a rather embarrassing situation, the process is carried out discreetly and with the neutrality also shown by doctors in handling the more intimate parts of the body.

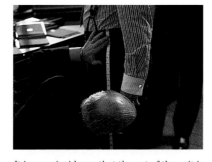

It is no coincidence that the cut of the suit is discussed before measurements are taken. After all, the cutter must always know in advance how high on the hips the trousers are to rest. If the customer wants traditional trousers kept up by suspenders, the outside leg length must be longer than if the trousers will sit on the hips.

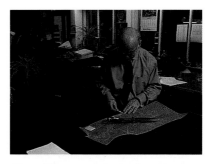

After taking measurements, the cutter, Peter O'Neil, draws the shape of jacket, trousers, and vest on brown paper. He uses a cleverly devised calculating system and the instinct he has developed over the years. This cutting is the architectural plan of the suit.

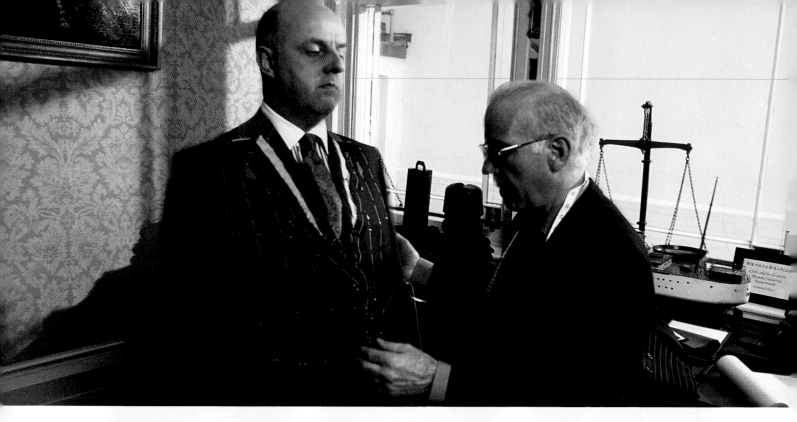

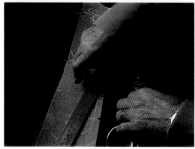

The separate parts of the suit are first cut out in paper and then laid on the fabric to form a pattern.

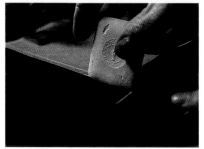

Next the cutter draws on the fabric around the edges of the pattern with tailor's chalk.

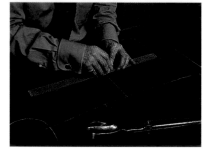

In working he must make sure that as far as possible the patterning of the fabric matches exactly at the seams when the suit is made up.

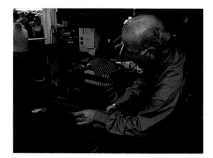

The cutting is done with shears, and of course by hand. Like the taking of measurements, this is an important moment in making a custom-made suit. The cut will be adjusted again after fitting.

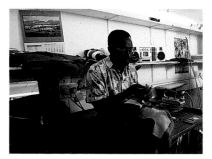

Sewing up the separate parts of the jacket, trousers, and vest is the job of the coat maker, trouser maker, and waistcoat maker. They baste the pieces of the suit together for the first fitting with white cotton thread.

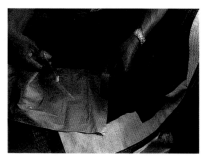

The first fitting could theoretically take place only a couple of days later, but famous tailors like Gieves & Hawkes usually have long waiting lists, and it is generally several weeks before the customer can come in for his first fitting.

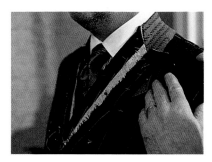

At the first fitting the customer sees the material he has chosen taking shape as a suit for the first time. This is an exciting moment, since up to now the suit has existed only in the minds of the customer and the cutter. At this stage everything about it can still be altered.

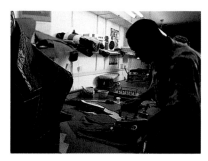

The suit is now taken apart again and goes back to the various tailors – in this picture, to the coat maker Albert Nelson. They make up the second version of the suit, including the alterations agreed at the first fitting.

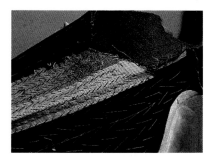

To give the suit its shape, interlining canvas, cotton, felt, or horsehair are sewn into the material itself with countless small stitches. The process takes much less time in mass-produced jackets, where the interfacings are glued into place, but the result is nowhere near as good as when the work is done by hand.

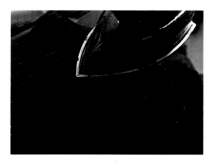

During the process of sewing the tailor constantly presses the fabric with an iron. He dampens the fabric first and then presses it into shape with the hot iron. The pressing and the interlinings give the suit its three-dimensional shape. The elastic nature of horsehair helps to build curves permanently into the fabric, for instance over the chest or in the lapels.

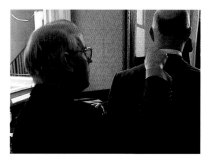

In Victorian times tailors apparently needed up to a dozen fittings before a suit was properly adjusted. Neither the tailors nor their customers have so much time to spare today. As a rule, it takes three fittings before the suit can be made up. But that is only on the first occasion; on going back to the same firm later, a customer will usually need only one fitting.

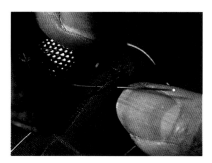

After the measuring and cutting, making the buttonholes marks another decisive stage. Only when the suit is to the customer's satisfaction are the buttonholes added. Again, it is a labor-intensive process. It takes several hours to stitch around all the buttonholes with silk thread.

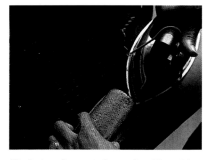

The last craftsman to have a hand in making the suit is the presser. He gives the suit its final form with the iron. No one but a professional presser should iron the suit later when it is badly creased or when dry cleaning is necessary.

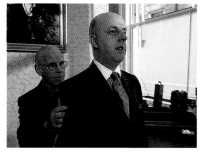

Once the suit is properly pressed the customer can come for that long-awaited final fitting. If he now thinks the suit is right and expresses his satisfaction, then the job is done. After weeks or even months, the customer can go home wearing his new suit.

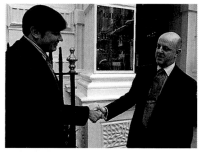

Although in fact, as they apparently say at that other legendary Savile Row institution Anderson & Sheppard, if the suit looks obviously new out in the street then the tailor has not done his job properly. The suit should look like a natural part of the customer.

Chester Barrie

Many a visitor to Savile Row who does not live in England will look wistfully at the display windows of the "bespoke" tailors. A weekend in London does not give him enough time to put his custom in the hands of one of these helpful establishments. It takes some days, if not weeks, for the suit to be cut out and basted together ready for the first fitting, and it will be another few days again before all the alterations have been incorporated. Only after the second, "forward fitting" can the suit be made up – always supposing no further fittings are necessary. This slow process is part of the pleasure of owning a custom-made suit, but it is a nuisance when you are short of time. Luckily, two numbers up the street from Anderson & Sheppard there is a firm that can help out, offering suits ready for you to take away at once, even though their cut and tailoring is of good Savile Row quality. This savior in your hour of need is Chester Barrie at 32 Savile Row, a firm that has been making suits, jackets, trousers, and coats for the demanding customer in a hurry for over 60 years, ever since 1937. The garments are made in Crewe, a town in the north of England. The original workshop soon proved too small, and in 1949 the firm rented more space from the Air Ministry, on premises where Rolls Royce used to make cars. In 1961 Chester Barrie expanded again and moved into a purpose-built factory, although even today it is less like a factory than a huge tailors' workshop where the garments are still 80 percent hand sewn. Chester Barrie has only one thing in common with ordinary ready-made clothing: cutting is to a system of sizes and not individual measurements. But if you have a certain amount of time and want a better idea of the final result in advance, the Chester Barrie cut can easily be adjusted to your own measurements. This method is still some way removed from "bespoke" tailoring, but it does produce the best

ready-made clothing available. Bespoke tailors themselves have the separate pieces of the suits they have cut made up by specialists, who often work for several different tailors. At Chester Barrie the cutting is still done by hand, although to average measurements rather than from a pattern designed for the individual customer. For a man with an average figure, Chester Barrie can thus provide clothes which will fit very well after some minor alterations, and so far as quality of workmanship goes the firm offers very high standards for a relatively low price.

You might think that the founder of this firm was a Mr. Barrie, but you would be wrong. Chester Barrie is an invented name: Crewe, the location of the factory, is near the city of Chester. However, the name was well chosen, for after more than 60 years it sounds as "genuine" as Barbour, Church, or Brigg – at least to customers from the continent of Europe or from America. In fact the man who really founded the firm came from the United States, and was a New Yorker called Myron Ackermann. Long before anyone else thought of it, he hit on the truly brilliant idea of producing ready-made menswear of very high quality by using the traditional methods of the tailor's craft. To this day there are fewer than ten similar firms all over the world, and in principle they all work to the system that has shown its worth at Chester Barrie ever since 1937. Looking through the brochures of these rival firms, you will find they echo the descriptions of the Chester Barrie method almost word for word: careful choice of fabric, the exclusive use of natural materials, cutting by hand with shears, making up mainly by hand, the incorporation of high-quality flexible interlinings, careful pressing to shape and meticulous final checking. In England Chester Barrie is an emergency solution; men with the money and the time will still prefer to go to a bespoke tailor. Italy also has some outstanding custom tailors, but much of the demand is supplied by ready-made clothing of high quality, such as the items made by Kiton, Brioni, or d'Avenza. Germany has only one firm of anything like comparable quality, Regent, and in fact the majority of German customers demanding high standards will buy in England and Italy.

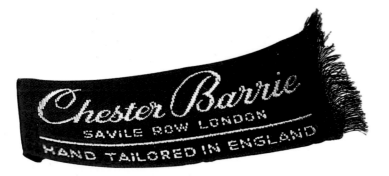

In 1981, after 44 years of producing goods of consistently high quality, Chester Barrie at last won something like recognition from its neighbors in Savile Row, or to be precise from the firm opposite at No. 11 – the premises of H. Huntsman, known as the most expensive tailor in Savile Row and a bastion of the highest standards of quality, standards guaranteed by exclusive in-house production. This venerable institution sold its first off-the-rack suit in 1981 – and the suit was made by none other than Chester Barrie. To this day Huntsman still has all its ready-made clothing manufactured in Crewe, proof of the quality that Chester Barrie can supply, and an acknowledgment that the ready-made suit does have its place.

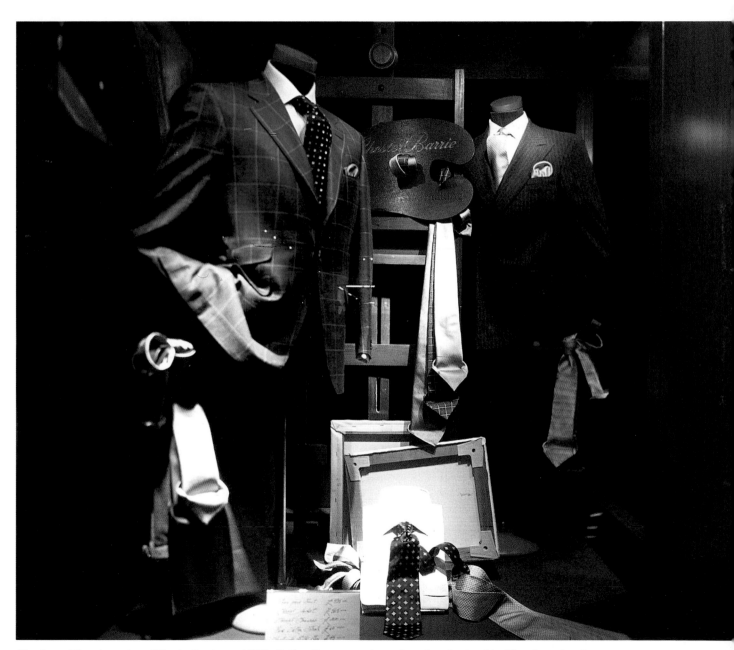

The air-conditioned premises of Chester Barrie are at 32 Savile Row. Here you can buy extremely well-cut and traditionally made suits, jackets, trousers, and coats at very moderate prices. A large sales operation is run from the basement, where the sales manager has his office.

Three Savile Row Customers

Men's fashion pages and illustrated magazines often mention that celebrities from the worlds of politics, the arts, or the media patronize a particular Savile Row tailor – information about as interesting as telling their readers that a billionaire drives a Rolls Royce, a Mercedes, or a Ferrari. Going to a Savile Row tailor is taken as much for granted by those who can afford it as buying an expensive car, living in a big house, or owning a gold watch. Every rich or even merely prosperous man with an eye for good clothes will buy a Savile Row suit at some time or other, although that does not mean he will not also patronize Caraceni in Rome, Charvet in Paris, or Knize in Vienna. However, he is always happy to return to Savile Row, where he can get something unobtainable anywhere else: a genuine Savile Row suit. As a result the lists of customers who patronize these tailors read like an international *Who's Who*, and the catalogue of famous names includes luminaries such as rock stars and politicians, kings and actors, billionaires and painters, musicians and dictators, dandies and the discreetly well dressed, writers and ministers, new money and inherited wealth. The celebrities mentioned here are just three of the many thousands who have sought out the luxury of a Savile Row tailor. It seems inconceivable that Savile Row will ever lose its appeal for such people.

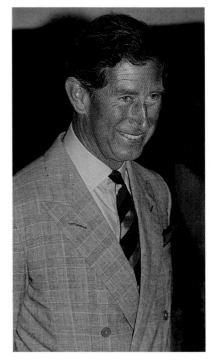

At first it may seem surprising that Bianca Jagger, like her ex-husband, is a Savile Row customer. Together with many of his colleagues, including Elton John, Eric Clapton, and Paul McCartney, Mick Jagger has appreciated exquisite tailoring since the 1960s, although for him tailoring has to have that certain extra touch of fashion. Tommy Nutter fitted out the stars of the swinging sixties with the broad lapels, flared trousers, and narrow waists of that decade. Bianca Jagger liked her husband's suits so much that she ordered one of her own from Tommy Nutter, setting off a revival of gentlemen's tailoring for ladies, just as Marlene Dietrich did before her when she ordered tailored suits from Knize of Vienna. Ordering Savile Row suits was as natural for Mick Jagger as buying a country house or an expensive car, since anyone who can afford it will want custom tailoring at some point in his career – and that is as true of a rock musician as of anyone else.

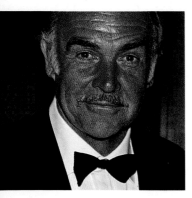

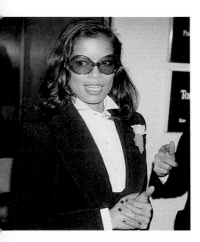

Sean Connery is known to have patronized several tailors, both privately and in his most famous film role as the British secret agent James Bond. Terence Young, director of the James Bond films *Dr. No*, *From Russia With Love*, and *Thunderball*, had Sean Connery's wardrobe made by his own tailor, Anthony Sinclair of Conduit Street. Sinclair created the unobtrusive and rather military style of the early James Bond, and it is still popular today. The character's shirts came from Turnbull & Asser, probably the most famous shirtmaker in Jermyn Street. In his private capacity, Sean Connery has gone for years to Dimi Major, previously in partnership with Douglas Hayward, who like Major specializes in show-business customers. Douglas Hayward also created the wardrobe for the later James Bond as played by Roger Moore.

Experts agree that Prince Charles now has his suits made by Anderson & Sheppard, but there will be no official confirmation of the claim from either St. James's Palace or the firm of Anderson & Sheppard itself. As a schoolboy and university student he was dressed in the old upper-class tradition by Colin Edmonds of Billings & Edmonds. He then went to Teddy Watson of Hawes & Curtis, Prince Philip's tailor. Like many heirs to the throne before him, he subsequently left his father's tailor, and went to Anderson & Sheppard. His uniforms used to be made by Johns & Pegg, but are now supplied by Welsh & Jeffries. There are also persistent rumors that Prince Charles is a customer of Kiton, although this seems improbable since the heir to the British throne can hardly wear anything but an English suit, if only for political reasons. And if Prince Charles does have a liking for Neapolitan tailoring, the Palace would never admit it. A gentleman may indulge himself, but he keeps quiet about it.

The King of Style

Even while he was still Prince of Wales the man who later lived in exile as the Duke of Windsor enjoyed experimentation. In the 1930s he gave the royal blessing to a double-breasted dinner jacket with a shawl collar, and it was apparently the Prince's idea to order a tuxedo in dark blue instead of black, because in artificial light that color looks "blacker than black." He and his shirtmaker also created the modern evening shirt with its soft turndown collar, double cuff, and pleated shirt front, which he wore instead of the starched dress shirt, in line with his general dislike of all formality as well as his preference for taking off his jacket and rolling up his sleeves at the first opportunity. He also introduced new fashions in sportswear. In 1922, as captain of the Ancient and Royal Golf Club of St. Andrews, he wore a colored Fair Isle pullover, and wrote later, "I suppose the most showy of all my garments was the multicoloured Fair Isle sweater with its jigsaw of patterns." On his journey around the world between his accession and his abdication he often wore gray double-breasted chalk-striped suits, and made them very popular. We also owe it to him that it is now considered correct to wear brown suede shoes with a blue suit – always an interesting look, and one he is said to have introduced. The name of the pattern known as Prince of Wales check, however, has nothing to do with the fact that Edward VIII often wore it while he was heir to the throne. The sporting pattern is called after his grandfather Edward VII, who often chose this particular check for casual suits when he himself was Prince of Wales. Also typical of the Duke of Windsor was his skill in mingling patterns, both in his choice of sporting

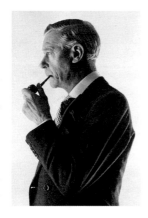

outfits and in his combination of suit, shirt, and necktie. For instance, he would wear socks with horizontal stripes with shoes in two colors, seersucker trousers with a check shirt, or Argyle socks with Madras check trousers.

By comparison with other members of the British royal family, in fact, his style could be said to be positively eccentric. From a modern viewpoint his philosophy of fashion may be called rather avant-garde, and many of his ideas anticipated the fashionable menswear of today.

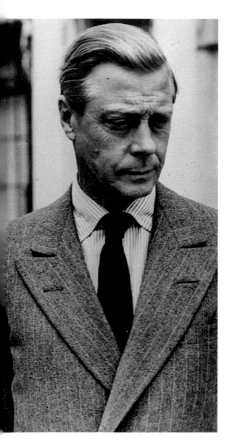

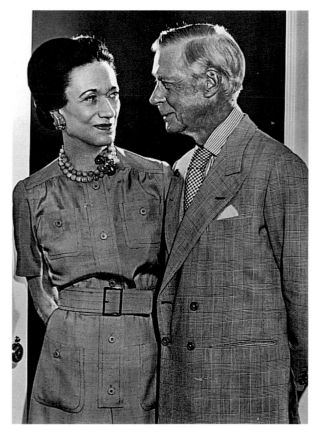

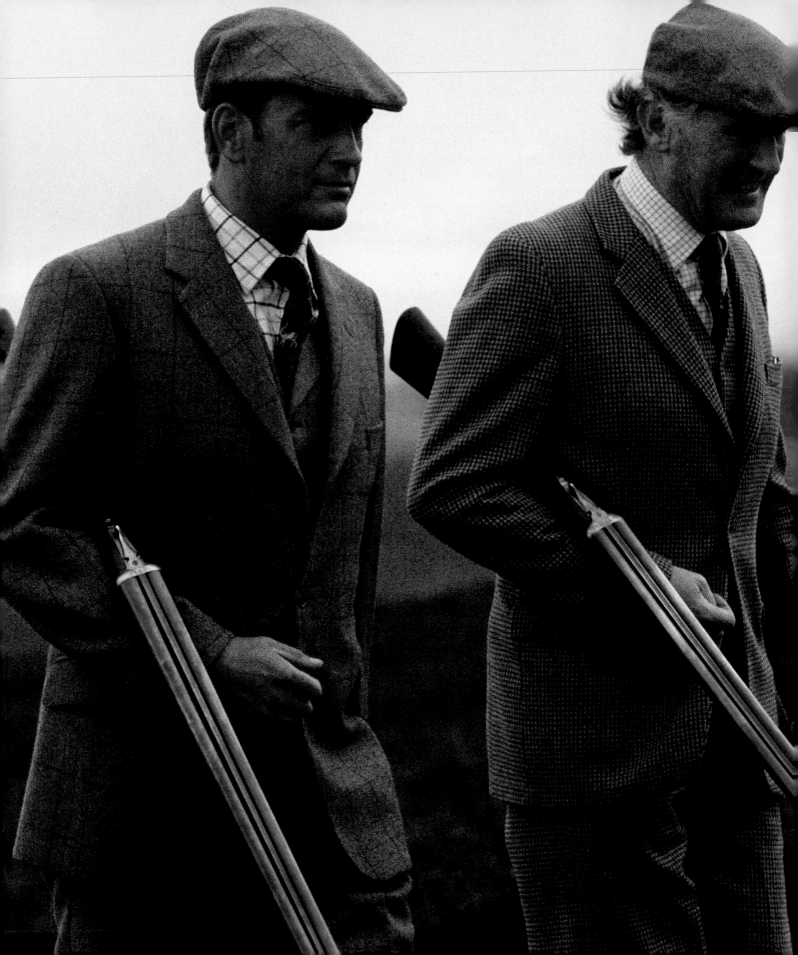

The Right Kind of Tweed Suit

Until quite recently British troops were still stationed in Germany, and gave anyone who was interested a chance to get to know the British way of life outside the United Kingdom itself. In questions of men's fashion, British officers in particular made excellent subjects of study, belonging as they often did to the "Sloane Rangers" type, a group dressing according to certain rules derived from the dress code of the aristocratic English upper classes, which prescribed a certain kind of outfit for every occasion. A horse race meeting in Hanover, for example, could provide a rare opportunity to see a tweed suit worn outside Great Britain – in the wild, so to speak – and at first sight it was obvious that it was a long way from the continental interpretation of this British speciality in cut, weight, and the feel of the fabric. This impression is confirmed by research in the tweed suit's native land, for instance at the traditional gentlemen's outfitter Cordings of Piccadilly.

The genuine tweed suit is heavy, rough, and stiff, and thus very good for keeping out cold winds, rain, mist, or even frost.

Continental tweed suits in the English style are softer and smoother, with rustic leather patches at the elbow, leather buttons, and sometimes fully lined trousers to keep the wearer's legs from contact with the scratchy wool. The cut of a continental tweed suit is also very different from the original British style, since a genuine tweed suit has three buttons, a vent at the back of the jacket, sloping pockets, and narrow, unlined trousers without pleats. The material is usually a greenish brown coarse tweed with a windowpane check. To be honest, it feels rather like a carpet square, but it is as tough as carpet too and will thus hardly let any wind or damp through.

Since these suits are mainly worn out of doors or in cold country houses, they are not so suitable for heated rooms. But toned-down versions of the genuine tweed suit can also be found in Great Britain, as weekend wear in the city, or on men who do not have to wear blue pinstripe suiting at work – academics, people in the creative professions, or freelances.

Ask for a tweed suit in the United Kingdom, however, and you will usually get the sturdy original, which is very much at home on cold racecourses, in drafty fields, and out shooting. If you want a suit for such occasions you can find nothing more suitable than genuine British tweed.

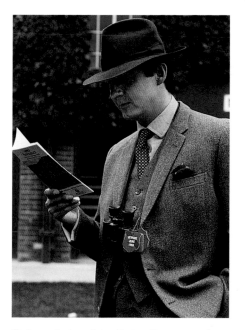

Race meetings and shooting parties are occasions when the gentleman may wear a tweed suit. It is not correct for city wear in England.

The Italian Suit

If we may allow ourselves a generalization here, it is hard to imagine a greater contrast than that between an Englishman and an Italian. They are irreconcilable opposites, particularly in matters of fashion. On the one hand we have British understatement verging on self-effacement, on the other a liking for display that can sometimes become outright vanity.

These attitudes are expressed in the very different suit-making traditions of the two nations, the only countries that really set the trend in classical gentlemen's wear. The Englishman, if another generalization may be permitted, expects his suit to show that he belongs to a certain class of society and is "one of us." "We" are the people who wear Savile Row suits and know just what is right and what is not in matters of clothing, lifestyle, politics, and religion. Since the Englishman still sees himself as part of a whole, his suit must not express individuality; instead, it must follow the traditional rules precisely so that it looks just like his father's and grandfather's suits. And indeed he will still wear those suits if they fit, and if they do not he will get them altered.

The Italian, on the other hand, wants to show off; he is sure of his own individuality and importance, a feeling impressed upon him by his mother and the rest of his family. His suit is to set off his individual nature, not through loudly proclaimed extravagance but by means of a certain elegance, something that does not generally much interest the Englishman, who simply wants to be dressed correctly. Classical elegance is among those Renaissance ideals that Italy is always trying to revive. The Italian looks for elegance in his clothing and his lifestyle, and the Italian suit is therefore first and foremost elegant, select, and refined. Its elegance shows in its lightweight, soft fabric; its select nature in its color and design; its refinement in the cut and excellent workmanship. The Italian suit is also a requisite of the Italian tradition of passeggiata, the leisurely stroll during which a man shows off his real or would-be prosperity to rivals of his own kind, naturally with the help of elegant clothing. Such points should be borne in mind as we look at the craft of Italian tailoring, which undoubtedly produces the most elegant gentlemen's fashions in the world. Unlike in England, Italy has several centers of good tailoring, as can be seen from the map on the facing page. With their help a journey in southern Europe can turn into a pilgrimage to the holy places of gentlemen's fashion.

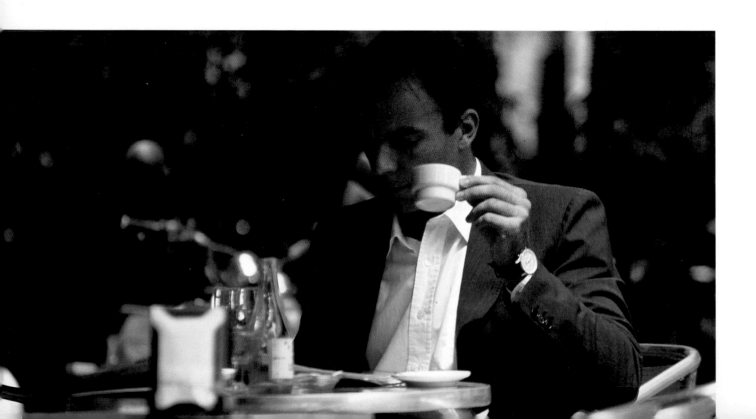

Who's Who in Italy

Caraceni

There are three tailors continuing to uphold the tradition of the name of Caraceni in Milan. A. Caraceni, at 16 Via Fatebenefratelli, can be relied upon to do justice to a famous name. A man who is looking for the most distinguished tailoring will find it there. Both cut and craftsmanship are of the highest standard.

Belvest

Belvest is still something of a well-kept secret, for relatively few people know about this firm, which derives from the traditions of Venetian tailoring. Its late founder Aldo Nicoletto, like his better-known colleagues, aimed to supply the best possible ready-made garments. At Belvest methods of manufacturing are still employed in pursuit of that aim. Most of the work is carried out by hand, and the making of a pair of trousers alone involves some 80 separate maneuvers.

D'Avenza

D'Avenza was founded by Myron Ackermann in Carrara in 1957. The firm's methods were then and still are like those of a traditional tailor's workshop, but on a larger scale. When founded, it was ahead of its time and of many of its Italian colleagues. Over the past 40 years and more this manufacturer of ready-made clothing has earned itself a reputation for good, sound work – not, perhaps, in the avant-garde of fashion but providing outstanding quality.

Angelo

If you are looking for an outfit that exudes Roman style you have a choice of four addresses in the Eternal City: Caraceni, Cifonelli, and Brioni, or you can go to Angelo. The store at 34 Via Bissolati was founded by the late Angelo Vittucci. He left Brioni in 1963 and opened a firm of his own that soon became very successful. It is still run by his family today. Among his customers in the 1960s and 1970s were several famous American actors, and there are Eastern noblemen who like to order from the firm today. If you appreciate personal service from a relatively small business, you will like Angelo.

Cifonelli

Like Caraceni, Cifonelli was founded before the end of the Second World War, and his firm too has a legendary reputation. However, there was no such power struggle at Cifonelli as in the Caraceni family. While Caraceni has to compete with the other firms of that name in Milan, Cifonelli of Paris is a legitimate offshoot of the headquarters in Rome. If you have no time to visit 68 Via Quintino Sella in Rome, you will still be able to get a genuine Roman Cifonelli at rue Marbeuf 81 in Paris. Connoisseurs recognize a suit from this famous tailor at once by the special cut of the shoulders.

Caraceni

Caraceni is a name that certainly inspires enthusiasm in aficionados of Italian gentlemen's tailoring. It owes its legendary reputation to Domenico Caraceni, a Roman tailor who began his illustrious career in the 1920s. After his death a power struggle took place in the 1940s among his descendants, all claiming the great Domenico's inheritance for themselves. Today there are four rival firms all bearing the Caraceni name, one in Rome and three in Milan. The Caracenis of Rome work where old Domenico did and claim, not just for that reason, to be the genuine article. Put yourself in their hands, and you will, without doubt, be in the best international company.

Brioni

As is frequently the case with other names originating in a custom-tailoring firm, one must distinguish between the garments ordered from and sold by Brioni all over the world, and those that are the product of its premises at 79 Via Barberini. Orders from the firm's branches in New York, Paris or Cologne will be made by hand in the Abruzzi, but simply made-to-measure – the craftsmen work from a basic if modified pattern. The workshop in Rome, on the other hand, also offers a traditional custom-tailoring service. If you want maximum individuality and a perfect fit, the headquarters are where you will order your Brioni suit, and in any case the place is well worth a visit.

Battistoni

Battistoni may not be the best Italian shirtmaker but it is certainly the best known, and differences of quality in those rarefied spheres where Battistoni moves are of a rather abstruse nature anyway. Objectively, you will get everything you can expect of a custom-made shirt here: a perfect fit; a collar adjusted to set off your neck, face, and figure to the best possible effect; handmade buttonholes; patterns matching perfectly between the separate parts of the shirt; and fabric of the highest quality.

Kiton

Kiton is famous throughout the world as a representative of the art of Neapolitan tailoring. The name of the firm derives from the Greek word chiton, meaning "garment" so there was never any Signor Kiton; the founder of the firm was Ciro Paone, who still keeps an eye in person on the quality of the products. His mercilessly keen eye will pass only the very best work – and his sense of touch decides the fate of fabric suppliers. In contrast to the Roman style, the shoulders of a Kiton jacket are typically Neapolitan, softly rounded and with hardly and padding. Kiton's ready-made garments are in excellent fabrics of very good taste, fitting extremely well, and made to high standards. Kiton also, of course, offers custom tailoring to the discerning gentleman.

Milan

Piazzola sul Brenta

Plave

Brenta

Po

Panaro

Carrara

Arno

Tiber

Rome

Naples

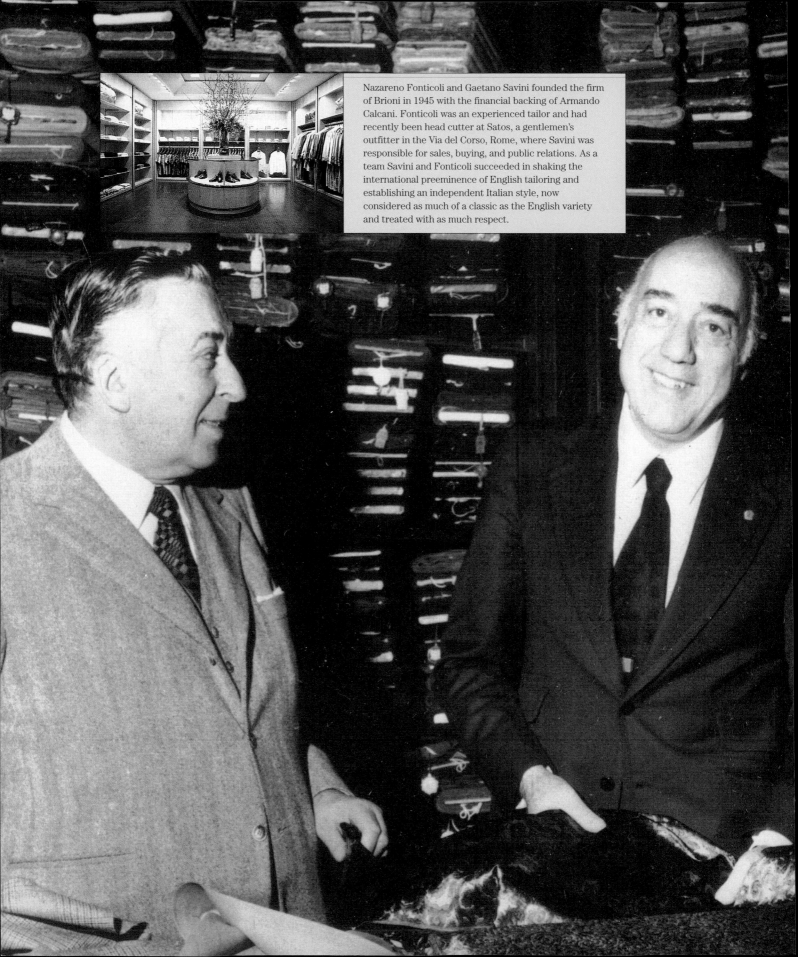

Nazareno Fonticoli and Gaetano Savini founded the firm of Brioni in 1945 with the financial backing of Armando Calcani. Fonticoli was an experienced tailor and had recently been head cutter at Satos, a gentlemen's outfitter in the Via del Corso, Rome, where Savini was responsible for sales, buying, and public relations. As a team Savini and Fonticoli succeeded in shaking the international preeminence of English tailoring and establishing an independent Italian style, now considered as much of a classic as the English variety and treated with as much respect.

Brioni – veni, vidi, vici

Nowadays everyone associates the name of Brioni with exclusive Italian gentlemen's outfitting. It is all the more interesting that the name properly has nothing to do with fashion. It is in fact the name of an island in the Adriatic just off the coast of former Yugoslavia. Before the Second World War it was a favorite resort of rich Europeans, and later on Marshal Tito used to vacation there. Nazareno Fonticoli and Gaetano Savini chose the name of this island for two reasons: first, even after the war the word "Brioni" still suggested something exclusive and luxurious; second, it did not sound at all English – and it was the declared aim of the new firm to create an entirely new style clearly distinct from English tailoring. The two founders did indeed soon succeed in making the name of Brioni known in Italy as an excellent tailoring firm and gentlemen's outfitters. It had the honor (and good luck) to take part in the second Italian fashion show in Florence in 1951, a presentation of Italian *haute couture*. At the third show in 1952, Brioni was already presenting 40 models specially designed for the runway. The buyers of B. Altman & Co., New York, subsequently took Brioni to the United States, and the way to becoming an international brand name lay open before the firm.

By the middle of the 1950s Brioni clothes could be bought in 22 stores on the American continent. The boom continued, and many American fans were even known to have crossed the Atlantic to the Roman headquarters of Brioni, to be measured for their Brioni suits in the authentic Italian surroundings.

With increasing demand, a factory was opened in Penne in the Abruzzi, Nazareno Fonticoli's birthplace. Here the traditional process of making up is divided among various specialists, each devoting his time to a single activity – cutting, basting, finishing the buttonholes, and so on. This has proved the best way to supply tailoring of good quality in the shortest possible time. It takes about 18 hours to make a suit by this method. (By comparison, a custom-made suit takes about 40 hours.)

Brioni also produces made-to-measure suits by the same method. The customer simply has to find a gentlemen's outfitter where he can select his fabric and cut, and then his measurements are taken and faxed to Penne. The suit will be ready three weeks later at the earliest, with no need for further fittings. But if you want a real custom-made suit from Brioni, then you should visit the firm's head-quarters in Rome, where about 500 suits are handmade every year on the very attractive premises at 79 Via Barberini.

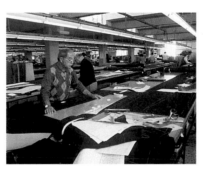

The Brioni factory is in Penne, a small town in the Abruzzi. However, the term "factory" should not be misunderstood. Since most of the work is done by hand, "manufactory" would describe the place better.

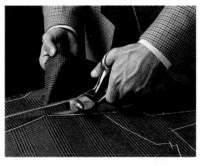

Cutting by hand is an important stage in making top-quality clothing. It makes the most economical use of the fabric and guarantees that the patterning will match.

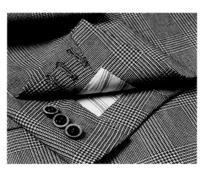

The sleeve buttons are not just for show in a Brioni jacket. You can undo them properly – but a real gentleman never undoes them all.

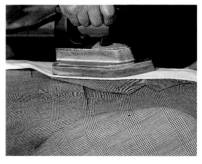

The suit is pressed throughout the process of making up. In Italy, as in England, the last pressing gives it its final shape.

Classics of Fashion

Brioni's international success began with its ostensibly revolutionary creations reintroducing color into men's fashions in the 1950s, and in photographs of the 1960s and 1970s Brioni was still coming up with models as far removed as many designs of today from easy-to-wear fashions and the classic style. In fact it is rather surprising that most people now think of Brioni as a firm with a very classic, even conservative image. Brioni's high reputation seems to be founded more on the quality of its tailoring, which is just as good as the quality of the past, than on its avant-garde creations. Looking around the Brioni department of a gentlemen's outfitter, it is quite hard to imagine that the firm used to design belted safari suits in black snakeskin, or tuxedos in a fabric called *brocatello* which looks much as the name suggests. Despite these excesses of fashion, Brioni has become a byword for classicism and tradition, for even its most daring designs in the fifties, sixties, and seventies were made with the same craftsmanlike precision as its classic suits made to measure for traditionally minded customers. Another reason is probably that the customer connects Brioni only with those garments that actually reached the stores, and presumably they were confined to the classic, easy-to-wear models appreciated by Brioni customers all over the world.

Brioni models of the 1960s and 1970s inspired designers again in the 1990s

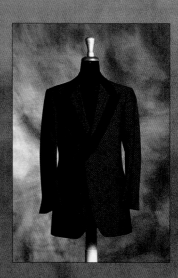

Once the Americans had tired of black tuxedos in the 1950s, Brioni attracted attention in the United States with evening dress in colored silk, velvet, and brocade.

The Hall of Fame

The list of Brioni customers is a long one, featuring buyers of ready-made suits as well as the custom-made variety. Gary Cooper, Clark Gable, John Wayne, Henry Fonda, Richard Burton, Peter Sellers, Robert Wagner, and many other stars figure in Brioni's Hall of Fame.

Today Armani is preeminent among gentlemen's outfitters to American stars of screen and pop music. His monotony of black and gray dominates the scene at film premières and Grammy award ceremonies. That will not trouble Brioni, since it would be impossible to meet the huge demand resulting from excessive popularity without relaxing the firm's high standards of quality. And once Brioni had come to the end of its avant-garde phase it was, after all, quality that ensured its still undisputed preeminence.

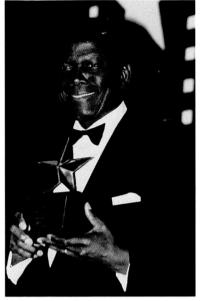

Sidney Poitier

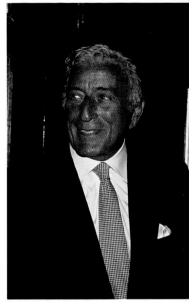

Tony Bennett

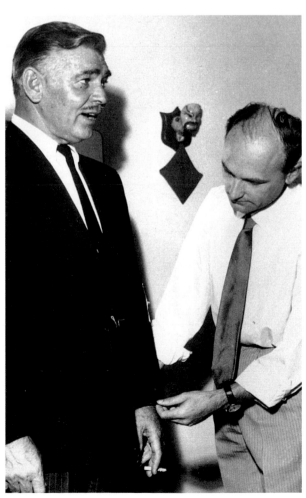

Clark Gable

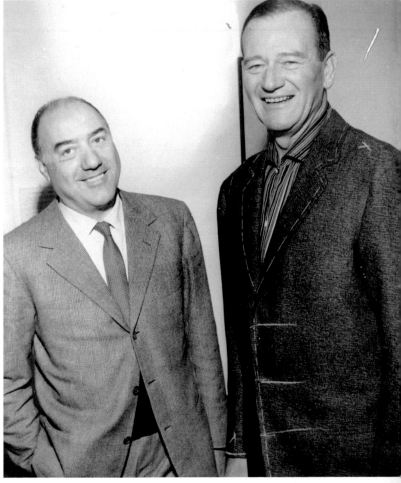

John Wayne (right)

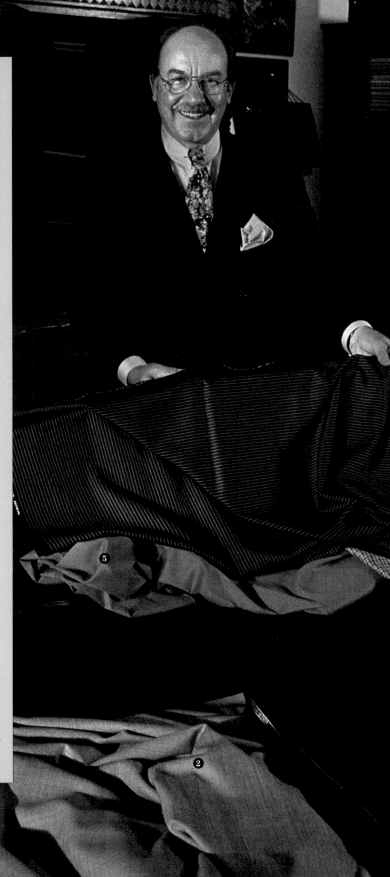

❶ If you think of cashmere only as a soft, warm, woolen fabric, then let your tailor show you lightweight cashmeres for summer. They are soft but still pleasantly cool to wear. Cashmere is not as hardwearing as merino wool, but keeps its shape better than cotton and considerably better than linen. At the establishment of the Dusseldorf tailor Heinz-Josef Radermacher the client can choose from a wide range of this noble cloth.

❷ Lightweight woolen fabrics have long been regarded as ideal for summer. Fabrics like "Super 100" or even lighter weights combine the good qualities of pure wool with the light, airy quality you want in summer. With very lightweight grades of pure wool you can get through the summer almost crease free.

❸ Many men find it difficult to think of silk as a suiting fabric, perhaps because most of them connect it primarily with the delicate Hermès scarves worn by their wives or girlfriends. But silk dyed in appropriate colors is an ideal material for summer suits. The Italians are masters of the production and working of this luxurious fabric.

❹ Mohair, like cashmere, is spun from the hair of a goat and then woven. It is an extremely elastic material and creases even less than merino wool, so it is ideal for formal summer suits. Most men think of mohair as the typical fabric for a tuxedo – in black or dark blue evening dress, the sheen of the weave is particularly noticeable. In fact this characteristic luster makes it harder to envisage mohair as

correct for daytime wear. In fact, it is used for suits to be worn in the daytime, but not many gentlemen have these in their wardrobes.

❺ Cotton is pleasantly cool to wear in summer and is therefore an ideal material for lightweight suits. However, the great disadvantage of these typically pale summer suits is that they crease easily, which is a particularly annoying feature because it affects the fit of the suit. Concertina folds inside the elbow and at the hollow of the knee, for instance, make the sleeves and trousers of the suit look too short. But many men either will put up with this drawback because of the pleasantly light feel of cotton in wear, or do not even feel that it is a disadvantage.

❻ Opinions on linen are divided. Traditionalists usually regard it as a material suitable only for white handkerchiefs. Others consider linen the ultimate summer fabric and think that its typical creases look distinguished. You could call it a marketing *coup* that an obvious drawback has been presented as a mark of high quality. Irish linen is considered the best. Linen for summer wear can be bought in many different weights, from heavy to very light.
Since linen creases even more easily than cotton, and the creases do not hang out, it is not used much in classic or traditional tailoring. The cut and fit of a linen suit does not aim to look good in spite of creasing, and so such suits fall into the province of ready-made designer clothing rather than good tailoring.

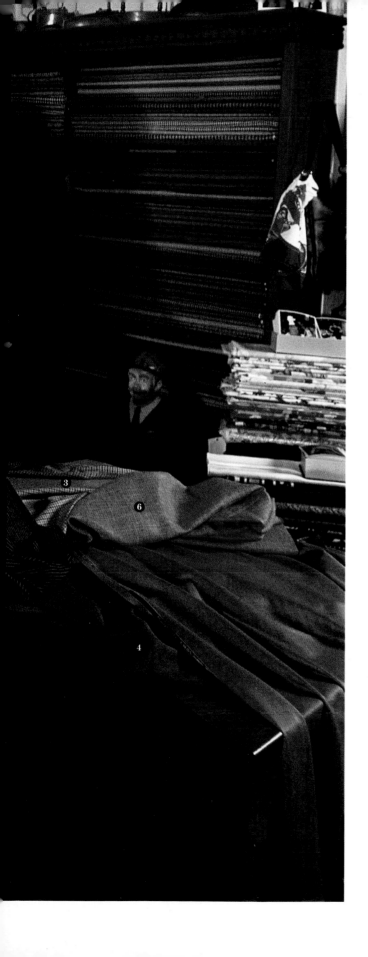

The Summer Suit

When you try on a very light, half-lined Italian summer suit for the first time you will be surprised that its lightweight fabric can be used for a suit at all. But if the suit fits well – whether because the right size is in stock, or you have ordered a made-to-measure suit, or you have had the suit custom-made from the first to your own measurements – you will be astonished to realize that this lightweight fabric hangs as well as the suit you wear in the fall. You can feel cool air around your legs as you walk, light actually seems to shine through the jacket, and the sleeves are so thin that the double cuff of your shirt seems heavy and stiff by comparison. When you look down at your legs you can see the ground through the fabric to right and left of your feet through your trousers. And note that we mean a woolen suit, although the wool is of so light a weight that it seems almost like shirting fabric – but unlike the cotton of a shirt it does not crease.

Of course summer suits can be made in other fabrics, such as cashmere, silk, mohair, and cotton. But a tropical weight of pure wool is the best material for a suit to be worn to the office every other day in summer. Mohair, made from the hair of the angora goat, is equally hardwearing. This grainy, elastic fabric is mainly made into tuxedos, but it can also be used for summer suiting, although not everyone likes the luster that is characteristic of mohair. Silk is also a typical summer fabric, and it was the Italians who reintroduced silk to the gentleman's wardrobe, like cotton and linen. Cotton and linen are certainly comfortable to wear in hot weather, but they crease badly, and a suit made of such fabrics soon loses its shape. In addition, the light weight of linen and cotton means that they do not drape so elegantly or hang out as well as pure wool – these materials just do not have the weight to pull the suit back into shape again as quickly.

These vegetable fibers, then, are to be recommended only if you do not mind creases in a suit, and if your suit will be given enough time between wearings for the creases to fall out again. The creases in linen suits are less likely to fall out than those of cotton suits, and so the wearer will have to be prepared to tolerate a somewhat crumpled look.

Brooks Brothers – New York Classics

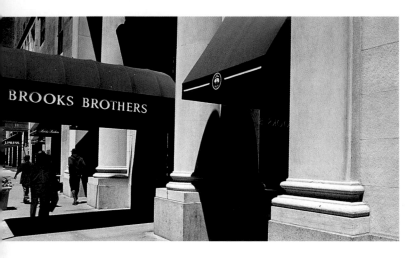

Brooks Brothers is not only the most famous gentlemen's outfitters in the United States but also an American institution. When Andy Warhol received his first check in 1955 for a series of advertisements for the shoe firm of I. Miller, he bought 100 identical white shirts from Brooks Brothers.

Brooks Brothers was founded in 1818, and can thus look back on as long a tradition as many European gentlemen's outfitters. Its history is closely linked with the history of America. For instance, on his second induction into office in 1864 President Abraham Lincoln wore a coat from Brooks Brothers. Nineteen years before this memorable event, in 1845, Brooks Brothers sold its first ready-made suit – a complete novelty in the United States at the time. It was the predecessor of today's Brooks Brothers suit in that it was a characteristic "sack suit" cut with natural shoulders, three buttons, and a vent in the back of the jacket and the top buttonhole was pressed in with the lapel. Typical fabrics are blue and gray pinstripes, gray herringbone, Prince of Wales check, plain blue, gray, and olive. Sizes range in single steps from 36 inches up to 50 inches, with jackets in up to five lengths – regular, short, medium long, long, and extra long – and trousers in regular, short, and long lengths. Alterations are made in the firm's own workshop. In addition, jackets and trousers can be chosen in different sizes, something that is not usually possible on the continent of Europe, and the trousers come either with or without pleats. Prices are lower than for European ready-to-wear suits of good quality. And if you do not need to buy suits off the rack, you can usually find something to suit you here

in the way of shirts, neckties, underwear, socks, and above all sportswear. Brooks Brothers supply the originals we are used to seeing in Ralph Lauren designer versions: check shirts, sweaters, rugby shirts, corduroy trousers, and chinos. The shoe department is worth visiting too, since the Brooks Brothers label sells, among other things, Alden's famous cordovan shoes, which can be recognized by the large eyelets for the laces. The great advantage of Brooks Brothers, however, has always been that if you like something so much you would rather not try anything else for a change, you can always reorder it. But today the firm displays traces of a modernizing trend regarded with some skepticism by old Brooks Brothers customers, who feel that it is diluting its style and quality and making unnecessary concessions to modernity. It is to be hoped that this will not lead to the loss of a sense of the firm's identity, since its charm and strength lie in its maintenance of tradition.

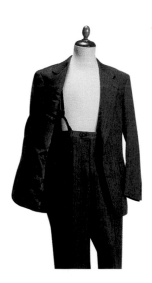

Brooks Brothers suits can be bought with either two or three buttons. In the three-button version the top buttonhole is pressed in with the lapel so that it cannot be buttoned up. You should never forget to point out this feature to your dry cleaner, or the buttonhole will be pressed straight.

The Brooks Brothers suit has natural, rounded shoulders, a feature which is responsible for the casual silhouette of the cut of the sack suit.

The back vent is a typical feature. It allows freedom of movement, and you can put your hands in your trouser pockets without pushing the jacket out of shape. The only drawback is that then the jacket opens up at the back, allowing a view of the wearer's behind – which is not always especially attractive.

The trousers sit high on the hips, and can be ordered with or without pleats. Although pleats went out of fashion for a time in Europe, at the end of the twentieth century many European men can scarcely imagine trousers without them. America, on the other hand, has a strong body of opinion against trousers with pleated fronts. Unpleated trouser fronts are therefore typical of the USA, and they are held up by suspenders for the sake of comfort rather than fashion.

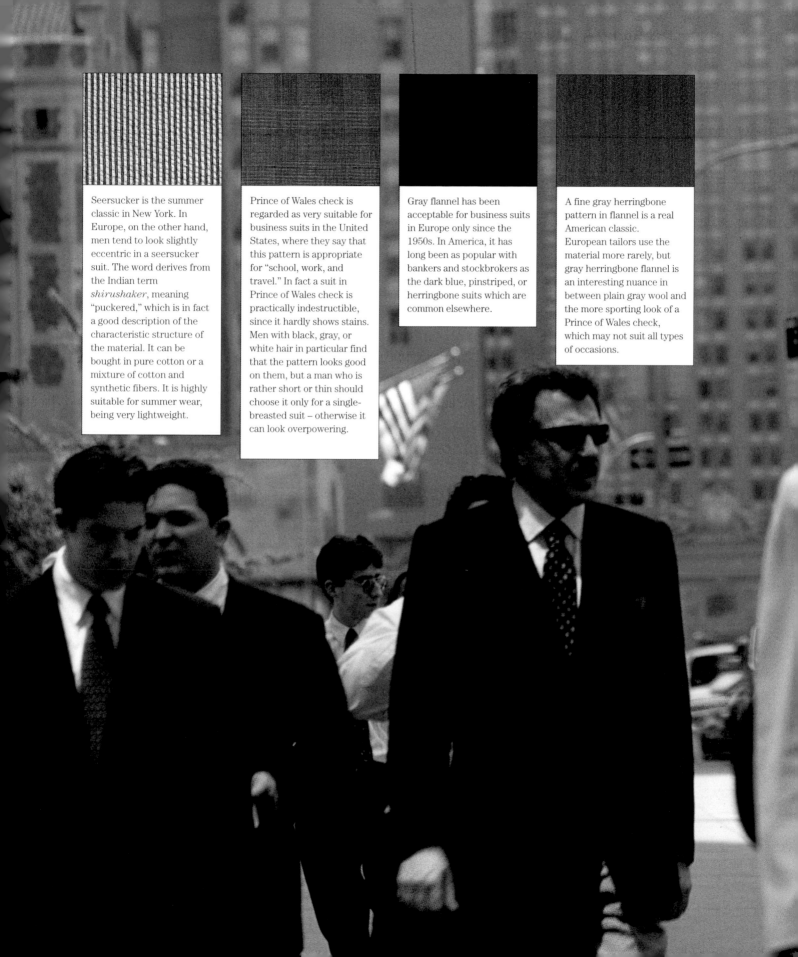

Seersucker is the summer classic in New York. In Europe, on the other hand, men tend to look slightly eccentric in a seersucker suit. The word derives from the Indian term *shirushaker*, meaning "puckered," which is in fact a good description of the characteristic structure of the material. It can be bought in pure cotton or a mixture of cotton and synthetic fibers. It is highly suitable for summer wear, being very lightweight.

Prince of Wales check is regarded as very suitable for business suits in the United States, where they say that this pattern is appropriate for "school, work, and travel." In fact a suit in Prince of Wales check is practically indestructible, since it hardly shows stains. Men with black, gray, or white hair in particular find that the pattern looks good on them, but a man who is rather short or thin should choose it only for a single-breasted suit – otherwise it can look overpowering.

Gray flannel has been acceptable for business suits in Europe only since the 1950s. In America, it has long been as popular with bankers and stockbrokers as the dark blue, pinstriped, or herringbone suits which are common elsewhere.

A fine gray herringbone pattern in flannel is a real American classic. European tailors use the material more rarely, but gray herringbone flannel is an interesting nuance in between plain gray wool and the more sporting look of a Prince of Wales check, which may not suit all types of occasions.

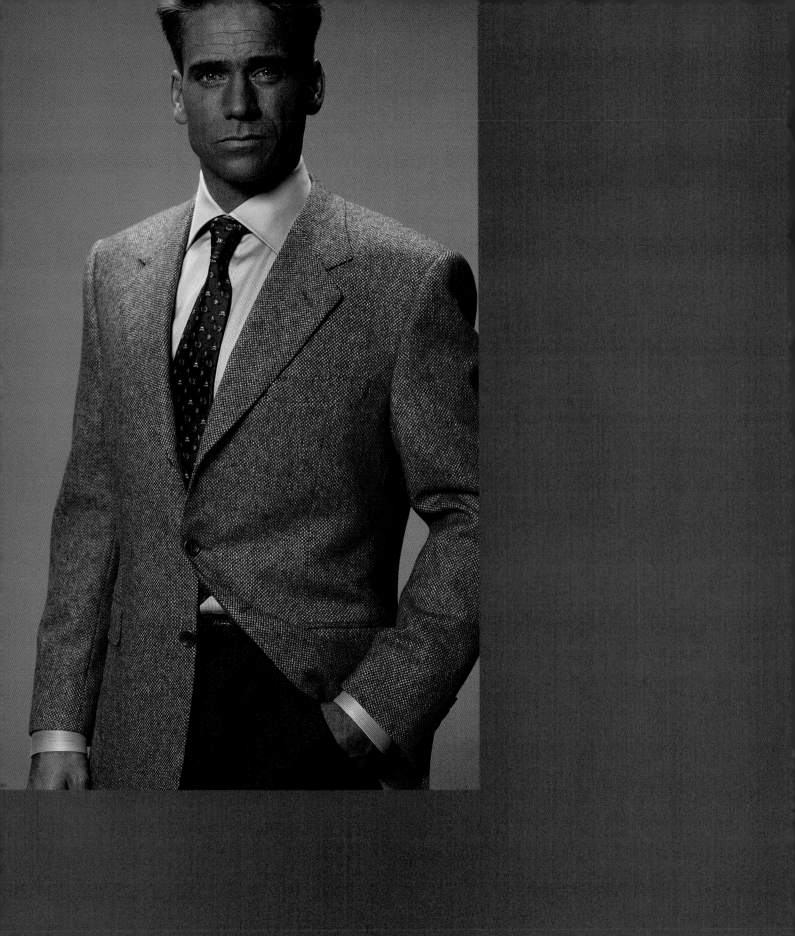

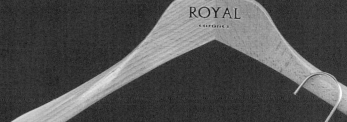

Smart Casual

The Sports Jacket

Fashion has gone down some strange paths since the end of the nineteenth century. Before the suit became the dominant mode, men used to wear morning coats with trousers of a different color. In fact the first suits were worn for sporting activities; later on, the suit gradually broke away from its association with leisure pursuits, and became socially accepted as correct business wear.

In the late nineteenth century, another combination of jacket with trousers of a different material came in, specifically for sporting activities, or more precisely for shooting. According to legend the new sporting look was first worn on the estates of the Duke of Norfolk; hence the term for this particular jacket, the "Norfolk jacket." It was made of tweed, with three or four buttons, a belt, pleats for ease of movement, and large pockets to hold cartridges and provisions. We have all seen this kind of jacket in movies set in Victorian England. It was especially made for shooting, and was therefore a real "designer jacket" in the sense of being designed for a particular purpose, according to the principle that "form follows function."

The Norfolk jacket was not just a suit jacket worn with the trousers of a differently colored suit, but an individual garment to go with pants that were not part of a suit at all. Jacket and trousers therefore represented a luxury; they were additional and for many people unnecessary items of clothing, but in any case clothes that had to be specially bought. Consequently, separate sports jackets were at first reserved for those who could afford to buy an extra jacket and pair of pants just for weekend wear. It was some time before the design of the sports jacket began to approach the cut of the traditional suit jacket.

It was not until the 1920s that the tweed jacket was made without the Norfolk jacket's typical belt and pleats to facilitate movement. Now it was no longer worn just for shooting, but for leisure pursuits in general, or as an alternative to the suit. Its cut derived from that of the riding jacket, and gray flannel trousers became popular with it. Flannel was soon in increasing demand with tailors' customers, as a soft, comfortable fabric that draped elegantly, and before long entire suits were being made from it. However, flannel trousers were still regarded as most appropriate when worn with sports jackets. And since fashion goes some strange ways, today the sports jacket has developed into an item of clothing somewhere between the suit and genuine leisurewear – and it sometimes seems to occupy a rather uneasy position in that capacity. Only in professions where it is no longer obligatory to wear a dark suit does it have a real function, as a more or less formal article of clothing that will allow you to wear a certain range of colors. The nature of those professions differs from country to country and from region to region. A glance through the many illustrated magazines on sale in Europe shows that in the south, politicians and captains of industry still wear suits, while the members of all other professional groups feel quite happy wearing sports jackets at work.

In England the suit is still obligatory in a number of branches of commerce and industry. In central and northern Europe, the sports jacket is widely accepted, and suits are still worn only in very conservative fields of business such as banking and insurance – and even in those fields, only at management level. The Americans, like the British, see the sports jacket as an informal garment, and consequently the models to be found in the USA are rather plain. If you like wearing a combination of sports jacket and flannels, you should look for them not in the United States, but in England or on the continent of Europe. The best place of all is Italy, where you will find the widest choice of beautifully tailored jackets, all of them able to compete with any suit in elegance.

The predecessor of the modern sports jacket – as well as the riding jacket – is the Norfolk jacket. This very sensible item of clothing, tailored exactly to its purpose, has very little in common with the sports jackets of the present day, but the Norfolk jacket is still a very appropriate garment for shooting or other outdoor activities. As this scene from a Sherlock Holmes movie shows, the Norfolk jacket can also be worn with matching trousers as part of a sporting suit.

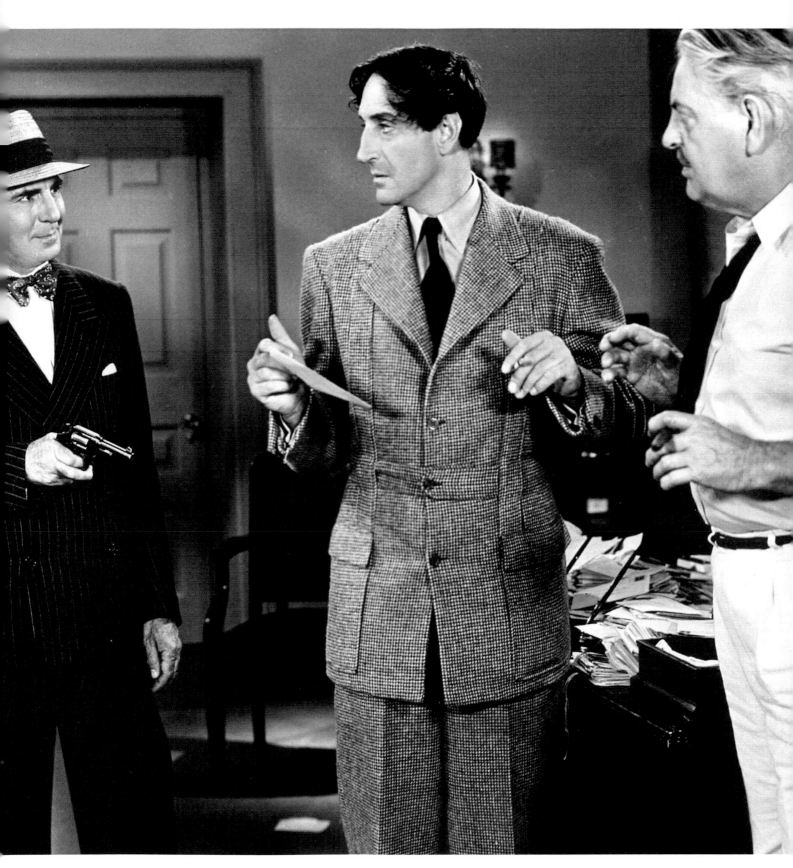

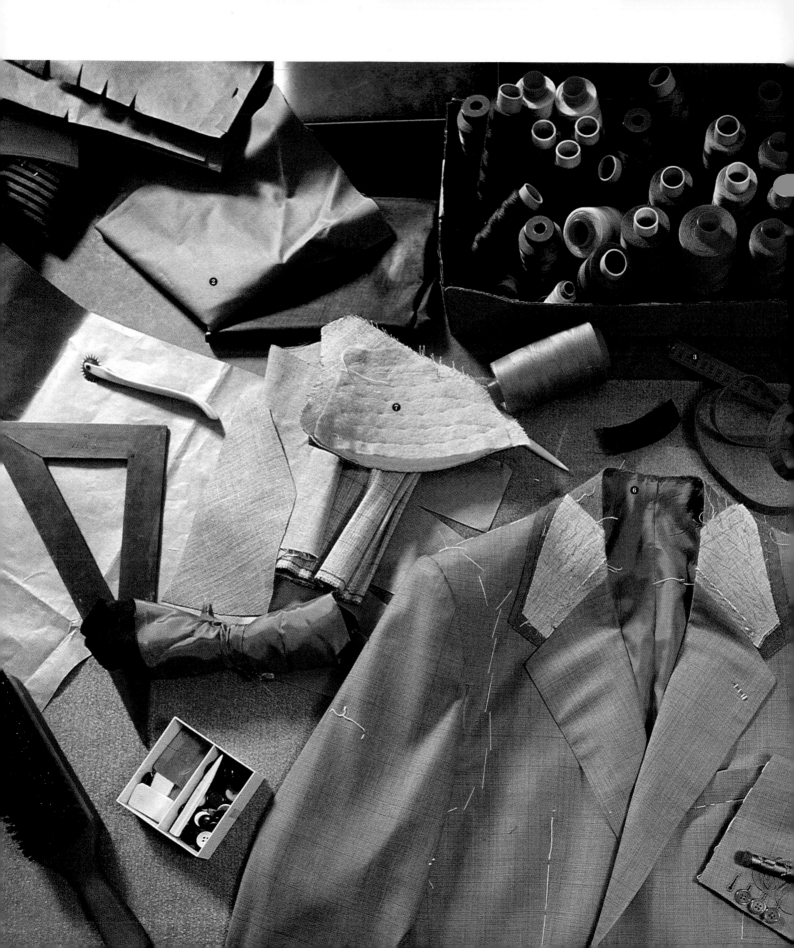

Needle and Thread

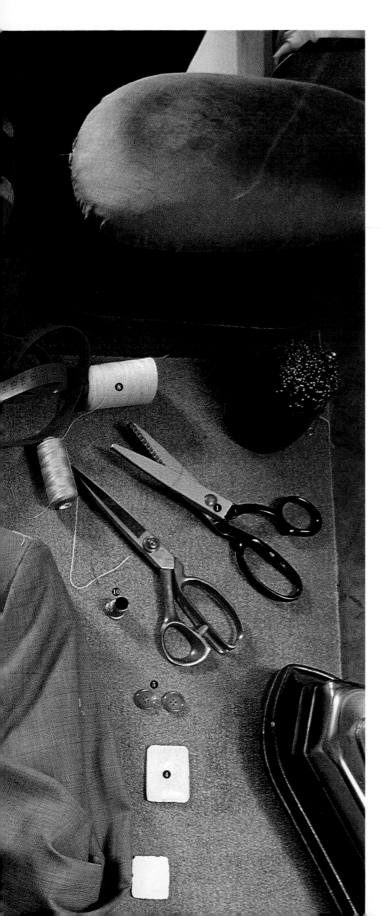

❶ The fabric for a tailor-made sports jacket is cut by hand, with *scissors*, which in Savile Row are called "shears."

❷ The "cutter" draws the separate pieces of the jacket on stout *brown paper*, to the measurements he has taken. This paper pattern will be carefully kept for subsequent orders. Old-established tailors often have thousands of such patterns stored away.

❸ The unknown inventor of the *tape measure* made a great advance in the craft of tailoring. This flexible tape enabled tailors to take precise measurements of the rounded parts of the body for the first time. The famous tailor's "yard," a rigid measuring stick, is really suitable only for measuring lengths of cloth.

❹ *Tailor's chalk* is one of the cutter's most important tools, since he can make marks with it directly on the fabric, thus passing his instructions on to the coat maker. At the first fitting the cutter marks any places that need adjustment or alteration, and at a later fitting he marks the position of the buttonholes and the exact length of the sleeves.

❺ *Horn buttons*, or buttons of some other natural material, are correct for a custom-made sports jacket. You can also get buttons covered with leather or the fabric of the jacket itself. If you are in any doubt, a good tailor will help you to make the best choice.

❻ The *lining* is sewn into the jacket by hand, as the irregularity of the distance between the tiny stitches shows. If the stitches were sewn by machine they would be perfectly regular. However, many manufacturers of ready-made clothing use machines that give a good imitation of hand sewing. But the Düsseldorf custom tailor, Heinz-Josef Radermacher, uses no such tricks, as anyone can see by glancing into his workshop.

❼ The shape of the custom-made jacket is largely determined by the materials concealed inside it. *Canvas*, horsehair, cotton, or felt are used in the substructure of the jacket, and it is these interlinings that give its most important parts their shape.

❽ Using *white cotton thread*, the coat maker bastes the jacket together with large stitches, ready for the first fitting. Then the separate pieces are taken apart again, to be fitted together once more, and more exactly. The white cotton thread can not only be torn out more easily than silk thread, but is more easily visible on the fabric.

❾ To this day, the workshop of a tailoring firm still smells of steam and singed canvas. That is because the tailor is almost constantly using his *iron* as he works. He shapes the fabric by damping and pressing it again and again.

❿ All tailors use a *thimble*. Without it, they could not keep pushing the needle through the material.

Tweed Plus

Donegal tweed is suitable for sports jackets of medium weight. Either woolen or silk neckties can be worn with this fabric, or alternatively neckties of Irish poplin, a wool and silk mixture. Because of the large amount of white in it, Donegal tweed also goes well with a Tattersall check shirt on a white ground, a combination often seen in Britain.

Shepherd's check is another popular pattern for a rather sturdy tweed, although it is a comparatively rustic one. It comes in various different colors and pattern sizes. The small check version in black and white is known as a Pepita check in the German-speaking countries.

When most people on the continent of Europe think of tweed, it is Harris tweed they have in mind. The fabric has a rough surface and is particularly hard wearing. Only wool woven into tweed in the Outer Hebrides can carry the coveted label. It is available in many strong colors, and is particularly suitable for sturdy sports jackets meant for country wear. Corduroy trousers are often worn with this rough fabric and the two garments together are highly suitablr for cold days.

Herringbone is a classic pattern for sports jackets. It is especially popular with American manufacturers, and is part of the Brooks Brothers standard range. It comes in various colors – typical shades are brown, dark to light gray, and green; it is also available in medium to dark blue. Gray herringbone looks good with a white button-down shirt of Oxford cotton. You can add either a black knitted necktie or a striped silk tie, either of which complement the ensemble very successfully. Herringbone is also very popular in continental Europe.

Another version of herringbone is known as "varied herringbone," and has additional colors woven into it, giving an even more complex appearance to the cloth.

Houndstooth is a rather busy pattern, and you must be careful when combining it with other colors and patterns. It is available in many colors, and is very suitable for sports jackets to be worn to the office. It is a classic design, but it may not be everybody's cup of tea.

Cheviot is a very hard-wearing – and very rough – worsted made from the wool of the Cheviot sheep. It is a typical fabric for British sport suits. Tailors often jokingly describe this heavy material as "bulletproof," although it may be wise not to put this to the test.

Covert fabric, with a small fleck, is another material typical of British country wear. It is mainly used for coats, and for the kind of riding jacket known as a hacking jacket. Covert fabrics come in greenish or brownish shades. Designers have recently rediscovered this classic fabric.

Bedford cord is a very warm, heavy wool, and in England it is made into jackets and suits for hunting and shooting. Its weight makes it appropriate for very cold surroundings; Bedford cord is literally unwearable in a well-heated office. Jackets of this fabric can be relied upon to outlive their owners. The optical effect of the weave will appeal only to real lovers of English country wear – but those who like it swear by this indestructible material. There is no doubt that it represents good value for money.

Two Tweed Jackets

The traditional English tweed jacket has three horn buttons. On the continent of Europe, manufacturers who want to make their tweed jackets look especially English more commonly use leather buttons. The slanted pockets, and the vent at the back, are reminiscent of the riding jacket. The fabric is rough, hard wearing tweed.

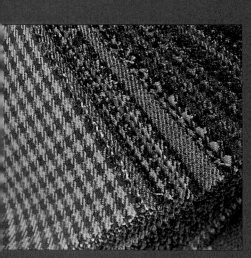

The range of tweeds offered by even really good gentlemen's outfitters is ridiculously small by comparison with the selection of fabric a tailor keeps in stock. Even a single swatch of samples from an establishment such as W. Bill or John G. Hardy contains a wide range of different possibilities for all tastes, occasions, and styles.

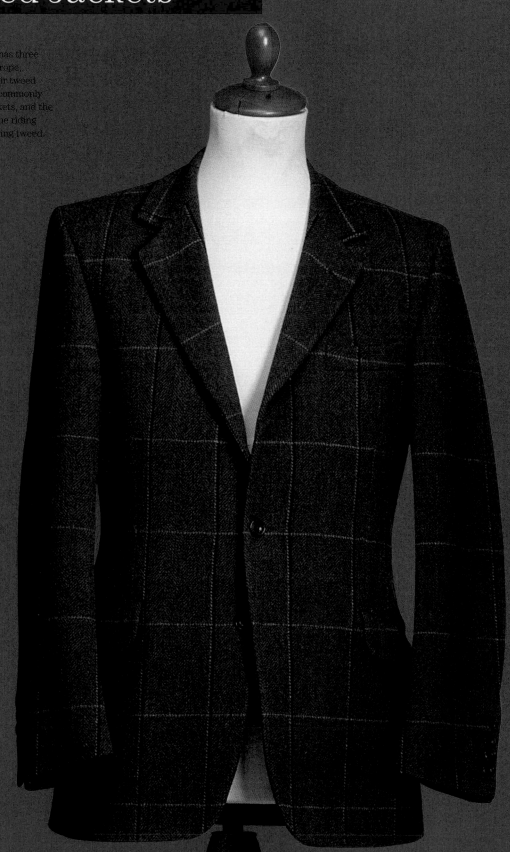

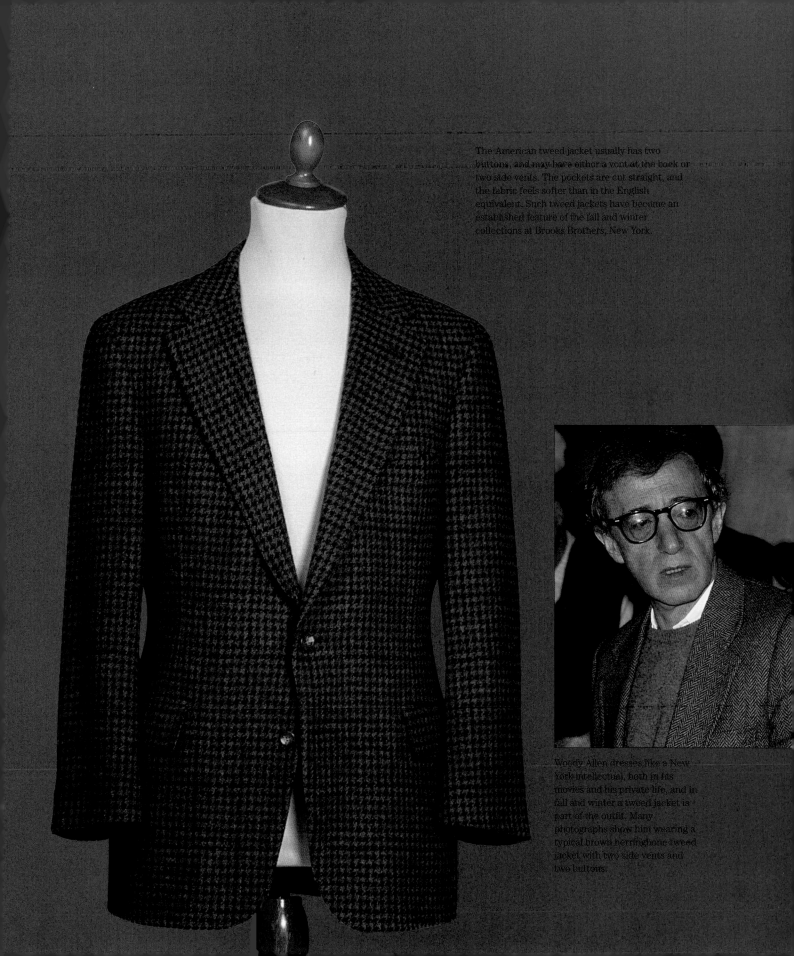

The American tweed jacket usually has two buttons, and may have either a vent at the back or two side vents. The pockets are cut straight, and the fabric feels softer than in the English equivalent. Such tweed jackets have become an established feature of the fall and winter collections at Brooks Brothers, New York.

Woody Allen dresses like a New York intellectual, both in his movies and his private life, and in fall and winter a tweed jacket is part of the outfit. Many photographs show him wearing a typical brown herringbone tweed jacket with two side vents and two buttons.

Today's Sports Jacket

The modern sports jacket has little in common with the English tweed jacket of tradition. For one thing, the sports jacket is available today in a much larger range of colors and patterns, and for another it has become increasingly light in weight over the course of time, not least through the influence of Italian tailors. Summer jackets in particular are made of light cashmere, thin worsteds, or silk and linen mixtures – in fact any kind of fabric that Italian, English, Scottish, and Irish weaving mills can supply. The Italians have no equal in the art of making up these soft, lightweight materials, and they also have a very good eye for pattern and color.

Italian tailors offer an international version of the English sports jacket, one that looks much more elegant and distinguished than the original. However, it is *not* the original; only English tailors can make that. If you feel happiest with the genuine English style you would do better to look for "your" jacket in Savile Row than Rome or Milan. Of course, you can get the lightest, softest fabrics in Savile Row too if you want them, but certainly not in the colors the Italians offer. If you are after a thoroughly British jacket, that is exactly what you can undoubtedly buy in London's famous street of tailors. But many men feel more comfortable in the internationally accepted Italian interpretation of the English sports jacket, whether because they prefer a more urbane, elegant cut, or just because they have a general preference for the Italian art of tailoring. An elegant sports jacket from Brioni, Kiton, or Barbera is evidence that it was the Italians who finally restored color to menswear.

One way or another, the quality of the predominantly or entirely handmade sports jacket is equally important in both English and Italian models.

An Eye for Detail

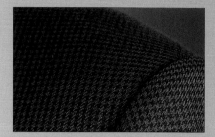

Basically, the art of constructing the shoulders consists of fitting a two-dimensional sleeve into a round armhole. This is as difficult as the long unsolved problem of creating a two-dimensional representation of the globe. The amount of fabric necessary to surround the circle of the sleeve opening must be pulled in and shaped so that there is no puckering where the sleeve meets the shoulder. In a well-tailored shoulder, the sleeve will fit smoothly to the armhole at every point.

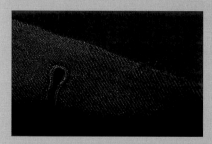

The edges of the lapels are pierced with a needle by hand before the seam is actually sewn. Hand working is the only way of ensuring the minimum of irregular distances between the holes. Since the fabric of the jacket will stretch or shrink to a small extent, depending on the humidity of the air, it may pucker slightly between the separate stitches at the edges of the lapels, but this is not a sign of poor quality. In fact the lapels of less expensive jackets have perfectly smooth edges where the fabric has been turned in and invisibly stitched.

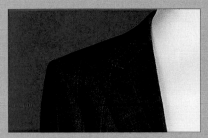

In a good quality jacket, the pattern must match neatly at as many of the seams as possible, particularly around the breast pocket. There should also be the minimum of discontinuity in the pattern between shoulders and breast. However, there are technical limitations to matching up the pattern. As it cannot run continuously at all the seams, a tailor will try to make the front of the jacket at least look all of a piece.

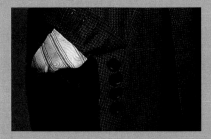

In Italian ready-to-wear jackets like those made by Kiton, all the sleeve buttons can be undone. Custom tailors are generally content with cutting open only the two lower buttonholes. That way, the length of the sleeves can always be altered later without any difficulty.

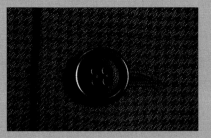

The buttons are made of natural materials, usually horn. The choice of buttons is the task of the "trimmer" in England. He selects all such items as buttons, interfacings, thread, and lining materials. If the customer expresses no particular wishes to the cutter, the trimmer will decide on these important details. Young tailors train their eye for style as trimmers. In garments of good quality, the buttons are sewn on by hand.

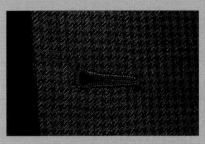

A custom tailor will always stitch around the buttonhole by hand, and the best of the ready-to-wear manufacturers do the same. There are various different ideas about how the buttonhole should look. Kiton, for instance, has a very individual shape. Normally, the buttonhole should close smoothly, leaving room for the shank of the button only at the end.

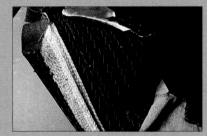

Interlinings are cut from canvas of different thicknesses, and sewn to the main fabric with tiny stitches. Horsehair, a very elastic substance, helps to give the jacket a permanently three-dimensional shape, for instance over the chest or at the curve of the lapels. In making ready-to-wear jackets, a substantial length of time is saved by fusing the interlinings into place.

The lining is sewn into the jacket by hand. The illustration shows the typical method used by European tailors. They use big stitches at the lower hem, leaving the lining material a certain amount of room to "give." For instance, if the wearer's movements put a strain on the lining, the seam will stretch slightly. This method also compensates for any stretching of the lining caused by body heat. English tailors, on the other hand, generally sew the lining to the lower hem with the same stitches as they use at the front, although here again there are various different procedures. In suits made by famous tailors like Henry Poole, for instance, the lining is sewn into every suit in a different way, depending on which coat maker has been working on it.

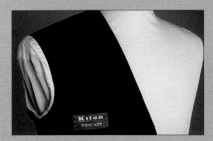

The lining is made of Bemberg silk (a soft cotton), or even of genuine silk. Summer jackets are often only half lined, at the shoulders, chest, and back. If the shoulders were not lined it would be difficult to slip the jacket on smoothly over your shirt.

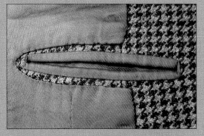

The inside breast pockets are usually edged with the fabric of the jacket, a traditional detail added solely for the benefit of the wearer, since almost no one else will ever get to see it.

Fabrics for Trousers to Go with the Sports Jacket

The sports jacket is a versatile item of clothing. Depending on the pants you combine it with, you can create a whole new outfit. The sports jacket is at its most formal with flannels or cavalry twill. However, it is only on the continent of Europe that a sports jacket and flannels really count as a formal outfit – corduroy and moleskin, on the other hand, are rather like the gentleman's version of jeans. If you are in London on business, it is wisest to wear a suit. For instance, in John le Carré's novel *The Tailor of Panama* a member of the British Secret Service is dismissed for venturing to deliver a message to his boss in the Grill Room of the Connaught while wearing a tweed jacket and flannels – a *faux pas* to be avoided at all costs, especially in conservative England.

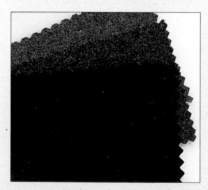

Not all grays are the same, and if you like gray flannels you can choose from a wide range of color gradations, depending on what goes best with your jacket.

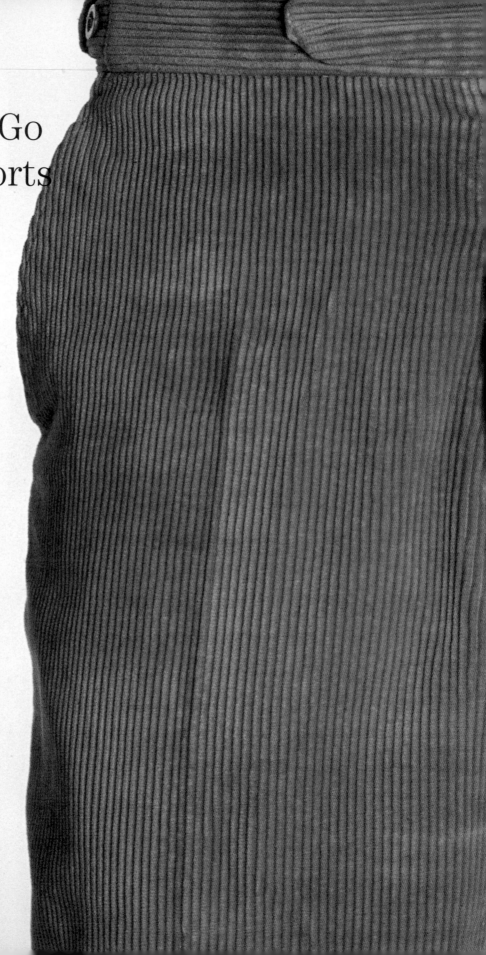

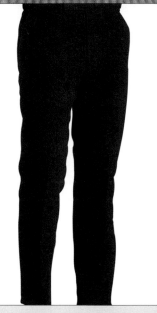

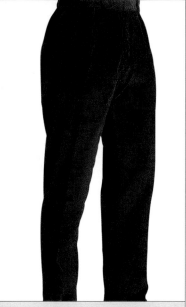

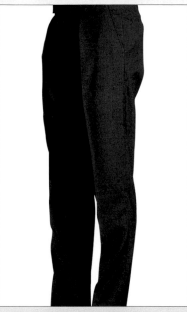

Moleskin is a fabric that really does feel like the skin of a mole, soft and smooth. You have probably felt moleskin in the pockets of a Barbour jacket when you warm your hands in them. The material is hard wearing, and it can be machine washed. It can come in various colours, and the above picture shows a particulary striking example.

Corduroy, with flannel and cavalry twill, is the third classic fabric for trousers worn with a sports jacket. Classic English cords are cut narrow, with an adjustable belt and buttons for the suspenders. Typical colors are russet, dusty pink, moss green, or corn. The last-named color, however, seems to attract dirt as if by magic.

Pure wool trousers are best with a summer jacket. Woolen fabrics both look and feel different from flannels, which are too hot for summer wear, but they make a good substitute for classic flannels, in color as well as feel – although flannels themselves were originally summer wear, and some tradionalists still wear them then.

Gray flannel trousers are the classic accompaniment to a sports jacket. However, the soft surface of flannel mixes well only with jackets in materials of a similar structure – something not too coarse and rough. The dark gray version, part of the standard range at outfitters like Cordings, is now regarded as a classic. Gray flannels with two front pleats to each leg can be obtained from any off-the-rack outlet on the continent of Europe.

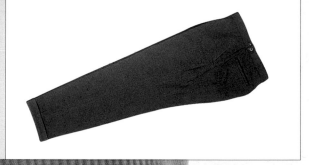

Cavalry twill is a classic when worn with the English sports jacket, but today this hard-wearing material appeals to fewer and fewer men. It may be because of the color – cavalry twill is usually eggshell, beige, or fawn – or because trousers in cavalry twill can look like the trousers for driving made of synthetic fibers, and regarded, not unjustly, as downmarket, and therefore hardly the correct apparel for a gentlemen.

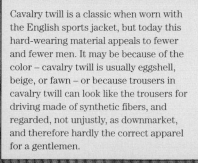

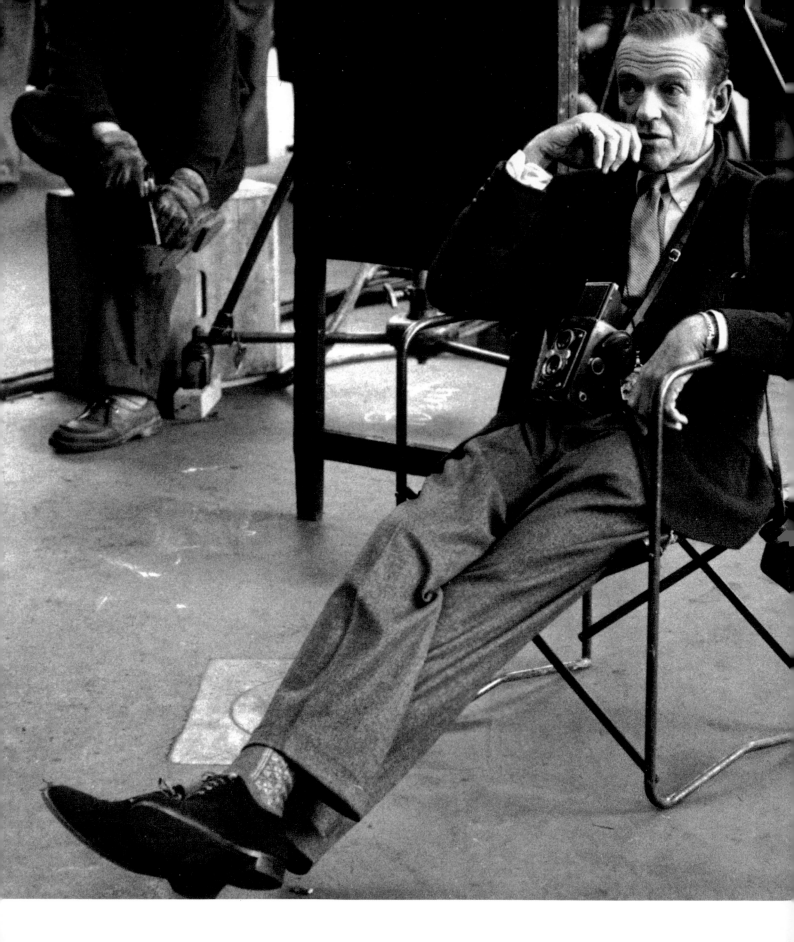

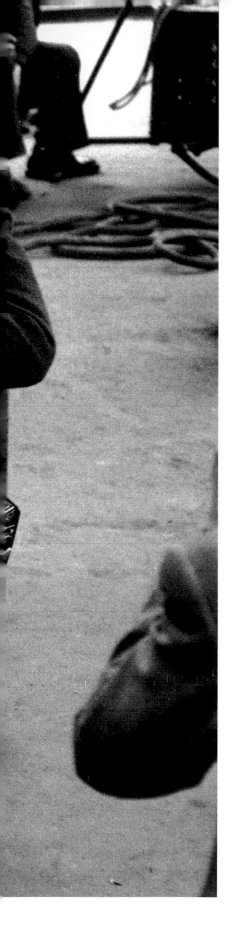

The Gray Eminence

If, for some mysterious reason, all gray flannel trousers and anything resembling them were suddenly to disappear off the face of the earth, we would be able to observe a very interesting phenomenon: no one would buy any more sports jackets. For gray flannels (and all their lookalikes made of wool or mixed fabrics) are still the best companion garment for a sports jacket. They are both formal and casual, elegant and sporty, and their color, that slightly flecked pale to dark gray, makes the perfect background for the material of your sports jacket. There is no limit to the ways in which you can combine gray flannels with the rest of your wardrobe. A shirt and pullover with flannels make an outfit that is semiformal but still comfortable. A long-sleeved polo shirt, a sports jacket, and flannels are ideal for a weekend visit to a restaurant. Sports jackets and flannels are always the perfect combination, and one that has been around for 80 years. While gray flannel trousers may go briefly out of fashion now and then, it is impossible to imagine the classic style without them.

The word "flannel" originally comes from Welsh, where the term gwalen means something made of wool. The smooth, soft nature of flannel is the result of a special manufacturing procedure. Fine merino wool is put through the fulling process until it felts up (merino will felt quite quickly), and in fact the surface feel of flannel does suggest that of a soft felt hat. At first flannel was used for summer trousers, but by the end of the 1930s flannels had become acceptable wear all the year around. If you look through illustrated books of the period, you will see a man wearing flannels in almost every photograph. At the time, flannel pants combined with sports jackets were worn by the younger generation, and flannels were positively "hip." That may be hard to imagine, now that flannel trousers are regarded as such a classic and conservative style. However, flannels will surely survive – questioning their future would cast doubt on the whole concept of wearing a shirt, necktie, jacket, and trousers. The unexpected revival of the suit at the end of the 1990s, ironically enough at the fashion shows of rather avant-garde designers, shows that classics in gentlemen's fashions will always reassert themselves. And whether gray flannels happen to be in fashion or not, devotees of the timeless international style will wear them anyway, as they have for over 80 years. There is just nothing better, and nothing could possibly replace them. It is perhaps unlikely that they will again become truly fashionable – although even this is not impossible – but within the classic gentleman's wardrobe they will always have their place.

Gray flannel trousers were Fred Astaire's trademark. Audrey Hepburn had a frame specially covered with gray flannel made for the signed photograph of the star that she owned.

Khaki Couture

It takes some time for an item of clothing to be accepted into the select company of classics – in the case of chinos, a whole century if you count back from the 1950s to the year 1848. In that year, so the story goes, Sir Harry Lumsden, commanding officer of a British regiment stationed in India, had the brilliant idea of dyeing his men's white uniforms with a mixture of coffee, curry powder, and mulberry juice, to disguise the inevitable soiling they suffered from the ever-present dust. Sure enough, the new yellowish brown color proved very suitable for everyday army life in India. The Indians themselves called this color "khaki," meaning "dust colored" or "earth colored". Even if the story is not true, it makes a pleasing anecdote, and is always told when the subject of these favorite cotton trousers for summer wear comes up. The word "chino," however, was not used for trousers of this characteristic color until the twentieth century, and there is another story of the way in which that happened. Apparently a consignment of cotton pants made in Manchester was sold to China. The businesslike Chinese in turn exported them to the Philippines. That group of Pacific islands was under American rule from 1934 to 1946, and the American soldiers stationed there liked the trousers. They took them home to the United States, and called them "chinos" because of their origin. There is no historical evidence for this story, but it can be read as it is told above, or with slight variations, in several sources, which tends to suggest there is something in it. It is certain, anyway, that after the Second World War chinos reached the continent of Europe, and became really established there in the 1980s.

In the United States, chinos are regarded as more formal than jeans – but quite informal by comparison with flannel trousers or a suit. These comfortable pants are often combined with a shirt, necktie, and jacket, but are never worn on very formal occasions, where the suit is still a must. With a Brooks Brothers shirt, a striped necktie from the same outfitter, a single-breasted blazer, and saddle shoes or boat shoes, chinos are part of the favorite outfit of students at the top American universities. It is a look copied by Ralph Lauren, and he has sold it all over the world as his own creation. Some years ago the combination of a navy-blue blazer with chinos also became increasingly acceptable in London, at any rate in circumstances where suits are no longer obligatory wear. Cotton trousers are now kept in stock throughout the year by such well-known English outfitters as Cordings.

Internationally, then, chinos are now generally accepted as trousers for leisurewear, and are a good choice when jeans seem too casual and flannels too formal. Chinos are still made in the traditional khaki color, but trousers described as chinos can now be found in a variety of different colors. It is a sign of style if the classic appearance is retained.

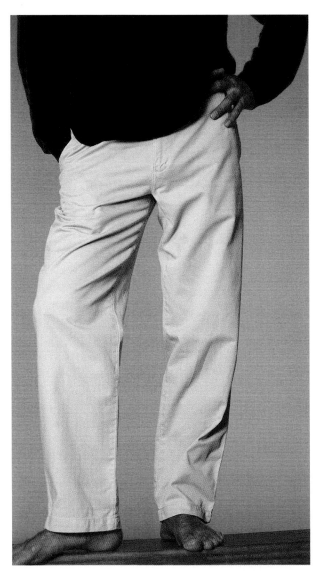

Chinos are ideal as summer pants. They can easily be combined with almost anything, and as they are washable the pale color presents no problems.

Shorts

However handsome your legs, however hot it is, and even if everyone else is wearing shorts, they are still a very dubious proposition stylistically, inappropriate except on the beach and in the privacy of your own yard. The exceptions are sporting occasions when shorts are worn for practical reasons, for instance to play soccer, rugby football, or tennis; for cycling, marathon running, and so on. It is very bad form to wear shorts in the office or the city, and is evidence of your poor taste. But even men who feel sure of their sense of style commit this *faux pas* repeatedly – and have done so with increasing frequency in recent years. Perhaps we should remember that it used to be a great moment in a boy's life when, on reaching the age of 13 or 14, he acquired his first pair of long trousers, and from then on his clothes showed that he was grown up. Just to repeat it: shorts are comfortable on the beach, on safari, on your patio, and in your yard, and of course they are suitable wear on the sports field. Everywhere else they are incorrect. But if you do find an occasion when it is right to wear shorts, it is best to choose a pair in classic khaki, cut quite wide, and ending just above the knee. In South Africa, New Zealand, and Australia, they are worn with knee-high socks and lace-up ankle boots, the footwear being a protection against ticks and poisonous snakes lying in wait in the grass.

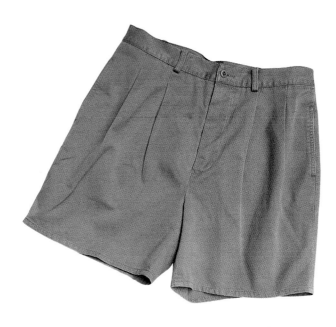

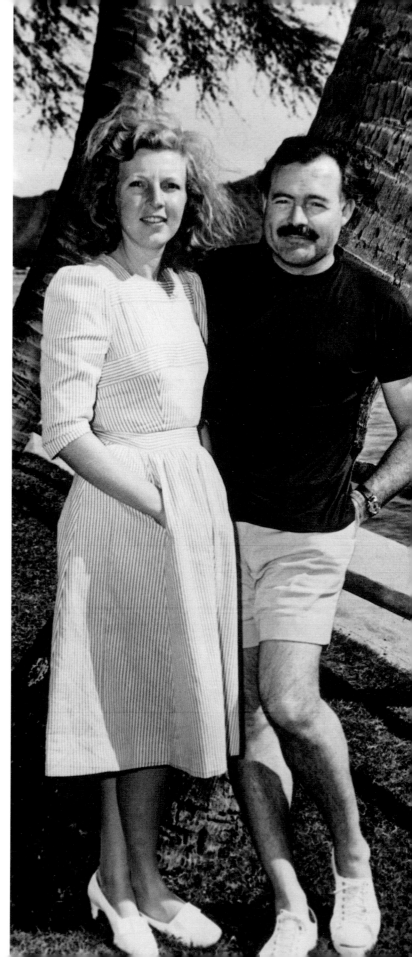

The Right Sort of Jeans

Since they first originated in the United States in the nineteenth century, jeans have undergone two major changes of image that are probably unique in the history of clothing. Initially devised by the founder of the firm of Levi Strauss as tough, hard-wearing work trousers, they became the cult object of the rebellious young in the 1950s. Studded blue jeans shocked the parental generation in post-war Europe even more than in the United States, where jeans had been around for a long time as cheap, nondescript trousers; while the idea of inexpensive, robust, washable pants that could be bought in your local drugstore or supermarket was entirely foreign to Europeans. For the young people of a continent shattered by war, these jeans, like other everyday products from the United States, came to symbolize liberty, adventure, and a new start.

The second change of image – from a display of rebellion to a socially acceptable item of designer clothing – began in Europe in the late 1960s. Jeans were always more expensive in Europe than in their country of origin. Even today Americans are amused to find that people in France, England, or Germany are prepared to pay three to four times the price in the United States. The high price was not the result of the high cost of the fabric or the manufacturing process, but was because of import duties. Jeans made in Europe would therefore offer a chance of good profit margins, and at this point the designers came on the scene, realizing that they could corner a large share of the market in blue jeans by producing superior versions. The idea of designer jeans then went back from Europe to the United States in the 1970s. Fred Segal led the way with his store in Los Angeles, where more designer jeans are still sold than anywhere else. Later on, a European trend centered on the fashion for 501 jeans. Trendsetters of the early 1980s had shrink-to-fit 501 Levi's imported from the United States, some time before they became the "in" thing again in the 1990s. They were worn with Kiton sports jackets and expensive English shoes. Jeans therefore became established in Europe, slowly but surely, as an indispensable part of the leisure look among well-to-do young people. It became increasingly important to have the "right" sort of jeans, and the only right sort were shrink-to-fit Levi's 501s. In the 1980s their straight cut was in great contrast to the wide-cut trousers with front pleats that were popular at the time. And long before trousers without front pleats became fashionable again, 501s showed that straight, narrow trousers could be very comfortable.

The 1990s finally set the stamp of approval on jeans. Who knows anyone without a pair of jeans in the closet? Today, they are worn by people of all ages, and on almost any occasion. Only the world of the office is still largely resistant to jeans. The combination of jeans, sports jacket, and necktie has never made the leap into the "conservative" working world, where jeans are still reserved for leisure time – that is, apart from professions such as fashion, the media, and advertising, where the dress code does not stipulate a suit, and even a sports jacket is felt to be formal. Here, 501s are universally accepted as hard-wearing trousers for work. And so, in a sense, another change has taken place – back to the origins of jeans.

Whoever wants to keep his 501s in their pristine blue should not machine-wash them but send them to the dry cleaners.

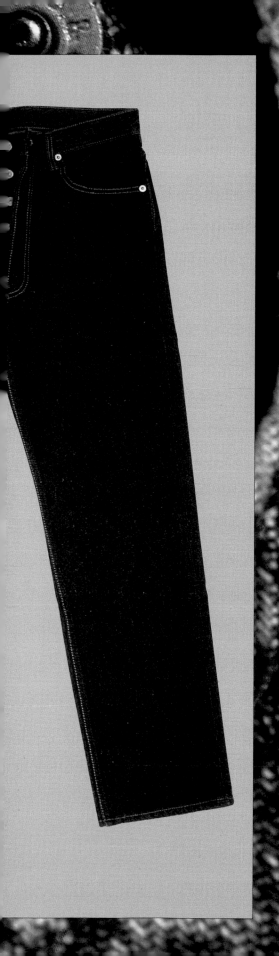

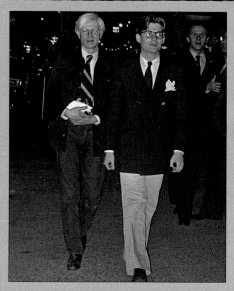

Levi's 501s are indisputably regarded as the best jeans today, partly because of one of their most famous fans, Andy Warhol, seen here with his assistant Vincent Fremont. He combined them with a check shirt, a necktie, and a blue blazer, creating an entirely new look. Or so the legend has it, anyway, but Bob Colacello, formerly editor of the magazine *Interview*, and a writer for *Parade*, and *Vanity Fair*, claimed in his book *Holy Terror – Andy Warhol Close Up* that it was not the pop artist himself but his colleague and friend Fred Hughes who first combined jeans with a suit jacket, creating a look that Andy Warhol copied later. This claim sounds very credible, since in questions of fashion Hughes certainly knew more than his friend: "Everything he wore was English: handmade suits from Tommy Nutter, handmade shirts from Turnbull & Asser, handmade shoes from Lobb's. His cologne was English – Penhaligon's Blenheim Bouquet. Even his Levi's 501s looked as if they'd been altered on Savile Row – the seams were never crooked and there was no extra fabric on the thighs – but maybe that was because he had them washed and pressed every day. Fred was the first to wear jeans with suit jackets, but when Andy adopted the style as his uniform it became known as the Warhol Look." It was perhaps inevitable that the combination would not be known as "the Hughes look", as Hughes hardly captured the public's attention as much as Warhol.

The Cut

Most men think that the cut of a pair of trousers depends on the vicissitudes of fashion. Sometimes they have pleats, sometimes they do not. Sometimes trousers are cut wide, sometimes flared, sometimes tapering. In fact the details of the cut of a pair of trousers vary from season to season, and in addition the basic cut changes about every ten years. We all remember the flared trousers of the 1970s, the large front pleats of the 1980s, and the narrow trousers of the late 1990s. But if we look at the trousers worn by men who do not follow every whim of the ready-to-wear clothing industry, we will see that they all wear certain very individual types of trousers, cut to suit their own proportions rather than the dictates of fashion.

Crucial points affecting the cut of a good pair of trousers are the size of the wearer's stomach and behind, the length of his legs, the desired height of the waist, and the width of the trouser bottoms. The last named must be measured so that the trousers leave the front third of the shoe uncovered. In other words, the width of the trouser bottom is about two thirds of the length of the shoe, never mind whether your shoe size is 8 or 12. However, you can depart from that general rule if you have very large feet, since the bottoms of your trouser legs would then have to be very wide to make up two thirds of the shoe length. It is advisable to avoid flares, and best in any case to let the trousers simply fall straight. You need not worry about putting your big feet on display – just relish the fact that you can show more of your favorite shoes than men who have feet of a "normal" size.

The size of the stomach is another factor. If you have a flat stomach you have a wide choice in the cut of the waist area. Slender men who do not like front pleats will look good in a pair of trousers cut to fit close to the stomach. If they do opt for pleats, one pleat to each trouser leg is best. The pleats will ensure that the trousers are still comfortable when they are sitting down, and will conceal anything they have in their pockets. Traditionalists prefer a pleat turned inward; the opposite is the kind known as a reversed pleat.

If you are rather large around the waist, then a pair of trousers tapering slightly downward will be best,

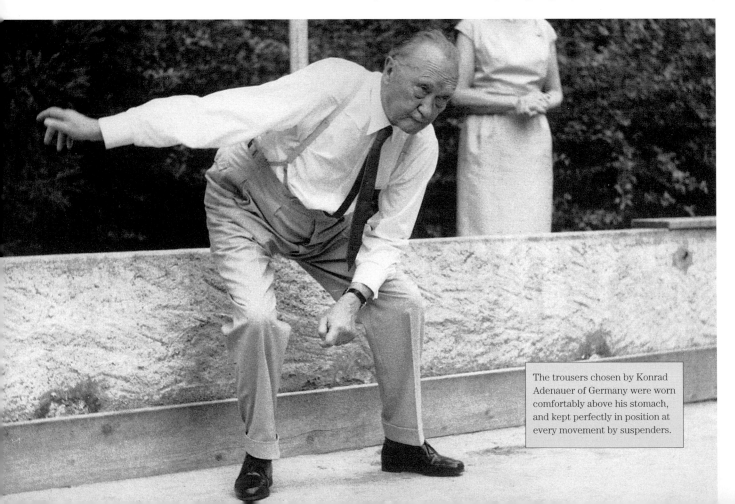

The trousers chosen by Konrad Adenauer of Germany were worn comfortably above his stomach, and kept perfectly in position at every movement by suspenders.

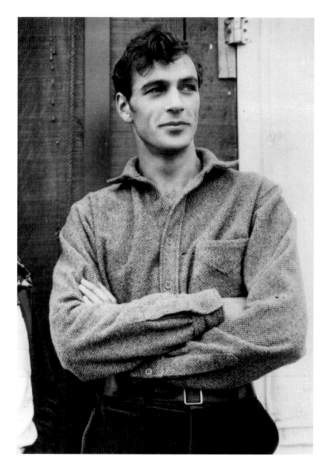

High-cut trousers without front pleats look best on men with flat stomachs, like the young Gary Cooper in this photograph.

How Trousers Got their Cuffs

The sources do not agree on the inventor of the trouser cuff. Most of them attribute its invention to King Edward VII, grandfather of the trendsetting King Edward VIII. Some time in the second half of the nineteenth century, he is said to have been the first to have had the idea of turning up his trouser legs to protect them from dirt and damp. In fact men with their trouser legs turned up like cuffs can be seen in photographs dating from the early years of the twentieth century. In later years too, it has sometimes seemed a "modern" look to turn up your jeans rather than cut them to a shorter length. However, no one really knows who was the first to order a pair of trousers with cuffs from his tailor – and it is a matter of no great importance.

Almost any kinds of pants can have cuffs. They look appropriate with suits, sports jackets, and blazers alike. The exceptions are morning coats, tuxedos, and tailcoats; trousers to go with these coats never have cuffs, and nor do the trousers of military uniforms. It is often thought that cuffs are *de rigueur* with double-breasted suits, but that is not really so. If you do not like cuffs, there is no need to have them on the trousers of a double-breasted suit, particularly if you prefer trousers without front pleats, since these look better without cuffs in any case. It is inadvisable for rather short men to wear trouser cuffs, which will make their legs look shorter. But if you do want cuffs, choose very narrow trouser legs and have the trousers made rather short, to compensate for the shortening effect of the cuffs. Trousers with cuffs are sometimes worn so short that the hem does not touch the shoe. A basic principle with trousers – as with the sleeves of jackets – is that slightly too short is better than slightly too long, especially if you are not a giant. Socks worn with slightly shorter trousers need to be fairly long, so that, when sitting down, no bare flesh is visable between socks and cuffs.

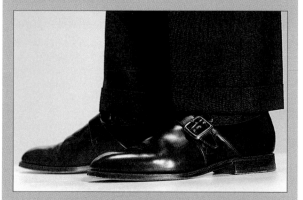

Wearing slightly short trousers is a youthful look, and seems to make the legs of short men appear longer. Continental tailors would think this length incorrect, and they measure trousers so that the hem will just brush the heel of the shoe.

since straight-cut trousers will quite obviously end in disproportionately wide trouser bottoms. And you have to decide how high you want to wear your trousers – that is to say, whether the waistband should come below, above, or on your stomach. Trousers doing up above the stomach are the most comfortable to wear. They are cut very high, but do not need suspenders, since they sit above the curve of the belly and cannot slip down. However, if you think this cut looks too much like the garb of a circus clown, you must reconcile yourself to wearing suspenders – or live with trousers that keep slipping.

The Waist Area

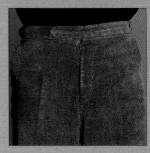

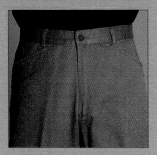

This classic English cut goes best with rather waisted, quite long jackets. Then the narrow trouser legs will look very elegant. Trousers of this type are really an English specialty, but since the middle of the 1990s they have frequently appeared on the runways of international couture. The originals, however, are still to be obtained only in England. There are buttons inside the waistband for traditional suspenders.

Cross pockets are traditional for riding trousers. A horizontally placed pocket has the great advantage that it is difficult to lose your change or keys out of it. However, as such pockets can be fitted only on trousers without front pleats, they went out of fashion entirely during the 1980s. On the continent of Europe, only a few gentlemen's outfitters offer them to their customers, so if you want horizontally placed pockets it is advisable to visit England – or a custom tailor.

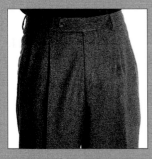

If you cannot quite manage without pleats, but you want trousers with a narrow cut to wear with an English sports jacket, try trousers with only one pleat to each leg. The London gentlemen's outfitters Hackett make trousers of this kind in flannel, cavalry twill, and cord, or as chinos. Since they have an adjustable waistband, they can be worn with suspenders.

Continental Europeans prefer a more generous cut, with at least two front pleats. These trousers look better while you are standing than pants without front pleats, although they can look baggy when you sit down. They are recommended wear with the rather wide-cut jackets made by Italian tailors, under which narrow pants can look rather lost.

The Trousers in Detail

In a good pair of trousers the pockets are made of stout, firm fabric, and sewn with many small stitches.

Trousers of good quality are lined down to the knees. In an English suit, however, even a good one, do not be surprised if you feel the fabric itself next to your skin. The British consider long trouser linings an unnecessary luxury even for a rough tweed suit, and a sign of effeminacy.

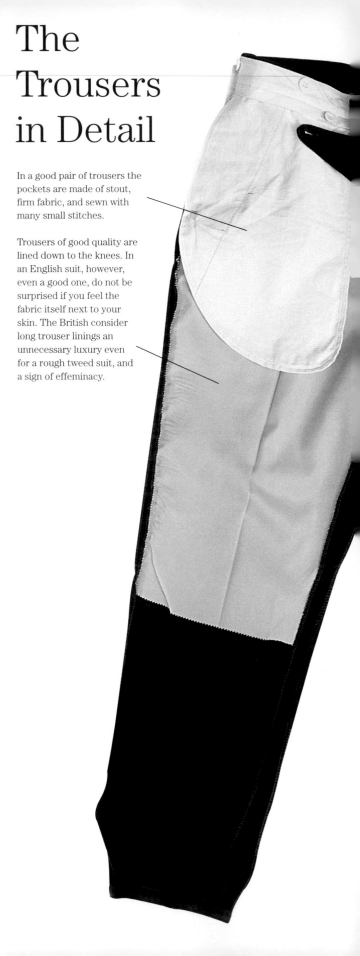

Other Countries, Other Trousers

The waistband is carefully lined, and the lining divides at the back so that the trousers can be taken out or in without too much difficulty.

The hems of the trouser legs are edged with tape. The edging tape must protrude by a fraction to prevent the hems from being worn by contact with your shoes. Edging tape also serves to give the hem of the trouser leg slightly more weight, so that the fabric will drape better. In very light summer suits, the edging tape may be confined to the back of the hem, since half the usual edging is enough to give weight to such flimsy materials.

If you try on suits by Kiton, Chester Barrie, and Ralph Lauren successively, you will notice a striking difference between the design of the trousers. Trousers made by the English manufacturer Chester Barrie are cut narrow and rather high, have no front pleats, and are not usually popular with female arbiters of fashion. The trousers of a suit by Kiton have front pleats, and sit comfortably just above the hip bones. The lightweight, smooth fabric falls elegantly to the shoes, and the back of the trousers is well cut. You may find that at first you do not like the trousers of a suit by Ralph Lauren, cut quite high in the English style but wider, because they somehow seem "too big." Americans in general obviously have rather larger behinds.

But whatever suit you decide on (and thus whatever type of pants), trying on clothes for purposes of comparison can tell you a great deal about the different attitudes to trouser making of English, Italian, and American tailors. The prime object of the Englishman (if we may be allowed to generalize) is to be correctly dressed in his suit. A suit is correct in the office because it is traditionally cut; he neither expects nor wants it to be "sexy." And since the jacket is best not taken off anyway, he does not mind what the trousers look like around the waist. An Italian, on the other hand, wants to look good in his suit, even or indeed especially when he takes off his jacket – in other words, when things are beginning to get interesting. The American sees the suit as a necessity showing that he knows how a successful man ought to dress. To him, the saying, "Dress for success," refers first and foremost to professional success. Once he has achieved that, success with women will follow naturally, and he will not need particularly well-cut trousers.

All about Suspenders

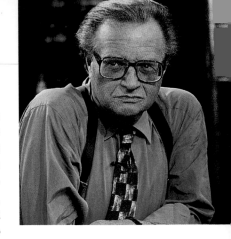

Suspenders (or in British English braces) are especially popular in the United Kingdom and the United States, for various reasons. In the case of the Americans, it may be their sense of what is practical and comfortable, and perhaps a feeling for nostalgia too. In Britain, by contrast, it is probably more a sense of tradition. Both the British and the Americans, however, tend to avoid excessive elegance to some extent. Italian ideas are very different. In fact, it is difficult to imagine suspenders worn with a Brioni suit, and actually appearing in front of an international audience in shirt sleeves and suspenders, as the CNN talk show host Larry King does every day, would be unthinkable to a style-conscious Italian.

However, on the continent of Europe, suspenders are worn mainly by ambitious salesmen in gentlemen's outfitters, and by Anglophile dandies. Of course, we mean genuine English suspenders buttoned to the waistband. Such suspenders are far removed from the very narrow examples in brown and white, or gray and blue, sold in the notions departments of many large department stores.

The great advantage of well-fitting suspenders is the way they keep the trousers securely in position.

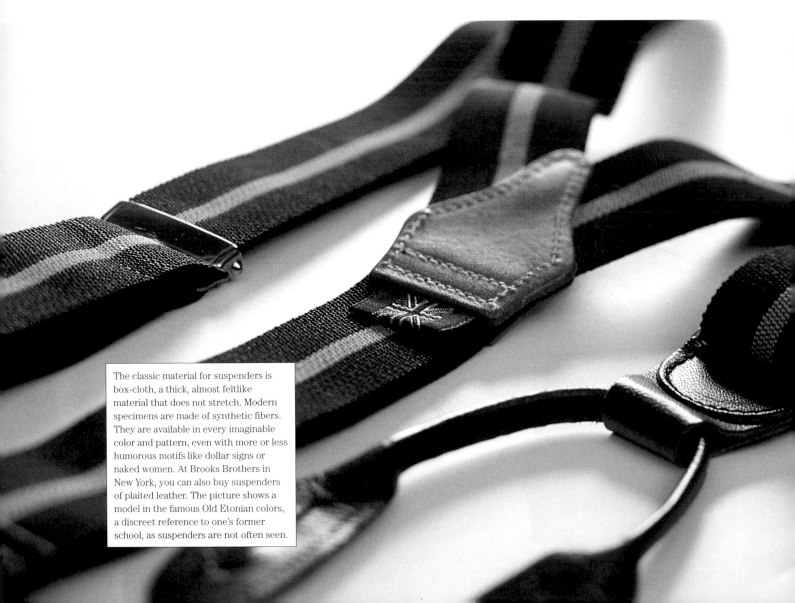

The classic material for suspenders is box-cloth, a thick, almost feltlike material that does not stretch. Modern specimens are made of synthetic fibers. They are available in every imaginable color and pattern, even with more or less humorous motifs like dollar signs or naked women. At Brooks Brothers in New York, you can also buy suspenders of plaited leather. The picture shows a model in the famous Old Etonian colors, a discreet reference to one's former school, as suspenders are not often seen.

Since they emphasize the vertical line, and thus have a lengthening effect, they are suitable to wear with high-cut trousers to make them look longer. They also let the air circulate freely between waistband and shirt, which is a good thing in summer. Many people even credit them with psychological advantages. If you are sure your suspenders will keep your trousers perfectly in position whenever you move, you will look more confident in general. There is something in this theory – at least, trousers that are always slipping certainly detract a great deal from your sense of well-being. Suspenders do feel rather warm on the shoulders, but if you like you can wear them under a light jacket. Originally they were hidden under the vest of a suit, but as the vest gradually went out of fashion, more and more men gave up wearing suspenders that were on show as soon as they removed their jackets in the office. Suspenders can also be a nuisance when you are sitting down, since they tend to slip off your shoulders, or stand out from the body in a rather unattractive way.

Suspenders must be right for the cut of your trousers, so that means you cannot wear them with trousers from Italy or Germany, which are cut so as to require a belt if they are in danger of slipping. These days, good ready-made English trousers are not usually designed for wear with suspenders either, but if you have your trousers custom made, then you will naturally get them cut and equipped for suspenders in the traditional way. Many old-established English outfitters provide their trousers with both buttons for suspenders and an adjustable waistband. Traditional American trousers, like those from Brooks Brothers, are ideal for suspenders, since they are cut high at the waist. England is the best place to buy the suspenders themselves. They are available in a wide range of colors and patterns from gentlemen's outfitters, tailors, and shirtmakers. But no amount of information about suspenders is a substitute for trying them on for yourself, and it is unlikely that you will have difficulty finding the right suspenders for you in London.

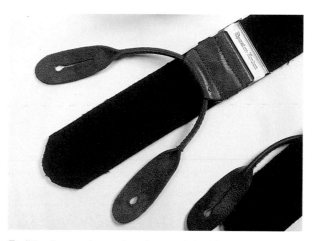

Traditional suspenders such as those made by Albert Thurston have buckles made of genuine hand-polished brass.

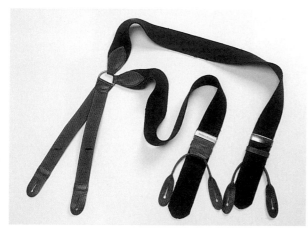

These box-cloth braces from Albert Thurston are the ultimate English suspenders, with real goatskin straps. Albert Thurston is the oldest manufacturer of suspenders; the firm was founded in 1820. Its customers have included famous Americans such as Frank Sinatra and Michael Douglas, as well as members of the British aristocracy. It is said that the Prince of Wales hates to wear suspenders, and in this he resembles his great-uncle, the Duke of Windsor, who disliked them just as much.

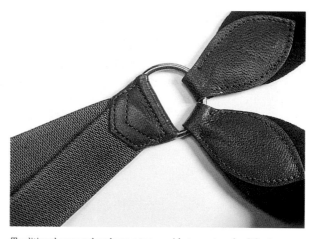

Traditional suspenders have a trapezoid strap at each of the two fronts, and two long straps at the back. The straps are sometimes made of white catgut, sometimes of brown, black, or white goatskin. White straps are usually worn with a business suit. They look good with either black or brown shoes, unlike brown or black leather straps, which should be worn only with shoes of the same color.

The Right Belt

Canvas belts are correct with chinos, cords, or moleskin trousers. They come either striped or in plain colors. However, canvas belts are incorrect with formal wear. And you should be careful that their colors go well with your shirt and trousers, and do not clash with strikingly patterned socks. Both leather and canvas belts should be color coordinated with your shoes.

Plaited belts are an attractive alternative to smooth leather belts, and can be worn with leisurewear, with a suit, or with the combination of sports jacket and trousers. However, you should make sure that the rather rustic look of such a belt does not overpower a fine suiting fabric. Plaited belts look good with American suits.

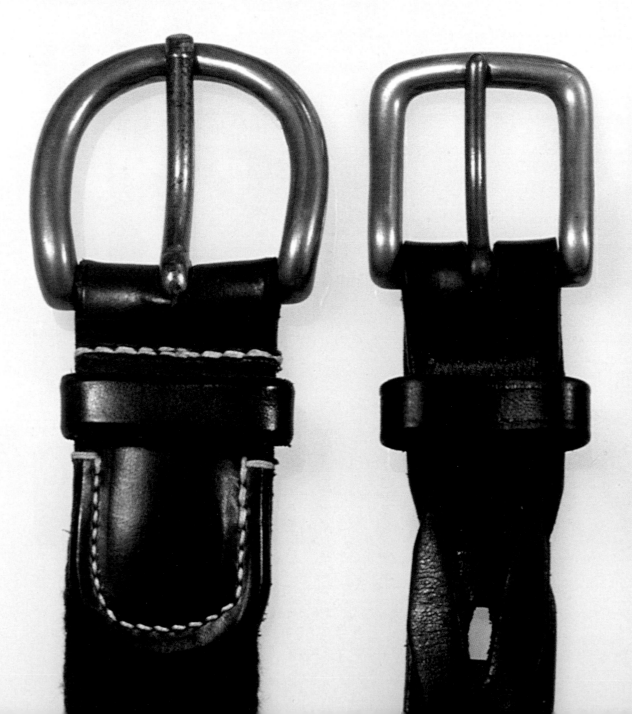

If you want something rather more striking, you can wear the classic reversible Hermès belt, with its H-shaped buckle made of gilded brass. These belts come in a large range of different leathers and color combinations, although you really need only brown and black. This belt is particularly effective worn with a really old pair of jeans.

You will need a plain black belt with a brass buckle as soon as you have just a single pair of black shoes in your closet. Broad belts with silver or mat silver buckles may look good with a fashionable suit, but a real gentleman does not wear them.

Below is the counterpart in brown, also with a brass buckle. It will take some years for it to acquire the right patina. Unfortunately the simple basic rule that your belt must match your shoes is still not generally known. Under that rule, brown belts are worn with all shoes that can be classed as brown, including wine red ones.

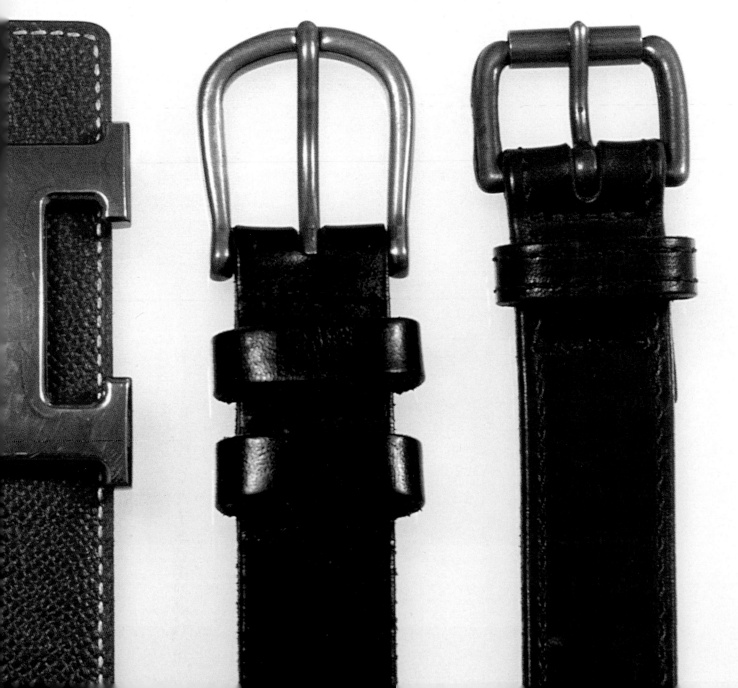

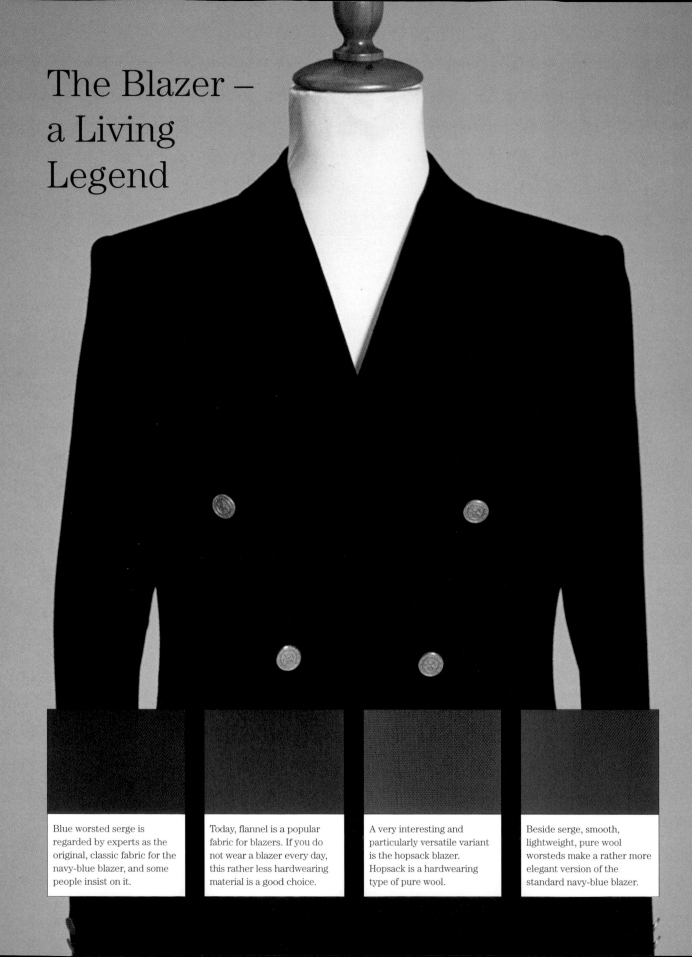

The Blazer – a Living Legend

Blue worsted serge is regarded by experts as the original, classic fabric for the navy-blue blazer, and some people insist on it.

Today, flannel is a popular fabric for blazers. If you do not wear a blazer every day, this rather less hardwearing material is a good choice.

A very interesting and particularly versatile variant is the hopsack blazer. Hopsack is a hardwearing type of pure wool.

Beside serge, smooth, lightweight, pure wool worsteds make a rather more elegant version of the standard navy-blue blazer.

Not all blazers are the same. The double-breasted navy-blue blazer is not of the same origin as the single-breasted blazer, which today is usually dark blue by association with the navy blazer, although it originally derived from the club jacket, and club jackets could be of any color. The navy blazer developed from the short, double-breasted jackets worn by the British navy in the nineteenth century. Its name is supposed to derive from the fact that the captain of the frigate HMS *Blazer* had similar jackets made for his crew to wear for the first time when Queen Victoria visited the ship in 1837. The new creation met with the royal approval, and this type of jacket soon spread to other ships. Today it is difficult to find out just how the blue jacket with gilt buttons made its way into civilian clothing, but maybe men who were not in the navy but liked ships and the sea had jackets made in the same style, as wear for sporting and maritime occasions. Or perhaps naval officers ordered blazers from their tailors as a civilian version of their uniforms, and they were then copied by other customers. Support for this theory comes from the fact that Gieves & Hawkes, traditional outfitters to the navy, are also the top source of navy-blue blazers. The origin of the navy blazer in the navy itself means that today it occupies a position midway between a sports jacket and a suit. Its attractive blue, and its bright gold buttons, make it more formal than a check tweed jacket, but by comparison to a dark gray suit there is something slightly stagy about it, suggesting some kind of Ruritanian uniform.

The single-breasted blazer, however, has no military background. It goes back to the club jackets of English rowing clubs in the nineteenth century. Dark blue is not necessarily its only color, although single-breasted blazers in other shades have never been really popular – leaving aside the American liking for blazers in bottle green, magenta, and yellow. The single-breasted blazer usually has three pockets without flaps, although today it is often sold with flap pockets, so that manufacturers of off-the-rack clothing can include it in their standard production line of sports jackets and suits. Since only a minority of men belong to clubs that can properly have their symbols on blazer buttons, most people wear blue

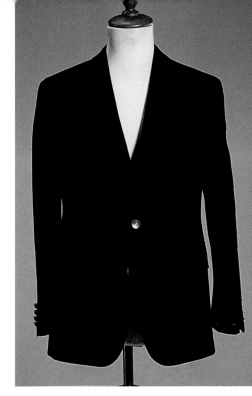

This bottle-green, single-breasted blazer from Brooks Brothers is a popular souvenir of New York. People may look at you curiously in Europe if you wear a jacket like this, but connoisseurs will immediately identify it as a classic from 346 Madison Avenue. Its dark green is a good addition to a classic international wardrobe. You can wear it with a white or pale blue shirt, a striped necktie, and gray flannels; or with beige wool trousers, which can be bought from Brooks Brothers at the same time as the blazer. It also looks very good with chinos and American check shirts. Try one on next time you are in New York and have a chance to visit the famous gentlemen's outfitters.

or enamel buttons on single-breasted blazers. Without gilt buttons, however, it is difficult to distinguish between a blazer and a sports jacket, and in fact the single-breasted blue blazer with blue buttons is simply a blue jacket that looks a little more formal than a sports jacket. Worn with gray flannel trousers or chinos, and brown shoes, this variant on the single-breasted blazer is particularly popular in France, Italy, and Spain, and is almost a uniform among southern Europeans, who wear it for both work and leisure.

The classic navy blazer, on the other hand, still occupies a halfway position. It is too formal for leisure, too much like something worn by a playboy for the office, too conservative for the young – and so it is waiting to come back into fashion, as it did in the middle of the 1980s, when it was worn to the office with a bright red polka dot necktie and white shirt. But the office is not where it really belongs, and anyone who wants to do his blazer and himself justice will wear it on occasions where it really looks good: at informal garden parties, for sporting occasions, on vacation, and on Saturdays and Sundays.

The classic navy-blue blazer is double breasted, and has six bright gilt buttons. It is always dark blue, and it always has two side vents. In addition it has a breast pocket and two pockets with flaps. It is really authentic only when made by English outfitters and tailors.

Blazer and Trousers

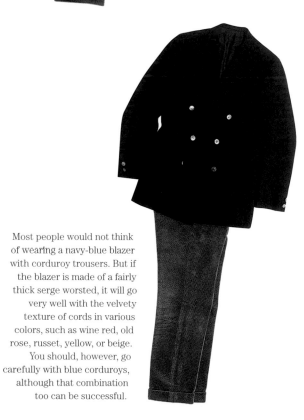

All over the world, pale gray flannels are regarded as ideal with a navy-blue blazer. A necktie should be worn with the outfit. Striped ties are often recommended, but dark-blue neckties with small motifs, ties in single colors, or Hermès ties look good too. However, you should remember that the buttons, which often have elaborate designs, can overpower a necktie with a small pattern, so you could try neckties made of thicker silk, or even knitted ties.

In many places, very dark gray flannels are much more popular today than the pale gray variant, perhaps because a good many men think dark trousers look more formal. In fact, however, the dark gray detracts from the effect of the blue blazer, so that the outfit as a whole can create a rather gloomy, unattractive impression. If you think pale gray flannels look too casual, maybe you would do better just to wear a dark suit.

Most people would not think of wearing a navy-blue blazer with corduroy trousers. But if the blazer is made of a fairly thick serge worsted, it will go very well with the velvety texture of cords in various colors, such as wine red, old rose, russet, yellow, or beige. You should, however, go carefully with blue corduroys, although that combination too can be successful.

A salesman in Cordings of Piccadilly, the old-established London gentlemen's outfitter, once described a navy blazer and cavalry twill trousers as the English uniform. In fact, this combination, although little known, is a real classic. In view of the fact that the navy blazer and cavalry twill trousers are both of military origin, one can see why they look so good together. Traditional cavalry twill trousers are darker and browner than the very pale models worn today. Many men from central and northern Europe think it is incorrect to combine dark blue with shades of brown, but there is nothing wrong with it. On the contrary, dark blue and brown look much better together than dark blue and black.

Navy-blue blazers with jeans are very popular among young people. They are just the outfit for going out in the evening, walking around town, or visiting museums. The combination was considered acceptable for office wear in the 1980s. Today it is seen as an undesirable compromise between formal and casual clothing. The best jeans to wear are Levi's 501s, but in any case they should be straight cut. The jeans with front pleats offered by many gentlemen's outfitters, on the other hand, are a stylistic *faux pas*, cited here only as a warning.

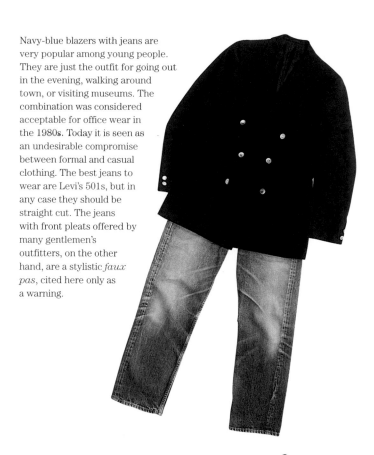

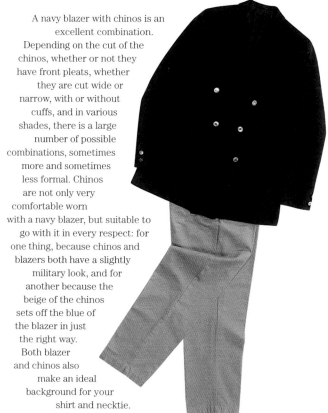

A navy blazer with chinos is an excellent combination. Depending on the cut of the chinos, whether or not they have front pleats, whether they are cut wide or narrow, with or without cuffs, and in various shades, there is a large number of possible combinations, sometimes more and sometimes less formal. Chinos are not only very comfortable worn with a navy blazer, but suitable to go with it in every respect: for one thing, because chinos and blazers both have a slightly military look, and for another because the beige of the chinos sets off the blue of the blazer in just the right way. Both blazer and chinos also make an ideal background for your shirt and necktie.

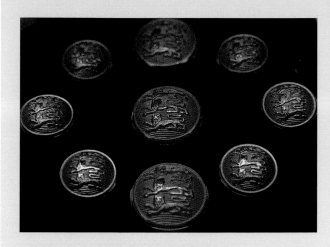

The classic navy-blue blazer has brass or gilt buttons. When you buy a blazer, however, it usually comes with temporary buttons showing the trademark of the tailor or manufacturer. Most gentlemen's outfitters offer a large choice of elaborately ornamented buttons in the naval or military style, or buttons enameled in various colors. There is also a thriving trade in antique gilt buttons from British army stocks, offered for high prices at auction or from specialist dealers. For instance, at an auction in Geneva in 1987, a little packet of ten provost marshal's buttons, three Coldstream Guards buttons, and several items of military insignia went to a buyer for £8,000. However, not everyone is keen on wearing buttons to which they are not really entitled. You can also buy gilt buttons made by manufacturers such as the London Badge & Button Company, a house in Jermyn Street with a long tradition behind it. If you do not like gilt buttons, but would still like to wear a navy blazer – although that is really a contradiction in terms – you should choose flat, blue enamel buttons to make it clear that you really are wearing a blazer, and it is not to be confused with a blue suit jacket. To make absolutely sure that such confusion cannot occur, brass buttons are really essential. Anyone who does not want to wear a jacket with brass buttons perhaps should not even consider wearing a blazer – there are after all, many alternatives.

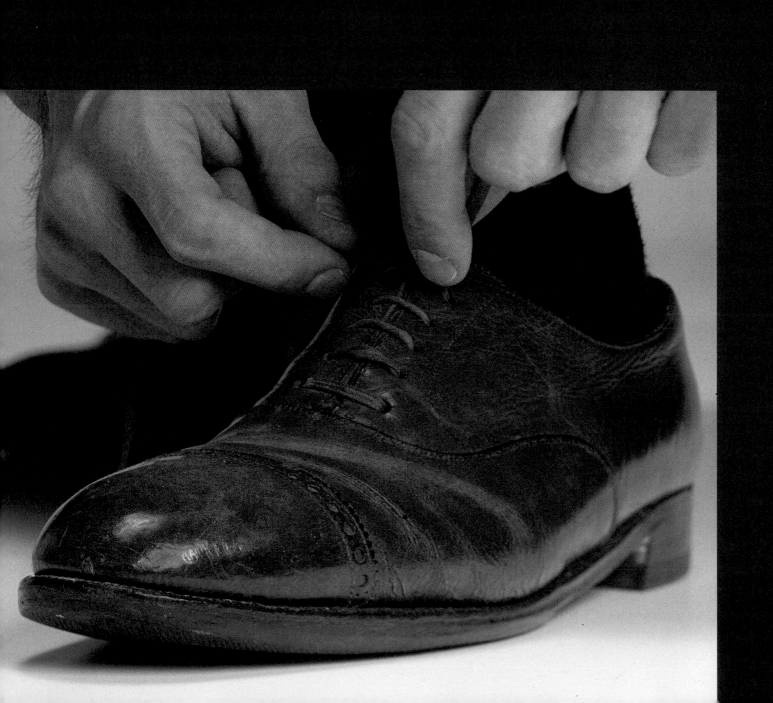

Shoes

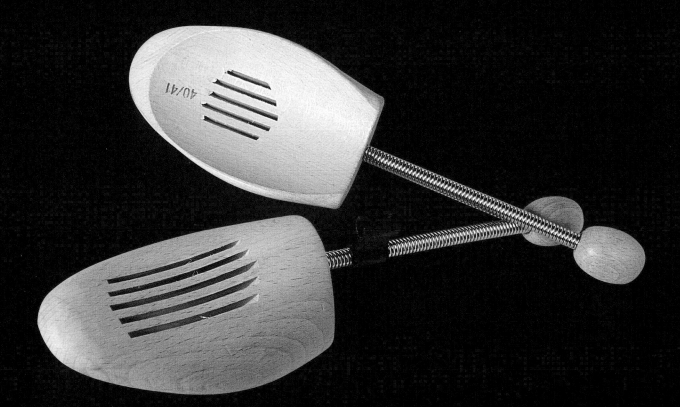

Good shoes

It is often said that a man's shoes are his most important item of clothing. They are. An otherwise perfect appearance is destroyed, irreparably and at a stroke, if a man has an ugly pair of shoes on his feet. It would be better to go through life barefoot or wearing just socks, citing religious reasons or the theft of one's luggage, than to lose face by wearing cheap shoes. Certainly, a good outfit and good shoes should go together – for not even the best shoes can be guaranteed to rescue a questionable wardrobe.

Some may find all this a little extreme, but it is just an exaggerated way of conveying how important shoes are. Anyone who is not in the fortunate position of being able to choose the best for every detail of his apparel should allocate his budget so that a generous chunk of it is earmarked for the purchase of good shoes. If a trainee or student has 600 dollars a year to spend on clothes, for example, he should plan to spend half of it on a pair of shoes. Better still, it should all be invested in shoes: he will need at least two pairs, for shoes ought to have at least a day or two to recover after every time they are worn.

But let's go back to the personal budget. A man who thinks it important to be elegantly or merely well dressed must accept that he will have to dedicate a substantial portion of his income and his leisure time to pursuing this objective. A sense of style will not simply fall into his lap, and vanishingly few of us grow up in an environment in which it is instilled as a matter of course, like everything else. And most of us are not fitted out with the best and most expensive of everything as soon as we learn to walk, so that we embark upon adulthood in possession of a wardrobe full of custom-made suits, custom-made shirts, the best neckties, and – above all – shoes. So anybody who is about to make a series of purchases, but who lacks unlimited resources, should make a plan – putting shoes at the top of the list. On very many occasions a man with a decent pair of shoes on his feet will find that his jeans and second-class shirts and sweaters will be benevolently overlooked. Suits, sports jackets, ties, and overcoats can be bought later. All that matters until then is to have a few pairs of well-broken-in, patinated shoes. But the lack of money is not usually the reason for the lamentable state of the footwear worn by a large number of our fellow men. Its main cause is the lack of a sense of style, combined with priorities which assign a high status to absolutely everything *but*

the most obvious items. For what could be more obvious than good shoes, that we have on our feet for half our lives and that give us such pleasure through the years? This naturally raises the question of what good shoes are, how it is possible to recognize them and where they can be bought.

Shoes are always good if they are made carefully, and to a large extent by hand, from the best leather. These criteria apply to all shoes – to moccasins just as much as to the welted models that cannot be beaten for soundness, comfort, keeping their shape and longevity. We shall consider later how good shoes are made, but first we should clarify the question of how a really good pair of shoes stands out from the rest, what particular characteristics make them what they are. It is by no means easy to distinguish a "fake" from a genuinely high-quality shoe at first sight, unless years of practice have given the purchaser an eye for this. And even then it is difficult to tell what the leather will look like in a year, in five years, in ten; or how things stand with the interior of the shoe; or by what process it was made. We must thus initially make do with two criteria: price and make.

Let us begin with the price. A good pair of welted calfskin shoes, made in a factory but nonetheless by craftsmen, costs about 360 dollars. Some makes come in somewhat lower, but buying them will always mean accepting minor compromises as regards the quality of the leather. The quality of shoes costing much more, conversely, will not be substantially higher – except possibly that they will be made from special types of leather. So this is a guide: the quality of a pair of frame-sewn shoes costing less than 240 dollars can at best be acceptable – never high. Where leather-lined moccasins with leather soles are concerned the price boundary is at about 200 dollars, since they are less costly to produce and use rather less material. Even so, good moccasins can easily be offered at 350 dollars – though here, too, the increase in quality is not necessarily proportional to the increase in price. Anybody unable or unwilling to spend that sort of money is recommended

Only when the pants of a custom-made suit fall onto a good pair of shoes can we speak of a perfect outfit.

to patronize end-of-season sales, where prices are reduced by anything up to 50 percent. But even here he should stick to shoes of a good pedigree.

That brings us to the second important criterion: the make. Contrary to popular opinion, a good make really is a guarantee of high quality. A customer will buy a poor make of shoes only once. The good makes have all been on the market for at least 20 years – and some of them for more than a hundred.

Before the potential purchaser starts looking round for shoes he should commit a few names to memory. For welted shoes the following makers are appropriate: Church's, Allen-Edmonds, Alden, Tricker's, Foster & Son, Edward Green, John Lobb Paris, Ludwig Reiter, Crockett & Jones, Cheaney, Lotusse. There are of course many more firms that make very good shoes, but these are the makes that can be found without difficulty in most of the world's major cities. The order in which they are given is not arbitrary, but represents a sort of rating. Crockett & Jones marks the start of the upper middle rank.

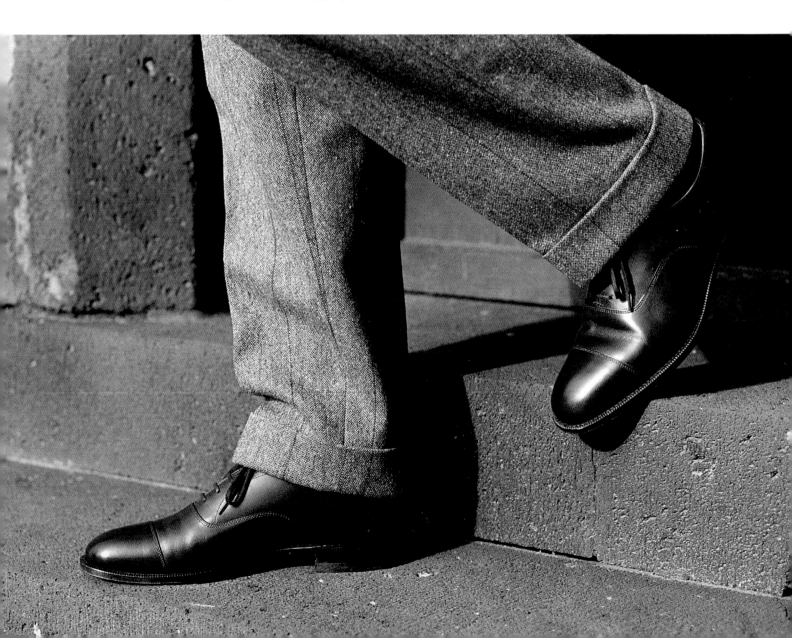

Where moccasins are concerned we must distinguish between American and Italian makes. American moccasins are really practical everyday shoes with no pretensions to elegance. Look out for these makes: Allen-Edmonds, Bass, Sebago, Timberland, and Florsheim. There are of course other makes in America, but they are not generally exported. Italian names worthy of attention are Gucci, Moreschi, Gravati, Fratelli Rosetti, and J. P. Tod's.

The man who comes across a make of which nobody has ever heard, and which is even unfamiliar to those of his friends who know about shoes, in a good shoe-shop, is entitled to be suspicious. There is a large number of small regional makes on the market that can be very good, such as J. B. Weston in France, Wildsmith in England, and Eduard Meier in Germany – but there is also a danger of ending up with a no-name product. It would be better to invest in a well-known make unless what is available is definitely a special offer, or you are absolutely certain you have been given an insider tip. In that case you can confidently stock up with three pairs, for nobody ever has enough shoes – and unworn shoes, if properly stored, will keep virtually for ever. Breaking down the makes by country of origin produces the following lists: USA (Allen-Edmonds, Alden, Bass, Sebago, Timberland, Florsheim), England (Church's, Tricker's, Foster & Son, Edward Green, Crockett & Jones, Cheaney), Italy (Gucci, Moreschi, Gravati, Fratelli Rosetti, J. P. Tod's), France (John Lobb Paris), Spain (Lotusse), Austria (Ludwig Reiter). This brief summary shows which countries attach importance to good footwear. Germany, interestingly, is not among

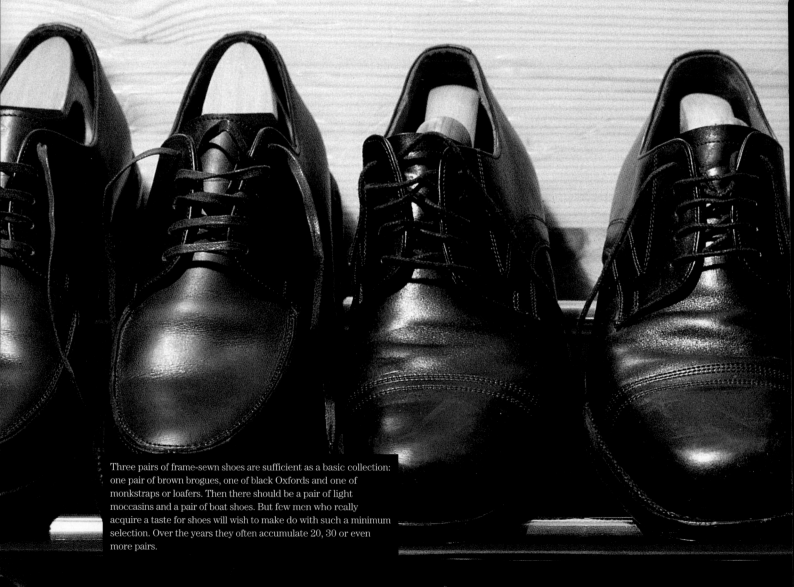

Three pairs of frame-sewn shoes are sufficient as a basic collection: one pair of brown brogues, one of black Oxfords and one of monkstraps or loafers. Then there should be a pair of light moccasins and a pair of boat shoes. But few men who really acquire a taste for shoes will wish to make do with such a minimum selection. Over the years they often accumulate 20, 30 or even more pairs.

them – and indeed, the leading German shoemakers stopped producing welted shoes in the 1970s. A glance at the footwear commonly worn by German men gives rise to the suspicion that they do not think it necessary to invest in good shoes: colossal expenditure on cars and houses seem to have priority. America, England, and Italy, in contrast, are major shoe nations – where wonderful shoes are not only made, but also worn with enthusiasm. Good shoes are highly valued in France, Belgium, and Spain. Hungary is once again on an upswing, for example with the ready-to-wear but hand-made shoes of László Vass. The far from inconsiderable prices and the long list of eminent names will be almost enough to put many a man off the idea of buying shoes at all. But the recommended antidote for anybody who feels this way is to visit a good shoe-shop. Take a pair of

Church's or Alden shoes in your hands and examine them really closely, and you will see the care and craftsmanship that goes into every detail. Often the owner of the shop, or even the salesman, will himself be wearing Church's, Alden or some other make of comparable quality – and with a bit of luck they will be old, but well cared-for and patinated, enabling you to see that it is in every respect well worth spending money on good shoes.

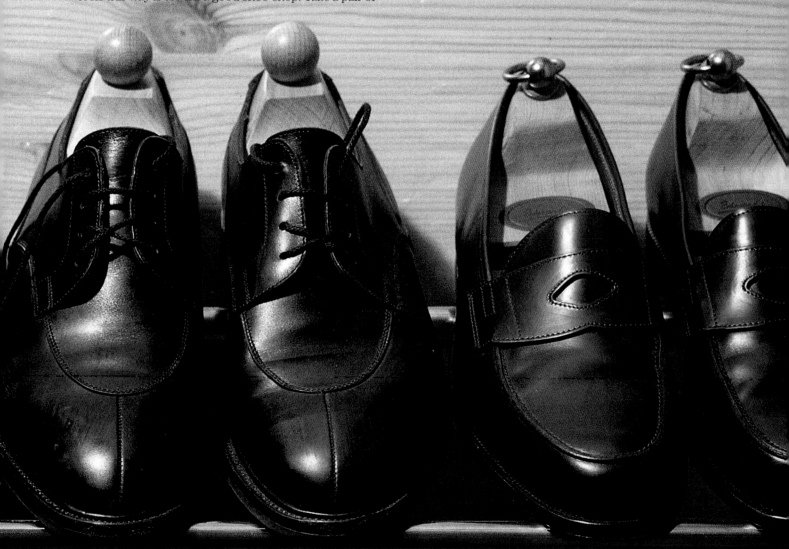

John Lobb

John Lobb is always the first name to be mentioned when the subject of custom-made shoes comes up. It would be wrong to consider him to be the only, or even the best, representative of this now rare craft. *Confrères* of this "shoemaker of kings and king of shoemakers," who also do excellent work, can be found elsewhere – both in London and in a few other cities around the world. But today most of the old names are kept alive by family members, descendants or former employees. You will not come across old John Lobb in London's St. James's Street – but nor, after all, will you meet a Signor Gatto in Rome. This is no more of a drawback than the fact that the great tailors of this world are now being run by the second, third or even fourth generation. Here, too, the art of the founders has been fostered and continued for generations. Unnoticed by the public at large, which must content itself with ready-made shoes and is only too happy to do so, there are still purchasers who insist on clothing and footwear being made specially for them. The extent to which custom-made shoes are a necessity is debatable, of course, but it makes no more sense to argue about it than to discuss the point of any custom-made clothing. For the purchaser to whom money means nothing but quality means everything, custom-made clothing almost always goes without saying, particularly where footwear is concerned. After all, it is the very foundation of our presence – literally as well as figuratively. The feet are subjected to a lifetime of strain, and it is the aim of the custom shoemaker to afford them maximum comfort and orthopedic support. Advocates of good ready-made shoes object that custom-made shoes are even harder to fit than a custom-made suit. The feet, they say, change so much – in the course of a single day, not just over the years – that a perfect fit is not really attainable, and shoes of average quality are generally sufficient as long as they are available in various widths. The advocate of custom-made shoes could certainly effectively refute this argument, but the factors above all others that speak in favor of custom-made shoes are the superior quality and durability resulting from the very expensive manufacturing process that is practiced only by the best custom shoemakers. Not even the best ready-made shoes ever involve the same degree of craftsmanship as custom-made shoes, and they are

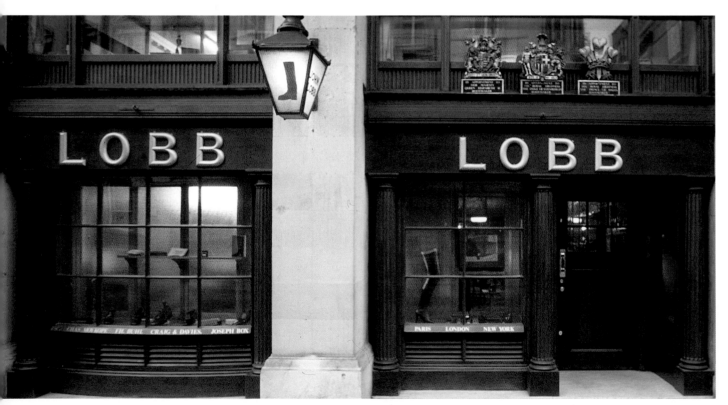

Number 9 St. James's Street in London is the home of the most famous custom shoemaker in the world. The unspectacular façade gives no hint that there is hardly a celebrity in the land who is not among this traditional company's illustrious clientele.

therefore the first choice for anybody to whom perfection of external form, subjective comfort and an objectively unequalled finish are all of prime importance. Unfortunately there has been a sharp decline in the number of really good custom shoemakers. Good ready-made shoemaking, once merely a substitute for and an imitation of custom shoemaking, has virtually supplanted that one true faith in most people's consciousness. Nonetheless there are still a few places left where the old craftsmanship is being maintained and developed.

The criteria for choosing a custom shoemaker should be similar to those governing the choice of a tailor. Ideally you should follow a personal recommendation or form a judgement on the basis of a "house style," which is most clearly expressed in the ready-made shoes often available as well as custom-made items. Experiments with the nameless shoemaker round the corner may culminate in success – or alternatively in utter disappointment. In the classic menswear cities of London, Paris, Rome, Milan, Vienna, Budapest, and New York, certainly, it is often worth seeking out the small one-man business that may perhaps be able to provide exactly what you have always been looking for. Anybody afraid to take this risk should put his faith in well-known names.

The manufacture of custom-made shoes always begins with the last, the equivalent of the patterns that the tailor draws out on paper. A preliminary trial shoe is then built around this last. This is equivalent to the suit that the tailor temporarily bastes together for the first fitting, and like that suit it is taken apart after a certain period of wear so that corrections can be made to the last on the basis of the impressions left in the shoe by the shape of the foot. Only then is the actual shoe made, by hand. Weeks or months pass before the first pair of shoes is ready. Subsequent orders can be placed by telephone, though there are custom shoemakers who advise that the last should be regularly adjusted to reflect how the feet change. Anybody who has acquired the taste for custom-made shoes will no longer be able to muster much enthusiasm for most ready-made shoes. But this is a fate that he is happy to accept.

John Lobb, incidentally, is the only shoemaker whose shoes are built without a fitting. Everybody knows that this works. Nobody knows how. It is one of the great mysteries of custom shoe making, and seems to have little bearing on customer satisfaction – at least, so it seems, as John Lobb is still in business.

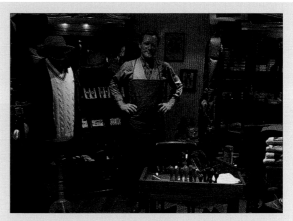

Benjamin Klemann learned his trade from Harai, the Hungarian shoemaker in Neumünster, Germany, and then worked for John Lobb and Foster & Son in London. His shoes can therefore be given a Hungarian or a London accent, as the customer chooses.

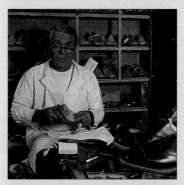

Gatto in Rome is one of the few remaining high-class Italian custom shoemakers. Here the discriminating customer can still find perfection in both finish and fit.

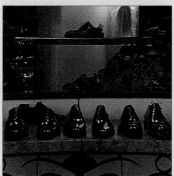

Berluti makes shoes of the classic London school, seasoned with Parisian elegance and Italian lightness. Berluti also makes exactly the right shoes to go with a Charvet shirt and a Cifonelli suit.

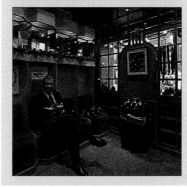

László Vass makes custom-made shoes squarely in the great Hungarian tradition; for the first time in many years the shoemakers of Vienna once more face competition from the east.

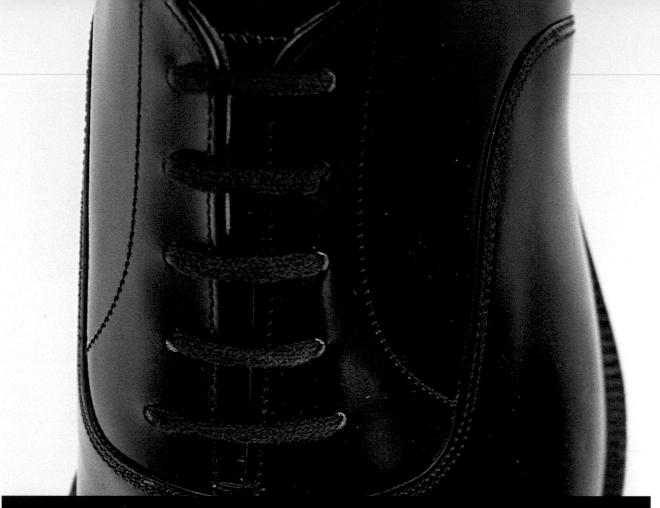

Formal shoes with closed lacing

Shoes can be divided very roughly into those with closed lacing and those with open lacing. The shoes on these pages have closed lacing, which means that the two sides of the upper that are drawn together by the laces are sewn under the front part of the shoe, and that they thus close over a tongue consisting of a piece of leather sewn on beneath the lacing. Shoes with closed lacing are basically a little more "formal" than shoes with open lacing: the feet simply look rather more "dressed." In America shoes with closed lacing are also called "Balmorals," or "Bals" for short. The most formal of all shoes of this type, the Oxford, dates back to the eighteenth century. In America they are known as "Balmoral Oxfords." Brogues became popular in the nineteenth century. They have their origins in the traditional footwear of Scotland, the characteristics of

which were initially adopted for ladies' shoes. Later the pattern of perforations was transferred to men's shoes, and hybrid forms between Oxfords and brogues developed. Because of their rural, folkloric origins brogues always make a rather more rustic impression than the urbane Oxfords. Even so, black brogues are quite acceptable in London. The curved toecap is typical of the full brogue, which is why these shoes are known in America as "wingtips." "Long wingtips" or "long wings" are brogues in which the sides of the toecap extend back to the heel, where they meet – a style popular with American makers such as Alden and Allen-Edmonds. The shoes shown here are made by Church's of Northampton, England, one of the most prestigious shoemakers based on what was once the shoe capital of the world.

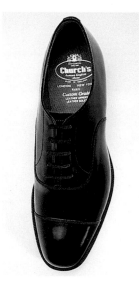 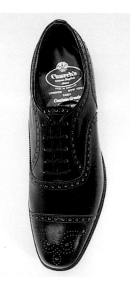 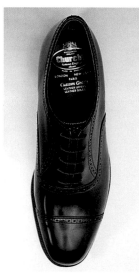 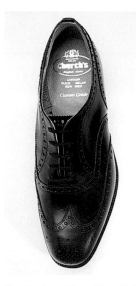

Black Oxfords like the Consul model are the most formal men's shoes. They can be worn in the office with a pinstripe suit, and they also go with a morning coat at formal receptions, weddings, and funerals. Though too formal to be worn with a blazer, in brown they go well with tweed suits and sports jackets.

Stylistically the Legate is exactly midway between Oxfords and brogues. It doesn't make quite such a formal impression as the sleek Oxford, nor is it as rustic as full brogues. A brogue is a shoe in which perforations have been punched. The term "brogue" is derived from "brog," the Gaelic word for shoe. Brogues are often also described as "Budapests" because very good shoes of this type are traditionally made in Hungary.

Here we have a pair of typical half-brogues. The textured surface of the Diplomat, in black, makes it a good match for softer or patterned suiting fabrics like flannel or Prince of Wales check.

The Chetwynd from Church's is the classic full brogue, an essential in every shoe cupboard – an ideal shoe, particularly in brown, for informal wear with tweed or flannel suits and corduroy or moleskin pants.

Their decorated toecaps make the Barcroft a touch less formal, thus rendering it unsuitable for highly ceremonial occasions. Otherwise it is worn like plain, sleek Oxfords.

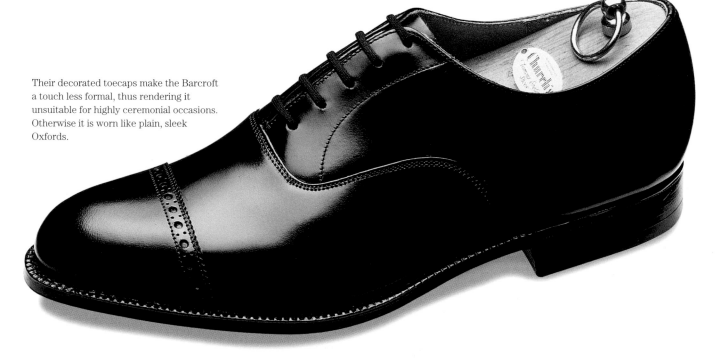

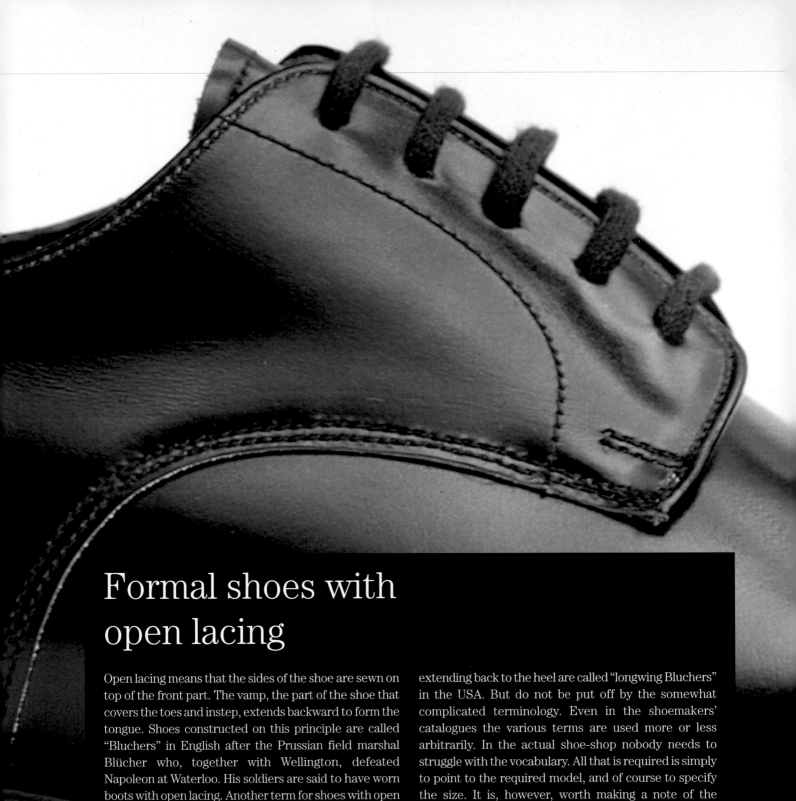

Formal shoes with open lacing

Open lacing means that the sides of the shoe are sewn on top of the front part. The vamp, the part of the shoe that covers the toes and instep, extends backward to form the tongue. Shoes constructed on this principle are called "Bluchers" in English after the Prussian field marshal Blücher who, together with Wellington, defeated Napoleon at Waterloo. His soldiers are said to have worn boots with open lacing. Another term for shoes with open lacing is "Derbys," which is also used in Germany. The term "Bluchers" is more common in America, however. If the vamp lacks decoration the shoes are called "plaintip Bluchers." Shoes with open lacing and toecaps are "toecap Bluchers." Brogues with open lacing and toecaps

extending back to the heel are called "longwing Bluchers" in the USA. But do not be put off by the somewhat complicated terminology. Even in the shoemakers' catalogues the various terms are used more or less arbitrarily. In the actual shoe-shop nobody needs to struggle with the vocabulary. All that is required is simply to point to the required model, and of course to specify the size. It is, however, worth making a note of the different styles for future reference, and to make sure that one has appropriate shoes for any occasion. A selection of styles is essential for any gentleman's wardrobe to ensure that the right shoes are available for formal and less formal wear.

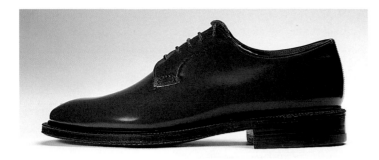

Derbys or Bluchers are suitable for anybody who is not compelled for professional reasons to wear elegant Oxfords. The Shannon in caramel brown is especially popular in southern Europe, where they are worn with flannel pants and navy-blue blazers, but they also go very well with corduroy pants and jeans.

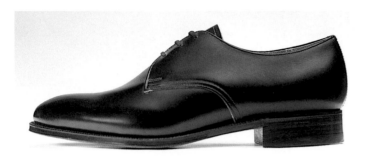

This black Derby is a good alternative to Oxfords, although it is not quite as formal. This is a shoe for those who believe understatement must extend to the feet. In brown this Gerrard is a slimmer version of the Shannon illustrated above, going well with lighter informal suits.

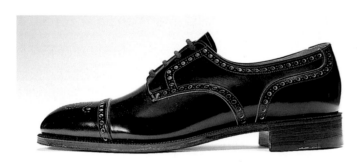

The Cromwell has the brogues' decorative punched perforations, the Oxfords' toecaps and the Derbys' open lacing, a mixture that makes their stylistic classification difficult. It would go best in brown with a check sports jacket and cavalry-twill pants.

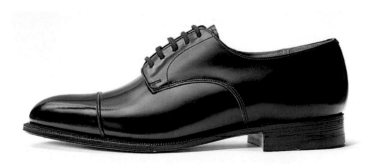

The Burford is normally only available in black. This means that its shape – which is a blend of Derby and Oxford – clearly makes it appropriate with a business suit. The open lacing makes it rather less formal than Oxfords.

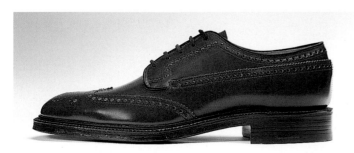

These "wingtip Bluchers," as Americans call them, are a successful mixture of brogues and Derbys. The open lacing goes well with the rustic extended toecaps and thick leather soles. These Graftons, as they are also known, are suitable for anybody who finds normal full brogues too formal and "plaintips" too plain. They are especially popular in Italy in sandalwood.

Loafers

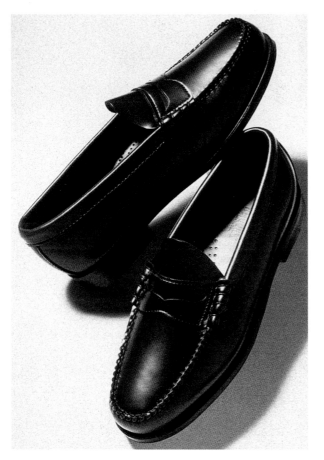

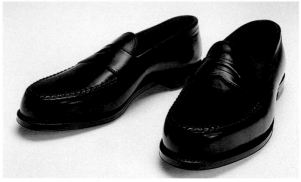

Welted loafers – tassel loafers and penny loafers – are the superior form of moccasins. Technically the term *loafer* no longer applies, except as an echo of these shoes' simple ancestor.

Weejuns from Bass can be regarded as the forerunner of all penny loafers. In black or burgundy, they have remained practically unchanged since their introduction in the 1930s. After a short breaking-in period the unlined uppers mold themselves ideally to the shape of the feet, and then these shoes are also very comfortable when worn without socks. They are called penny loafers because in the 1950s students at the Ivy League universities adopted the practice of putting a penny under the cross-strap for luck. The name "Weejun" is a corruption of "Norwegian," for the shape of these loafers is said to originate from the shoes that Norwegian fishermen used to make during the off-season.

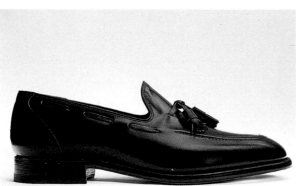

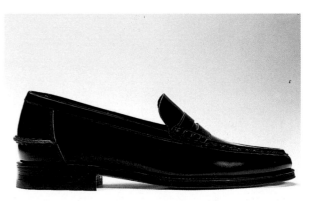

English shoemakers produce tassel loafers: these are cut higher than the American originals, giving them a rather more elegant silhouette. In terms of style tassel loafers are often compared with the navy-blue blazer, because they are just as versatile and just as difficult to classify. But to conclude from this that they can always be worn when it is acceptable to put on a navy-blue blazer would be to forget than in the USA tassel loafers in their classic form are an accepted item of "business wear."

The so-called Beefrolls are among the most popular loafers today, classically produced by American shoemakers Sebago. The name "Beefroll" refers to the thickened seams each side of the instep, reminiscent of beef olives, that are produced by giving the cross-straps a generous edging. Outside America these loafers are most popular in southern Europe, where they are often worn with a dark suit. The shoe illustrated is actually made by Church's, but even so it is a classic Beefroll.

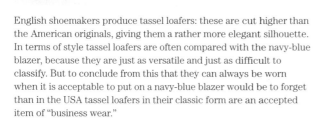

Loafers are shoes that are easy to slip on. This definition, as broad as it is brief, includes both moccasins and the various welt-stitched loafers. Loafers are generally less formal than lace-up shoes. When penny loafers first appeared in America in the 1930s, their effect on adherents of traditional lace-up shoes was genuinely as if the wearer had inadvertently gone out wearing slippers. But despite this, light loafers quickly became extremely popular: they relieve the wearer of the bother of tying and untying laces, and – in the original unlined version, at least – they are also cooler than lace-up shoes. Soon loafers in the original simple form were supplemented by welted versions. Today loafers have long been accepted as classics – but on really formal occasions lace-up shoes are still preferable.

Tassel loafers originate from the same design found today in boat shoes: the laces are passed once round the shoe through eyes or "tunnels" and tied in a bow on the instep. In the original tassel loafers the ends of the laces were decorated with leather pompons. The American company Alden claims that in the 1940s it improved this original design in that since the shoes were a perfect fit they needed no laces, the "tassels" serving only a decorative purpose. So anyone who wants the originals can get them from Alden.

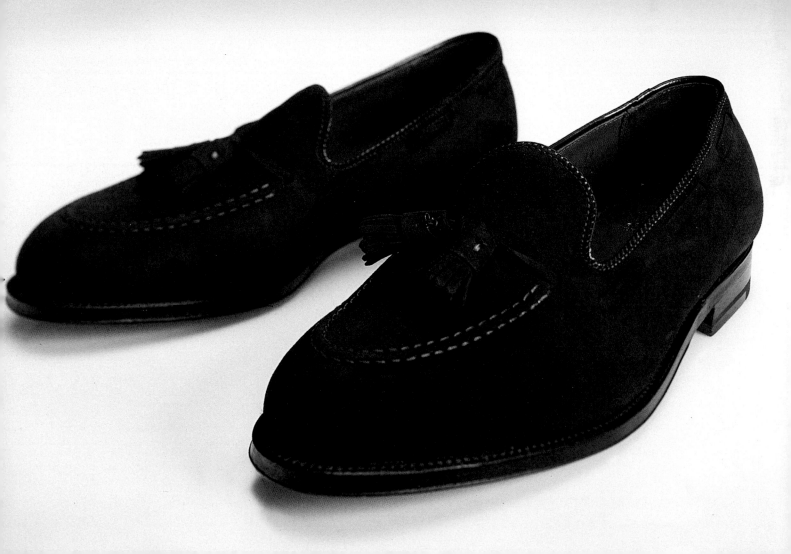

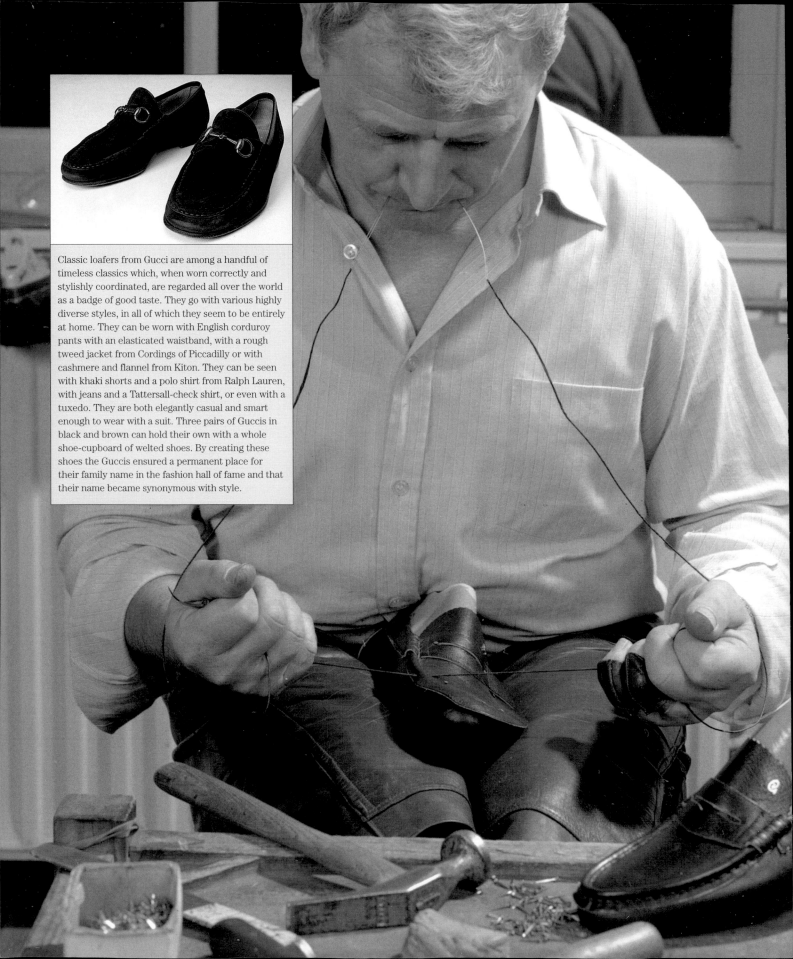

Classic loafers from Gucci are among a handful of timeless classics which, when worn correctly and stylishly coordinated, are regarded all over the world as a badge of good taste. They go with various highly diverse styles, in all of which they seem to be entirely at home. They can be worn with English corduroy pants with an elasticated waistband, with a rough tweed jacket from Cordings of Piccadilly or with cashmere and flannel from Kiton. They can be seen with khaki shorts and a polo shirt from Ralph Lauren, with jeans and a Tattersall-check shirt, or even with a tuxedo. They are both elegantly casual and smart enough to wear with a suit. Three pairs of Guccis in black and brown can hold their own with a whole shoe-cupboard of welted shoes. By creating these shoes the Guccis ensured a permanent place for their family name in the fashion hall of fame and that their name became synonymous with style.

Moccasins Italian Style

Until the First World War it was the English who set basic standards for men's shoes throughout the world, just as men's clothing – apart from slight local variations – conformed with English patterns and guidelines. Even the great Hungarian shoemaking tradition followed English stylistic guidelines.

Only the Americans introduced innovations: loafers, for example, which found their way across the Big Pond into European gentlemen's shoe cupboards. After the Second World War the new American shoe designs inspired the Italians to create an entirely new type of soft, light shoe that was a far better match for the innovative lines of Italian tailoring than the traditional English Oxfords, Derbys or brogues.

For their classic wardrobe men today may thus choose an international style with an English or an Italian accent. And where shoes are concerned this choice is exercised often and with pleasure. Many lovers of English footwear also own a few pairs of Guccis, which look much better with a light summer suit than traditional Oxfords. There are also men who have exclusive faith in the art of Italian shoemakers. They love the supple, glove-soft leather of southern moccasins, and are happy to accept the disadvantages of shoes that do not last as long and in which the feet tire more quickly, as long as they are as light and soft as slippers and make the feet look smaller. In their view the delicate stitching, thin soles, and leather that often feels like silk are the best possible match for the equally fine workmanship of Italian tailoring. What the Italian tailor strives to achieve is lightness and natural elegance – properties that are equally characteristic of the products of Italian shoemakers, whose ready-to-wear and custom-made shoes are both of outstanding quality. For a very long time Gucci loafers were the first choice. At present, however, these classic shoes are barely surviving in the Gucci footwear collections. The times when they were available in tomato-red or medium-blue suede would now appear to be long gone; this renowned Italian fashion house is now dominated by black, gray, and brown. But fashion is a fickle creature, and it is just possible that one day perhaps she will once more conjure up a pair of orange-red loafers in the Gucci range.

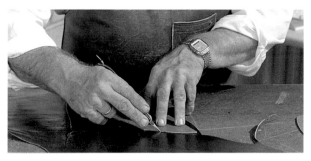

As with welted shoes, the first stage in making moccasins is to cut out the leather upper. In Italy and at Greve in Holland (shown here) this is done by hand.

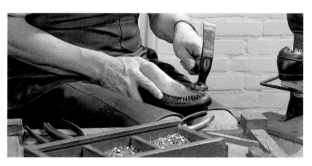

In the second stage the upper is stitched together and stretched from below over the last, and hence over the inner sole, and temporarily attached to the last. This picture shows the shoemaker at the Dutch manufacturer driving tiny nails through the upper into the last. In the next stage the upper is closed by sewing on the missing top. The nails can then be removed, as the upper now firmly encloses the last.

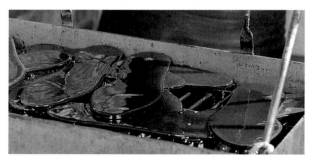

Moccasin soles are sewn on, the stitches passing through the inner sole and middle sole. The outer sole is then glued on, however; preparations for this are shown here. If a hole is worn in this sole the adhesive prevents it from being removed, and it has to be sanded off so that a replacement sole can be fitted.

Monkstraps – the Shoes with Buckles

Monkstrap shoes are so called because their buckle fastenings recall those on monks' sandals. This feature, which is actually very practical, has made shoes of this type just as many friends as enemies. Devotees like them for their firm fit and convenient buckles, which unlike laces never break at inopportune moments – while detractors find them affected and unnecessary. Every man must decide for himself whether or not he likes this half-way house between formal lace-up shoes and casual loafers. Objectively there is nothing to be said against monkstraps, if one or two minor drawbacks are overlooked. It is possible, for example, that they may affect the fall of the pants-legs, the hems of which may get caught in the buckles or rest on the protruding tongues. This is why shoes with buckles only really look right when worn with slim-cut pants-legs that are both narrow at the ankles and so short that they only just touch the shoes, if at all. This shows off the elegant features of the long vamp and the brass buckle to

Either you like these shoes or you don't. Their devotees are generally particularly fond of the Westbury, which is among the classics made by Church's.

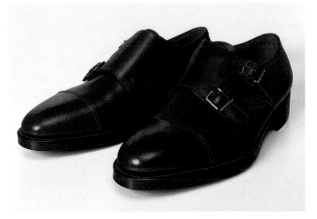

Those who can't get enough of the buckle go for shoes that have two of them. This style is especially sought-after by the French, above all because the double buckle spreads the pressure on the instep better and therefore offers much more comfort.

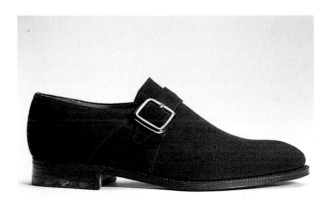

Most men prefer black buckled shoes. They are often seen in France, worn with dark gray pants and a blazer. Suede buckled shoes, like the suede Westbury from Church's, are only for advanced fans of this shoe design.

their best advantage, and you finally realize what these shoes actually remind you of: not of the shoes seen beneath a monk's habit, but of those worn by the Three Musketeers, which were also embellished by large and highly polished buckles. For better or worse, anybody who is not won over by this association must stick to lace-ups and loafers. The monkstrap type of shoe is popular in certain countries of Europe, particularly in France and Germany, but shoemakers in England produce some of the best examples.

The Other Word for Weatherproof

Welt-stitched shoes do suffer from one design fault: they are not waterproof. This is not generally a problem, as most welt-stitched shoes are worn in the city rather than for taking long country walks in the pouring rain. Such activities require shoes constructed by the Veldtschoen method. The name comes from the Afrikaans; "veldtschoe," or more accurately "veldtskoen," means field shoe, which conveys what these shoes are intended for: working in the fields, or – in the transferred sense – country wear. In the Veldtschoen method the upper is turned out and stitched together with the inner sole and the welt. To provide additional protection against the wet a synthetic or extra-thick leather sole is then stuck or stitched to the welt. Since the upper is turned out the rain runs off, and there is no way for it to penetrate the welt. If the shoe has open lacing the upper is also fastened to the quarters with a bellows tongue to prevent water from getting in under the lacing. Shoes like this can of course never be as waterproof as rubber boots or galoshes, but even so you can wear them for quite a long walk in the rain without getting your feet wet. Only very few shoemakers still make Veldtschoen shoes: Tricker's, whose Country Collection includes several Veldtschoen models, is an example. Joseph Cheaney & Sons in Desborough, a firm rich in tradition that was founded as long ago as 1866, is another maker of "veldts," as these waterproof shoes are often called. Indeed, the Cheaney Country Collection contains a good dozen different models of Veldtschoen. Unfortunately "veldts" made by Tricker's or Cheaney are virtually unavailable outside England, so if you have a need for footwear that can really cope with wet weather you should be sure to put these shoes on your shopping list next time you visit the United Kingdom. It is unsurprising that this country has made the production of such shoes a speciality, considering its climate, which seems to produce a great deal of wet weather. There are many occasions when an English country gentleman needs to be outside in inclement weather, and he will always require suitable shoes.

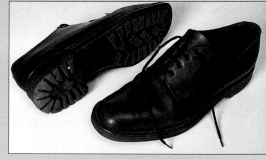

To make them entirely waterproof "veldts" are usually fitted with a treaded sole made of Vibram, which is flexibly stitched onto the leather sole.

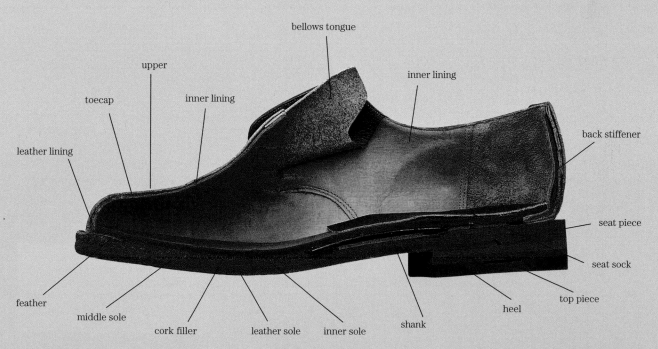

bellows tongue

upper

toecap

inner lining

leather lining

inner lining

back stiffener

seat piece

seat sock

top piece

feather

heel

middle sole

cork filler

leather sole

inner sole

shank

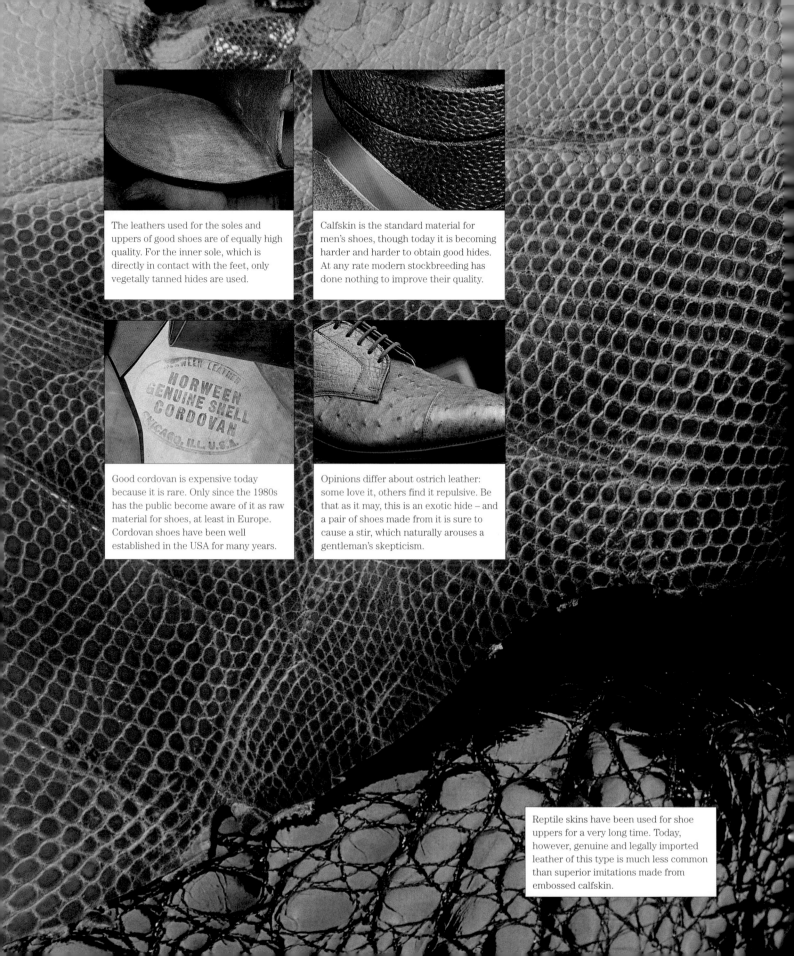

The leathers used for the soles and uppers of good shoes are of equally high quality. For the inner sole, which is directly in contact with the feet, only vegetally tanned hides are used.

Calfskin is the standard material for men's shoes, though today it is becoming harder and harder to obtain good hides. At any rate modern stockbreeding has done nothing to improve their quality.

Good cordovan is expensive today because it is rare. Only since the 1980s has the public become aware of it as raw material for shoes, at least in Europe. Cordovan shoes have been well established in the USA for many years.

Opinions differ about ostrich leather: some love it, others find it repulsive. Be that as it may, this is an exotic hide – and a pair of shoes made from it is sure to cause a stir, which naturally arouses a gentleman's skepticism.

Reptile skins have been used for shoe uppers for a very long time. Today, however, genuine and legally imported leather of this type is much less common than superior imitations made from embossed calfskin.

Leather Does not always Mean Leather

The term "leather" commonly denotes animal skin that has been rendered durable and supple by the tanning process. If a skin were removed and then allowed to dry without further treatment, it would merely become hard and brittle. This is prevented by removing the hair, epidermis and endodermis and exposing the resulting skin to certain tanning agents. These interlink the tissue fibers, thus making the hide stretchable, elastic and able to breathe. The most common tanning process for the uppers of high-quality men's shoes is chromium tanning using basic chromium salts. Leather for the soles is mostly tanned vegetally by the oldest known tanning process, which is called pit-tanning. It is also rolled or hammered to impart the necessary toughness. The classic leather for men's shoes is calfskin or "boxcalf," after London shoemaker Joseph Box. France traditionally supplies the best hides. Calfskin is used to produce smooth leather, the so-called "scotchgrain," and suede. Suede is obtained by mechanically roughening the reverse side of the leather to produce a more-or-less velvet-like surface. Roughened leather is also sometimes known as velour leather. The English name for this sort of leather is "reversed calf," but it is also often known by the name of "buckskin." A buck is the name for the male of various cloven-hoofed creatures such as deer, chamois, and antelope. Many people may be surprised that leather from these animals is used to make shoes, and that the distinguished-sounding word "chamois" means nothing but the skin of the chamois antelope, while the refined "chevreau" comes from the goat. Today, however, "buck" is often used only as a synonym for suede – and in America it is actually the term for a particular sort of light-colored summer shoe made from plain calfskin. As well as calfskin, welted shoes are also made from horsehide. Horsehide is particularly expensive, because only the skin from the horse's hindquarters is suitable for shoemaking. In order to avoid fakes, horsehide shoes should be purchased only from well-known makers – for example from the Alden Shoe Company or Florsheim, the world's leading makers of cordovan shoes. For Italian moccasins, besides calfskin and various soft buckskins, the skin of wild pigs is used: the so-called peccary leather, which has a characteristic grained texture. As well as the hides of various mammals, lizard and crocodile skin are also used for shoes – though not for any with a claim to be considered especially stylish.

Even the ostrich is called upon to give up its skin for human footwear, and there is no celebrated maker of custom-made shoes who does not include ostrich-leather shoes in its pattern collection. Frankly, however, we could very well do without this leather, for its esthetic value as footwear material is not great; it is too reminiscent, unfortunately, of the highly magnified skin of a plucked chicken.

This world's good makes of shoe are also distinguished by the fact that their products are not only well finished but are also made from superior leather. It is, of course, entirely possible for a manufacturer of ready-made shoes to have better contacts with the tanneries than the little custom shoemaker round the corner. A good, tried-and-tested make is often the best guarantee of good leather, as even an expert is often unable to judge the quality of the raw material by examining the completed shoe. It might be only much later, perhaps after months of wear, that deficiencies in the quality of the leather become apparent. No shoemaker of repute will want to be associated with suppliers of poor-quality leather, which could ruin a business built up over many decades. Of course, mistakes can occur, but one can generally be confident that a well-repected name will ensure a good quality shoe.

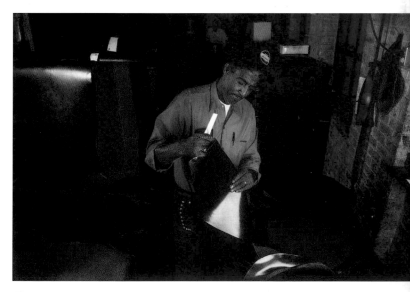

The American Horween tannery is acknowledged as the world's leading supplier of cordovan. All the well-known manufacturers obtain their supplies from this traditional firm.

The Center of the Shoe World

English men's shoes and Northampton are always mentioned in the same breath. And in fact at the end of the 1960s the town was still the home of more than a hundred small family firms making shoes in the traditional way. It was they who created the reputation of the region as the stronghold of the shoemaker's art. By the end of the 1980s barely 20 of them remained, among them Church's, Tricker's, Crockett & Jones, and Cheaney. Beyond the English borders Church's is undoubtedly the best-known of these four makes. This is due on the one hand to the fact that Church's started exporting early, with exclusive Church's boutiques in leading cities such as London, Paris, New York, Brussels, and Hong Kong. The two Church's shops in Brussels, for example, are strategically extremely well-placed, because their customers include not only the Belgians and their neighbors from France, Germany, and the Netherlands but also the personnel of the EU and NATO. On the other hand Church's offers a high standard of quality, a broad range of models with a large number of classics that have figured in the collection for decades, and above all an outstanding repair service which enables a pair of Church's to be sent to England for resoling from the nearest shop that stocks them. There the shoes are thoroughly overhauled in the factory, and three months later your favorite shoes are as good as new. Given the economic pressures of today, the smaller shoemakers simply could not afford the organization required by a service like that.

At first the other suppliers hardly differed from their great competitor in the way they worked. All of them were established between the middle and the end of the nineteenth century, when most shoes used to be made by shoemakers working at home. Only the upper components were cut to shape centrally, and were then sent to the individual specialists who each carried out a particular process in their tiny domestic workshops. Thus the shoes kept moving from one workshop to

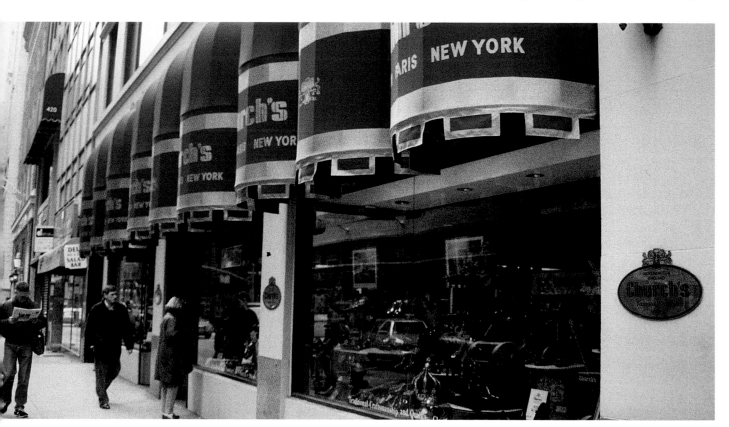

Church's shop on New York's Madison Avenue was opened as long ago as 1930. Initially the salesmen wore black jackets and pinstripe pants, which New Yorkers found sensational.

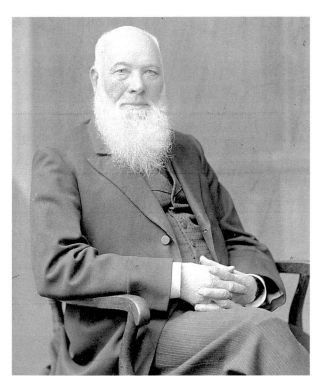

Thomas Church, born in 1826, was the father of Alfred, William, and Thomas Church, the founders of the company. In 1873, together with their father, the brothers opened the factory. Today, however, it no longer belongs to the family.

another, being gradually built up by various craftsmen as they went. Growing success meant that the shoe manufacturers could afford their own production facilities, where every process was carried out under one roof. Charles Goodyear's invention in 1872 of a special sewing machine, which made the difficult and exhausting job of stitching together the upper and the welt both easier and faster, made his name immortal. Church's installed this machine, and others, in its new building in Duke Street, Northampton, in 1873.

Church's new idea was to print the firm's stamp on the product. Around 1900 it had not occurred to most makers to market their shoes under a label of their own. They produced for men's outfitters and tailors, who sold the shoes under their own name. This practice is still common today. Edward Green, for example, sometimes used to make shoes for John Lobb Paris, and Crockett & Jones make welted shoes for Ralph Lauren and for Hackett, the English outfitters. But starting in 1921 Church's opened its own shops, first in London and then, in 1930, on Madison Avenue in New York. America remained the most important export destination for many years. Today it is Europe, and Church's shoes can be found in every major European city. For a make like Tricker's, which is no less traditional, it is hard to catch up with a competitor who has established such a lead in terms of distribution and renown. But for Tricker's and other smaller makers it is probably sufficient that they enjoy a more exclusive reputation than Church's at home: as a supplier to the royal household, for example, Tricker's is entitled to use the coat of arms of the Prince of Wales. Even if Church's has not yet been granted this mark of distinction (though there are apparently members of the royal family who wear Church's shoes), and even if there are shoes that are thought to be even more English, and perhaps better, for most people who know anything about shoes Church's is a byword for English ready to wear footwear.

Despite the contraction of the industry in the last thirty years, Northampton and other towns in the county retain a prominent position in the world of shoemaking. As long as Church's, Tricker's, Joseph Cheaney & Sons, and other firms continue to make shoes, Northampton will remain a byword for high-quality English shoes.

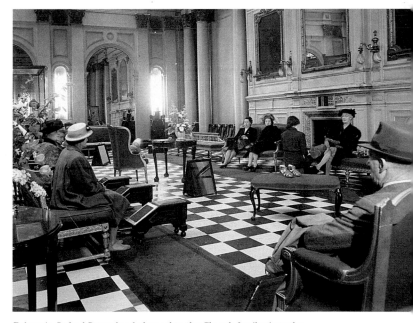

Babers in Oxford Street has belonged to the Church family since the 1920s. This particular store sells more Church's shoes than any other shoe-shop in the world.

The Shoemaker's Tools

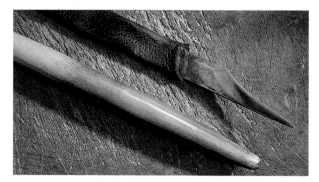

With this sharp knife the "clicker," or leather cutter, cuts out the individual components of the upper. The "clicker's" role in shoemaking is just as important as that of the cutter in tailoring: he has the responsible task of cutting up the valuable raw material. A single error here can cost the craftsman dear, particularly in the manufacture of a one-off pair.

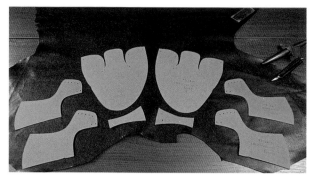

Each shoe model has patterns for each size and fit, so the number of patterns kept by a large shoemaking company is enormous. The "clicker" cuts round the patterns to produce the individual components of the upper. Custom shoemakers make individual patterns for each customer, just like the paper patterns of the custom tailor.

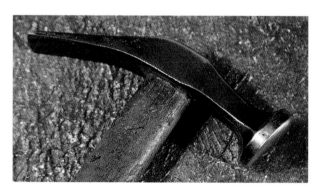

The "laster" is the shoemaker who stretches the leather over the wooden last and temporarily nails it in place. Later, when the upper has been firmly stitched to the welt, the nails are taken out again. The hammer is often magnetized to facilitate handling the many small nails.

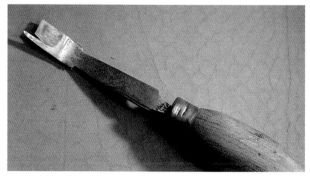

The "gouger," a sort of chisel, used to be used to cut a channel in the sole leather to accommodate the sole seam. Today this is done by machine, which replicates the manual process and thus helps to speed up production.

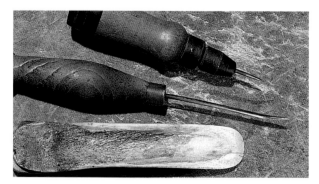

Thick leather cannot be stitched unless holes are made in it first, for which the shoemaker uses an awl. This tool is still used today for decorative embroidery on the uppers.

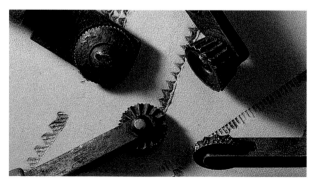

"Serrated stitch wheels" can be used to emboss decorative designs in the leather, for example to embellish the outer sole. In large shoemaking firms this is now done using machines.

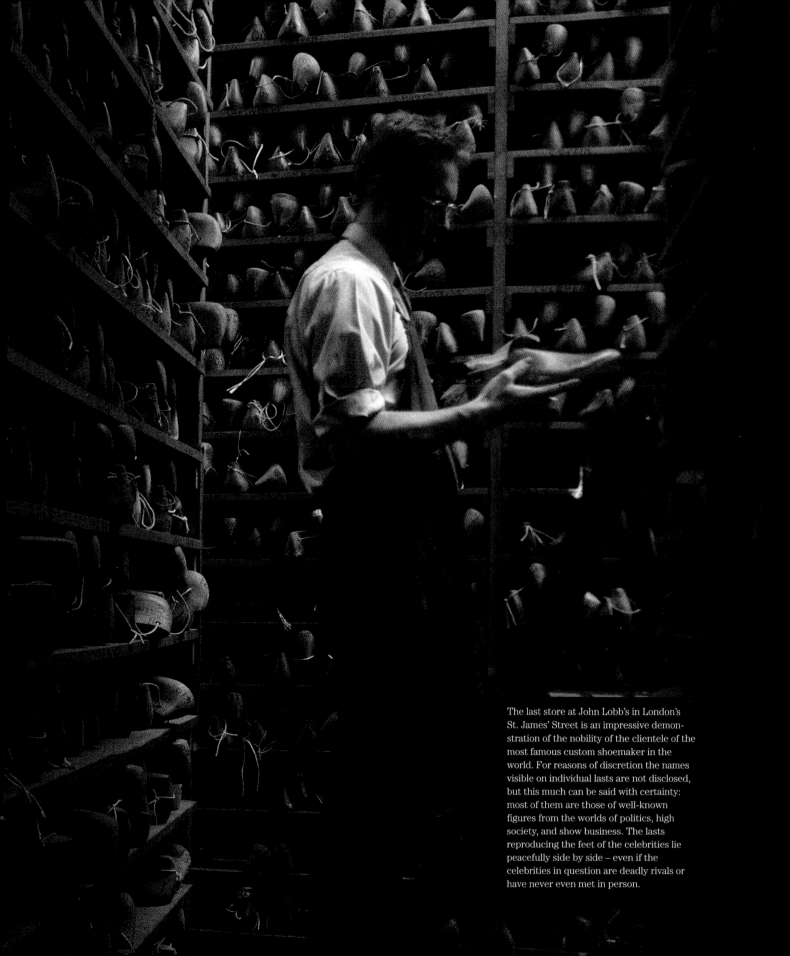

The last store at John Lobb's in London's
St. James' Street is an impressive demonstration of the nobility of the clientele of the
most famous custom shoemaker in the
world. For reasons of discretion the names
visible on individual lasts are not disclosed,
but this much can be said with certainty:
most of them are those of well-known
figures from the worlds of politics, high
society, and show business. The lasts
reproducing the feet of the celebrities lie
peacefully side by side – even if the
celebrities in question are deadly rivals or
have never even met in person.

How a Shoe Takes Shape

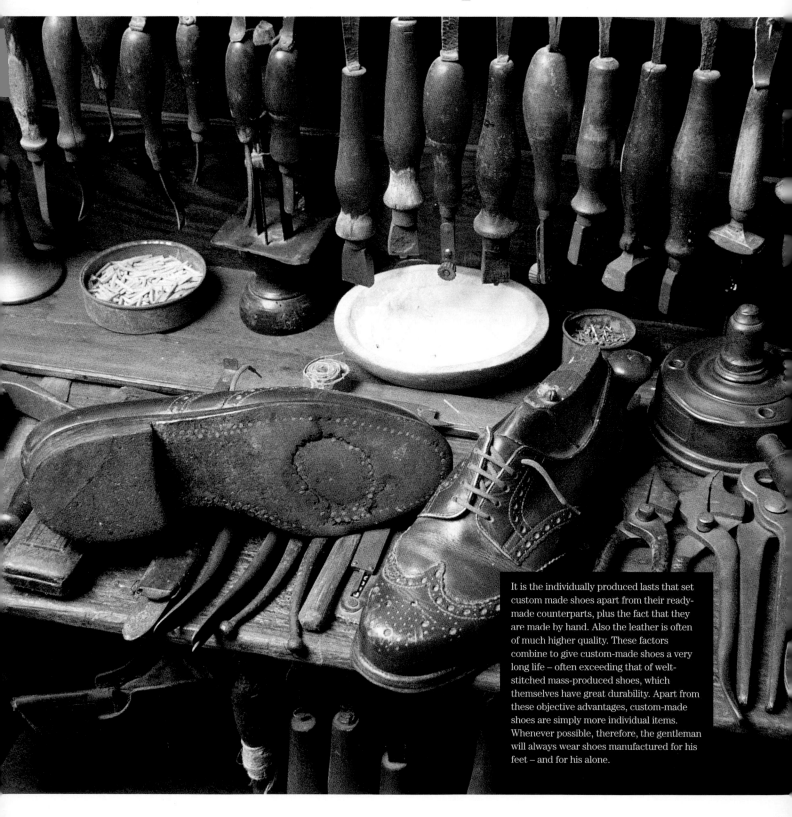

It is the individually produced lasts that set custom made shoes apart from their ready-made counterparts, plus the fact that they are made by hand. Also the leather is often of much higher quality. These factors combine to give custom-made shoes a very long life – often exceeding that of welt-stitched mass-produced shoes, which themselves have great durability. Apart from these objective advantages, custom-made shoes are simply more individual items. Whenever possible, therefore, the gentleman will always wear shoes manufactured for his feet – and for his alone.

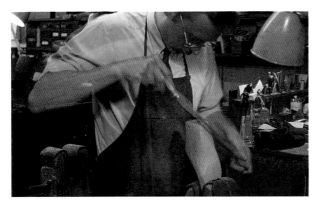

The last on which a ready-made shoe is produced can satisfy only average values – though admittedly with very adequate results. At Church's, for example, there are up to six widths per model. Most men will find one of them entirely satisfactory.

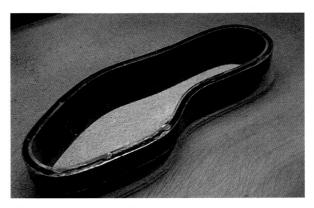

The inner soles of industrially manufactured shoes are stamped out to the correct size by a machine in order to minimize wastage. Custom shoemakers cut the soles individually to size.

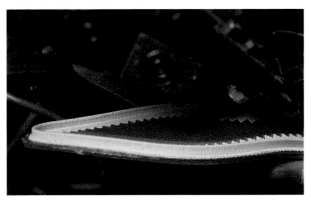

Once the inner sole has been secured to the last a narrow strip of leather is stuck on. This is the feather, to which the welt and the upper are later stitched. This gives welt-stitched shoes their stability and flexibility.

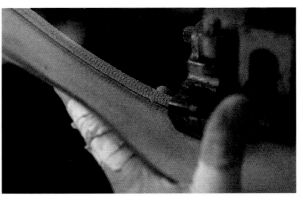

The feather can also be cut out of the inner sole. This is what custom shoemakers do, though they generally work without a machine, carving the feather out of the inner sole.

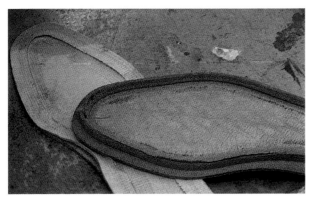

Two inner soles, one with a cut feather, the other with a raised feather. At Church's they can fall back on this alternative to sticking the feather on with adhesive.

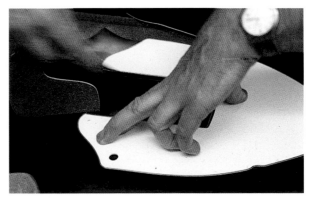

While the inner sole and the feather are being prepared, the "clickers" cut the components of the upper to size. For this they use patterns of the individual pieces.

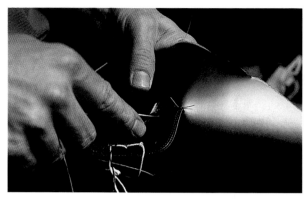

The "closers" stitch the components of the uppers together, execute decorative and backstitched seams – partly by hand – and fasten the upper to the lining, which in good shoes is made of goatskin or linen.

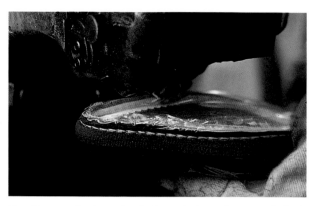

Once the upper has been stretched over the last and temporarily fixed to it, it is stitched together with the feather and the welt. This is the most important stage in the production of welt-stitched shoes, as this one seam holds the upper, feather, and welt firmly together.

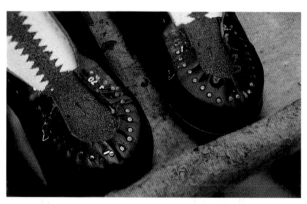

The seam that holds the upper, feather, and welt together does not extend to the seat. Under the seat the sole is therefore not stitched onto the welt, but nailed to the heel through the inner sole from the inside of the shoe.

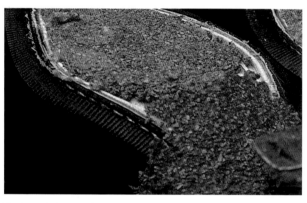

As the welt forms a frame round the inner sole, the resulting gap must be filled before the outer sole is fitted. This is done with mastic, a mixture of cork and resin, that will later mold itself to the exact shape of the foot.

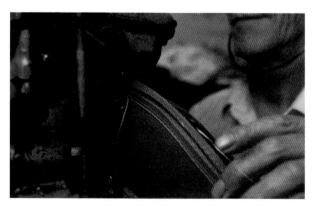

The outer sole is stitched to the welt by machine. Although it is this seam, which is visible under the outer sole, that holds the sole and the welt together, there is no danger that the sole will fall off when the seam is abraded.

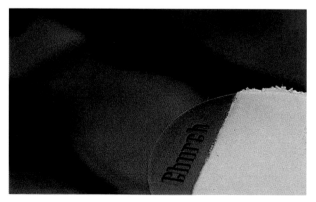

Depending on height, the heel of a welt-stitched shoe consists of four or five "lifts," pieces of leather placed on top of one another. A rubber lift is inserted between the last and next-to-last leather lifts, as this is the point of maximum wear.

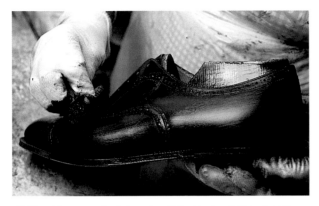

At Church's every pair of shoes is polished by hand. This gives the leather a distinguished patina that would otherwise take years to acquire. The alternative to this is the high-gloss bookbinder finish.

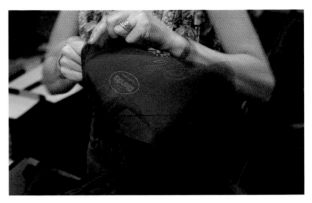

Church's shoes are supplied in cloth bags that come in useful when traveling. The bag contains maintenance instructions with a number of valuable hints – the most important of which is to give a pair of shoes a day to recover after each wearing.

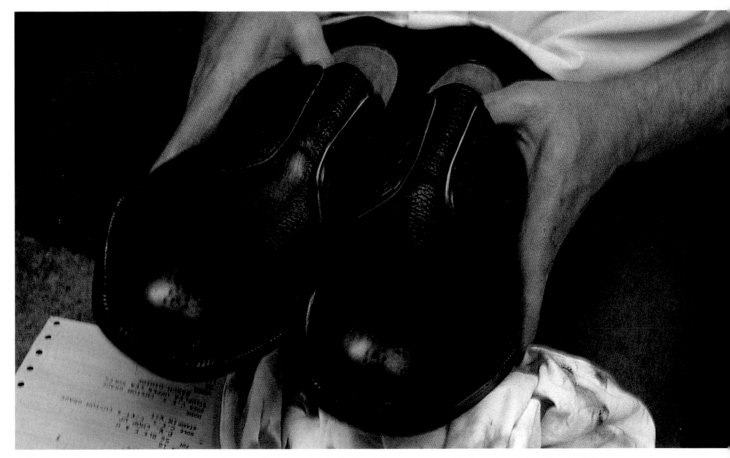

A final inspection makes sure that the shoes really are entirely free of defects. If not, they are returned to the relevant department – if the fault can be rectified, that is. Large, old firms like Church's are ultra-critical on this point, which is why they enjoy such a high reputation. Shoes with minor cosmetic shortcomings are sorted out and sold as seconds. Church's shoes with only the most minimal imperfections can be bought at extraordinarily low prices in end-of-season sales at Babers in London's Oxford Street.

The Other Word for Cordovan

When people speak of cordovan shoes today, they usually mean those made by American shoemakers Alden. In America they have long been a classic; the firm has been in existence since 1884. The term is somewhat misleading, for originally "cordovan" only meant that the leather came from the Spanish town of Cordoba – which used to produce extremely fine leather in various colors from buck and goat hides to be used for making shoes or binding books. We can no longer be sure how the term changed its meaning. Today "cordovan" means horsehide, that is to say the skin from the horse's hindquarters, which provides exactly two round pieces of leather sufficient to make two or three pairs of shoes. Tanning horse hides has become the exclusive preserve of the Americans, or rather of the American Horween tannery, where the hides are processed by a time-consuming and expensive method. Altogether it takes about five months to produce a piece of leather, mainly because of the protracted vegetal tanning process. Cordovan immediately calls to mind the distinctive red-

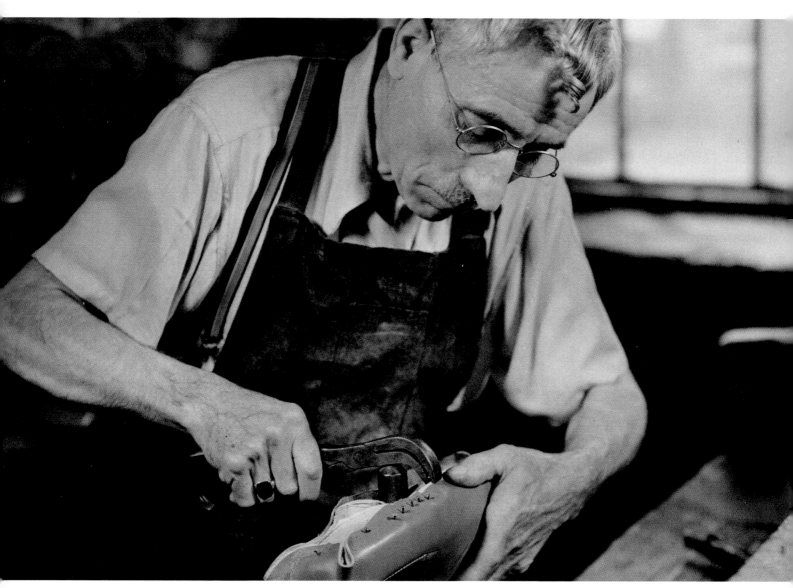

The times when the upper used to be stretched over the last by hand at Alden are long past. Today this process is carried out using a machine, but this has no effect on quality.

brown color that is typical of Alden shoes, but it can also be black or undyed. Regardless of the color, cordovan shoes are characterized by an exceptional gleam – which the use of shoe-care preparations will only destroy. Enough fat is infused into the leather during the tanning process, so that it later merely needs to be buffed up: no polish should be applied. Despite needing little care, cordovan shoes – provided they are properly treated – last an extraordinarily long time. They differ from calfskin shoes in two important respects: because of the elasticity and suppleness of horsehide it forms creases quite differently from calfskin, and over the years cordovan shoes develop a unique, unmistakable patina. The creases and wrinkles in a brown calfskin shoe grow perceptibly darker through the natural aging process and the use of excessively dark shoe polish, but in horsehide it is the smooth areas that gradually darken, whereas the points under the greatest strain actually grow lighter – particularly in the classic red-brown models.

Until 1980 or so cordovan shoes were virtually unknown in Europe; men who knew anything about footwear wore welted shoes from England or moccasins from Italy. Then cordovan shoes suddenly appeared in a few expensive gentlemen's outfitters and shoe-shops, and a small group of trend-setters made Alden a must-have make with the yuppies, especially in those countries – such as Germany, for example – where English shoes were not yet in a particularly strong position. One of these trend-setters that put their money on Alden at an early stage was Herbert B. Möller of Hanover. His shop in the exclusive Luisenpassage is among the best gentlemen's outfitters in the world. In Italy, where English shoes have an outstanding image, it remained difficult to interest customers in horsehide shoes until well into the 1990s. England itself is in any case dominated by its own makes of shoe, and anybody who considers foreign shoes chooses Italian moccasins in the first instance. So it is still the USA, where horsehide shoes have legions of devotees, that accounts for the lion's share of Alden's sales. Brooks Brothers included Alden's tassel and penny loafers in its product range as long ago as 1957, joining other classics like "plaintip Bluchers" and "wingtips." In the USA, in stark contrast to Europe, these shoes are seen as part of an extremely classic wardrobe: a role which in England and on the continent of Europe is still played by English shoes. Perhaps Alden will never manage to penetrate the English market.

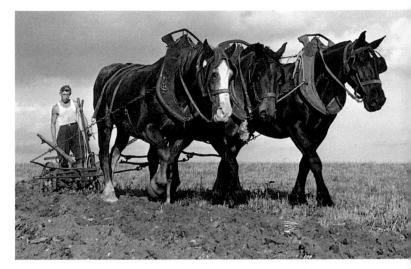

Making leather from horsehide used to be considered just as natural as using the hides of many other domesticated animals, and the innumerable drafthorses and carriage horses provided such huge quantities that this type of leather was not thought of as at all exclusive. It was mechanization that later made horsehide such an expensive rarity.

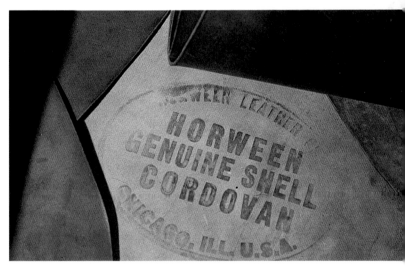

Cordovan shoes from Alden are made exclusively with leather from Horween, the acknowledged world specialist in horsehide.

Suede Shoes

Many men give suede shoes a very wide berth because they are not quite sure what to wear them with. These shoes also suffer from the prejudice that they are particularly delicate. But although it is true that they ought not to be deliberately put on for a walk in the rain, dampness does them no more harm than other shoes. After they have dried, the marks left by moisture can easily be removed with a brush or a special rubber eraser. And as for what to wear them with, there are only two things to bear in mind: the color of the shoes and their surface texture. Otherwise the rules are exactly the same as for all other types of shoe, because from the formal standpoint there is no difference between suede and leather shoes.

First let us consider color. Most suede shoes only come in brown – and quite right, because they ought only to be worn in brown. Black suede shoes have never established themselves, presumably because the casual aura of suede stands in crass contradiction to the formality of black. Brown suede shoes are worn with exactly the same clothes as brown leather shoes. They are not worn on formal occasions, so they are never paired with a morning coat; or for evening engagements, so never with a tuxedo or tails; nor are they worn with a business suit. Only in England and the USA, it must be said, does this last rule still apply in its strict form. However, if the tone within your company is still rather formal, brown shoes are best avoided. Otherwise suede shoes, like brown leather shoes, can be worn with gray, blue, green, and of course all shades of brown. They will go with a suit, a sports jacket, and a navy blazer. Of course, everyone must check in each individual case whether the particular brown really harmonizes with the rest of his ensemble. Basically brown and blue go very well together, and it is a very long time since combining these colors was considered a *faux pas*. But the preference for this combination is more marked in some countries than in others; brown is paired with blue by more French, Italians, and Spaniards than Englishmen and Americans, and it is really a mix that Germans and Austrians actively dislike. An outfit consisting of a blue single-breasted blazer, light-blue shirt, burgundy necktie, gray flannel pants, and dark-brown suede tassel loafers, for example, will be encountered very frequently in Italy but still rarely in Germany.

When deciding what other clothing suede can be combined with, its surface texture is even more important than its color. Suede that is hard and almost smooth goes better with light, summery new wool, while if it is heavily roughened and very soft it looks better with tweed and flannel. Surface textures which are too alike, on the other hand, can be boring; often it's the contrast that is interesting, such as between mat suede and a gleaming mohair suit. As long as you have properly thought through every facet of the question, and have the courage to experiment with new combinations, suede shoes open up some very interesting possibilities.

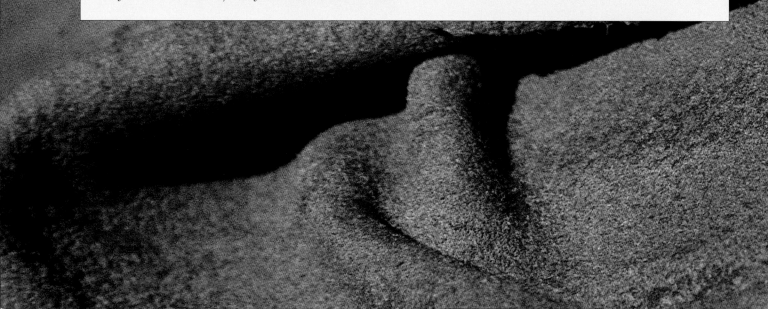

leisurewear. They even look good with a business suit if you have a gift for stylistic potpourri. A pair of black Tods would go perfectly well with a light Italian summer-weight suit in Super 180 wool, for example, or with knee-length socks in gossamer-thin wool or silk. Suede Tods go with gray pants and blazers. There are also designs with proper heels, not just knobs. Their price positioning is such that they look expensive to the average purchaser, whereas the target group used to good footwear, and to paying for it, will find them affordable, particularly in view of their high prestige value. It must be said, however, that their price-performance ratio is relatively unfavorable if you bear in mind how simple they are to produce. Nor does the "handmade in Italy" tag really justify the price. But, and it's a decisive but, J. P. Tods are now practically indispensable to the modern, international wardrobe – and they simply look so good that worrying about durability and price looks like nit picking. Tods will not last a lifetime. If you like them, you'll be happy to buy a new pair every season – and indeed, where the lightweight summer models are concerned, you'll have to. For unless you are unusually light-footed, walking on asphalt for a few sunny weeks will entirely wear them out. Once they are thus wrecked, fans of this cult Italian brand then finish them off completely in the garden or in the house. And every season Diego Della Valle can once more enjoy high sales.

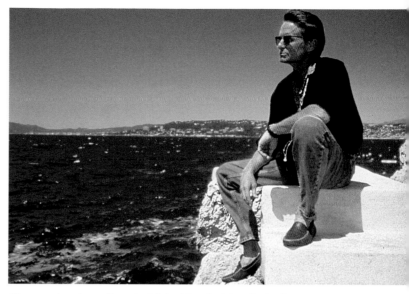

Like many Americans, film actor Michael Douglas takes absolutely no chances when he sets foot on the continent of Europe. He is always happy to be seen wearing Tods shoes.

Raincoats for Shoes

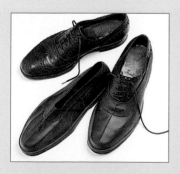

Many devotees of good footwear get rather nervous in the rain. They are afraid that the water may damage their shoes. Fundamentally, however, it doesn't. If shoes really do get thoroughly wet, they should simply be stuffed with newspaper and left to dry in a well-ventilated, warm room – though not directly in front or on top of a source of heat. Once they are totally dry the uppers should be cleaned and polished. But as it is not normally possible to take your shoes off at the office just because you happen to get caught in a downpour one morning, you should protect your shoes from rain and snow by wearing galoshes. People who drive their cars to work, of course, have less need for galoshes – which is why they are principally seen in major commuter conurbations like London and New York.

Galoshes are overshoes made of rubber or other synthetic materials that are pulled on – generally rather laboriously – over leather shoes. They provide ideal protection against water, and their nonskid soles also prevent slipping on wet sidewalks or on snow and ice. So if you are unwilling to give up your leather-soled footwear in the depths of winter, by all means use galoshes. At extremely low temperatures it is a good idea to adopt the practice of wearing warm boots for the journey to work, putting on your elegant shoes only when you get there. The effort of carrying an extra bag for these shoes will be rewarded when you are able to appear presentable at the office.

Socks – Getting the Combination Right

There is one golden rule about the male leg which is more important than any rules regarding colors and fabrics: always wear knee-length socks rather than ankle-length, so that your bare leg is never visible either when standing or when sitting. The sole exception is in summer when you are wearing boat shoes or loafers, when you should wear no socks at all. In other words, wear either knee-length socks or none.

Now for the question of color, pattern, and fabric. The basic principle is that the socks should be just as dark as the shoes, and on the other hand they should not contrast too strongly with the pants and your other clothes. But since the shoes must in any case be coordinated with your clothes, socks of a similar shade to the shoes will automatically match them. A few examples will show what I mean. If you wear a navy blazer with light-gray flannel pants, you might put on a pair of tassel loafers with them. You now have a number of possibilities regarding the socks. First comes dark gray, which is almost never wrong. But dark blue would be better, because that's the color of your blazer. Now let us assume that with the navy blazer you are wearing a light-blue shirt and a necktie in dark-blue and burgundy stripes. Again dark-blue socks would be right, because they would harmonize not only with the navy blazer but also with the shirt and the blue stripes of the necktie. Burgundy socks would also be a possibility, matching the other stripes of the necktie. If we remember the rule that the socks should be just as dark as the shoes, then burgundy is all right because burgundy and dark brown have a similar color value. Dark-blue socks are also just as dark as dark-brown shoes, and dark blue goes with dark brown, so this is also an eminently wearable combination. Black socks, although they are often recommended, would be too dark; they would contrast too strongly with the other color values of your ensemble. Dark brown is a possible color for socks to go with tweed suits tending towards the brown, but burgundy or bottle-green are generally better. So when choosing socks don't only think of the color of your shoes and pants, but also of your jacket, shirt, necktie, and dress handkerchief. No color can ever be "right" or "wrong" *per se*; it is always the combination that matters. This even applies to white socks, so often the object of contempt. If you spend time in the tropics or in the Mediterranean region, you might wear a white suit. If you choose to wear white shoes with it, you could certainly put on white socks; black would definitely be too sharp a contrast. If you wanted to wear black shoes with the white suit, black socks would be correct – though you should also bear in mind the color of your necktie and shirt. If the necktie is dark blue and the shirt light blue, you could also wear dark-blue socks with the white suit and white shoes. Black shoes would make it difficult, because black and dark blue do not go well together. If you want to wear black

To be on the safe side, choose plain socks; patterned socks require great sensitivity. There is a persistent legend that Albert Einstein never wore socks because he apparently thought them pointless. It is also said that this brilliant physicist owned multiple duplicates of all his clothes to make sure he always looked the same. It seems that some people will go to exraordinary lengths to preserve their individual style.

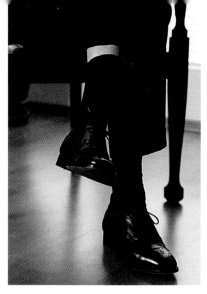

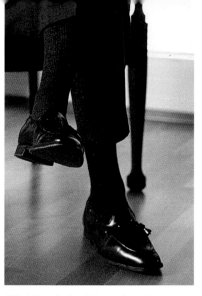

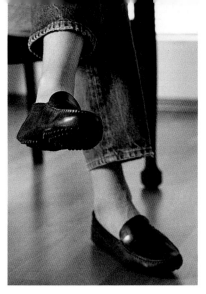

A sight considered distasteful in many parts of the world: the bare male leg. The dark sock makes the whiteness of the skin even more conspicuous.

This is how it should be: no bare leg is visible when sitting. This rule also applies in summer, when the recommended fabric is gossamer-thin wool or – of course – silk.

We have nothing against the male leg, except when it peeps out between ankle-socks and dark pants. In summer loafers should be worn without socks, if the occasion permits.

shoes, perhaps you ought to put on black socks, exchange the light-blue shirt for a white one and replace the blue necktie by one in black and red stripes. White socks are also acceptable with a white shirt, light chinos and black or burgundy Bass Weejuns – if you do not prefer to do without socks entirely in summer, that is.

Patterned socks require coordination skills of a slightly higher order than plain, as again you must naturally ensure that the pattern harmonizes with your pants, shirt, jacket, necktie, and dress handkerchief. If you suspect that you lack the talent to mix patterns it may be safer to stick to plain socks. You might, however, risk making Argyle check – which is generally mentioned in the same breath as the Burlington label – an exception to this pattern-teetotalism. It is easy to combine with jeans, chinos, and polo shirts, simply by matching the dominant color of the sock pattern with that of the polo shirt or with the plain color of a shirt or a sweater.

As for fabrics, the choice is between wool, cotton, and silk. Then there are various blends of these, together with alternatives with and without synthetic additives. Adding synthetic fibers has definite advantages: the socks fit better and keep their shape. Socks made of wool and wool blends come in various degrees of fineness, from light, almost transparent fabrics to heavy, tough winter weaves. What fabric you choose will depend mainly on the outdoor temperatures, but of course it must also go with the rest of your clothing. Silk socks ought not necessarily to be

worn with a sturdy Cheviot suit; they go better with light new wool or mohair. Medium-light woolen socks go with flannel pants; thick, ribbed woolen socks with tweed pants – though these are also a good alternative to smooth knits, as they break the surface up and add texture to it. Caution is again advisable, however, for a ribbed texture will not go well with delicate suiting fabrics. Anybody who takes even a slight interest in socks will immediately recognize that they must be chosen with the same care as every other item of clothing. At any rate it is worth investing in good, expensive socks, not only because you owe it to the rest of your costly wardrobe but also because good-quality socks last substantially longer. As soon as any of your socks become at all threadbare, get rid of them. Nothing is more appalling than discovering after an important occasion that one of your socks has a large, prominent hole in the heel.

It is wise to buy socks at the same time as buying other items of clothing, because you can then be sure of getting the right color coordination. Most gentlemen's outfitters and tailors also sell socks, as do some shoe-shops. Buying socks at firms making custom clothing or shoes will also guarantee a level of quality not found anywhere else.

Socks may seem such a minor detail in a gentleman's wardrobe, but they are are nevertheless very important in complementing an outfit. The wrong sort of socks can completely ruin an image and it is very important that they look right.

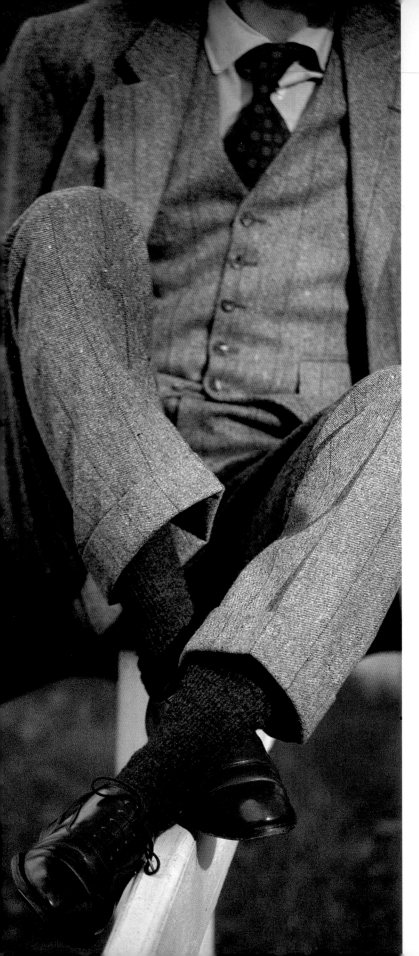

Shoes and the Rest

Skillfully coordinating shoes with the rest of your clothes is either hard or easy, depending on whether formal or esthetic criteria are applied. "Formal" means in accordance with social convention, such as choosing formal shoes – black Oxfords, for example – to go with a formal suit, and only wearing informal brown shoes with a casual outfit like a tweed suit, jeans, and a blazer or corduroy pants and a sweater. In order to conform to social convention, naturally, you must be familiar with it. Choosing your clothing according to purely esthetic criteria avoids this problem, but you must accept the possibility that you will attract attention – either approbation or censure. The esthetic was first adopted as a guideline in continental Europe, where no later than the end of the Second World War it was felt that upper-class standards had had their day. In Italy and Germany whether shoes should be black or brown was a question of fashion, whereas in England upper-class standards still decreed that only black shoes could be worn in London after 6 o'clock. On the continent it can therefore be quite acceptable to wear dark-brown suede shoes with gray flannel pants and a blue blazer, though when choosing shoes it is not just color that matters: the surface texture of the leather must be coordinated with the fabrics worn. More than that, account must be taken of the shoes' entire silhouette. Filigree Italian loafers will be simply overwhelmed by a heavy tweed suit, and the reverse is also true: thick-soled cordovan brogues will look unutterably lumpish with a feather-light suit in finest Super 180 wool. As is so often the case where clothes are concerned, shoes and suits are never wrong in themselves – all it depends on is the wearer finding the right combination.

The right combination of suit and shoes is a question of both style and custom. Brown shoes, for example, are the traditional choice when spending a weekend in the country.

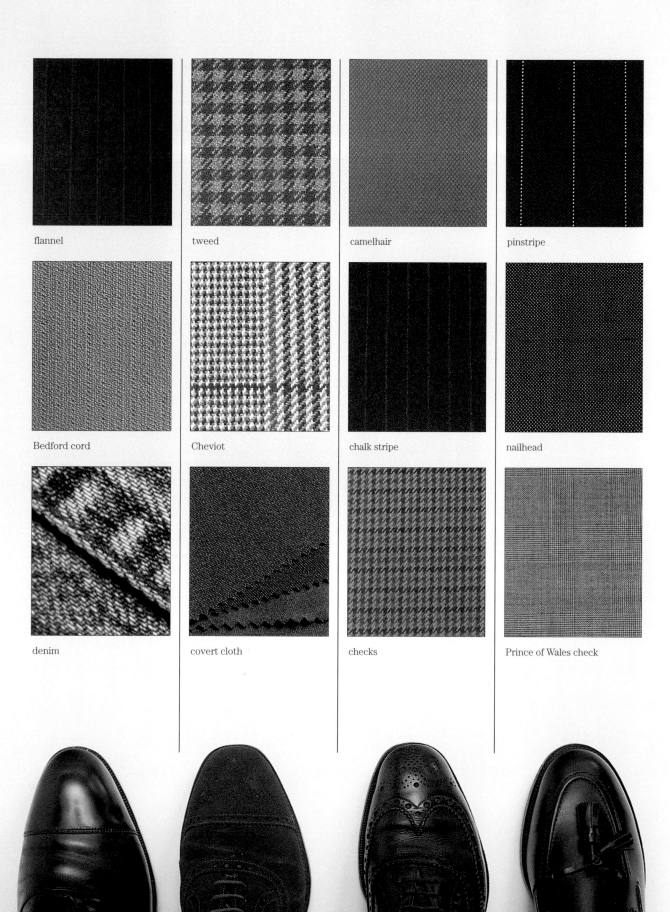

flannel

tweed

camelhair

pinstripe

Bedford cord

Cheviot

chalk stripe

nailhead

denim

covert cloth

checks

Prince of Wales check

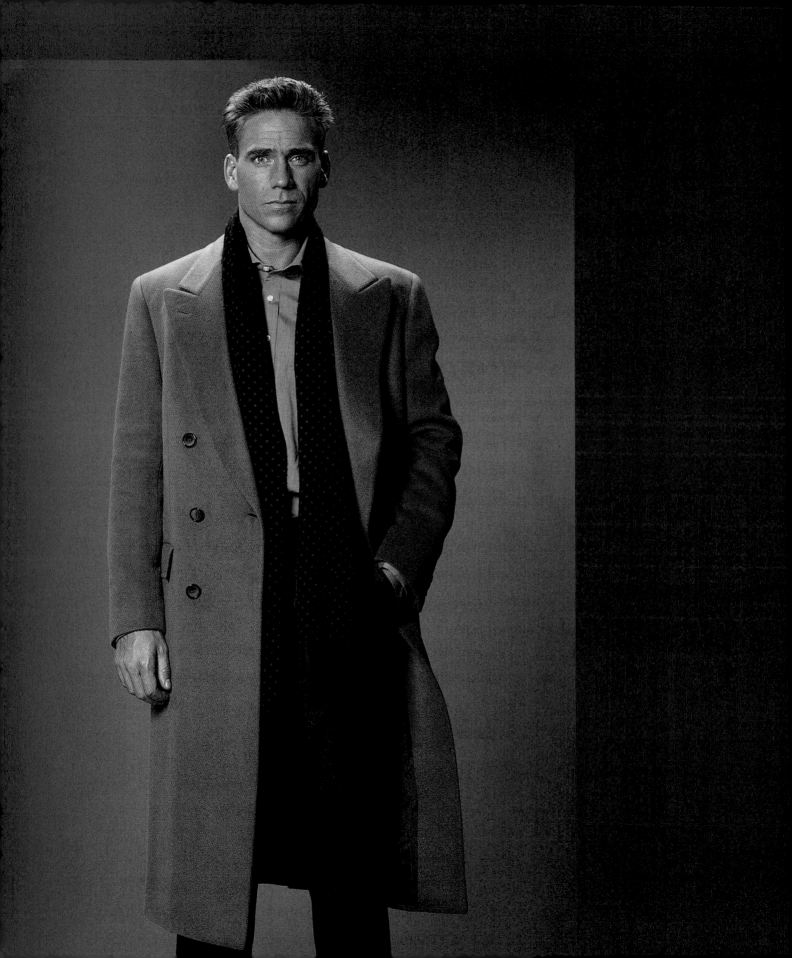

Overcoats & Jackets

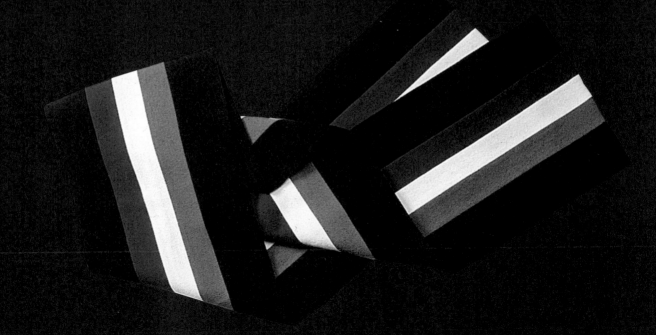

Overcoat Culture

Superficially the prime function of the overcoat is to protect its wearer from the cold, wind, dust, and rain. But it also demonstrates that he is on his way somewhere. By putting on his overcoat a man indicates his intention to leave. By taking it off he indicates that he has arrived. Only when he has been relieved of his overcoat does he begin to make his entrance. But the man who arrives without taking off his overcoat is signaling reserve, distrust, or just indecision. "Later the whole crowd went to a bar, where at first everybody stood around in their overcoats…" wrote Max Frisch in *Gantenbein* (also known as *A Wilderness of Mirrors*), outlining in a few words a situation that is as yet unresolved.

The protective function of the overcoat can also be understood in the transferred sense. We see it as a sort of wrapping, defending us against a sometimes hostile environment – it draws a line between ourselves and the outside world. Anton Chekhov describes this need in his short story *Man in a Suitcase*: "…in this man one could observe the constant and irresistible endeavor to wrap himself up in a cocoon, to create a suitcase to cut himself off, to protect himself from outside influences." And so Belikov, a teacher, always kept his overcoat on. We are all familiar with this reluctance to take our overcoats off when we find ourselves in uncongenial company or an uncongenial location.

This is why the overcoat figures in people's wardrobes in parts of the world where it is not really a necessity. Even in warmer countries people feel the need to have something to put on and take off. Italian tailors, for example, make very beautiful overcoats from the lightest worsted fabrics, which provide hardly any warmth at all but nonetheless isolate us from the outside world. The overcoat has the additional function – in all regions – of proclaiming the style of the clothing concealed beneath it. The protective overcoat thus gives away a great deal about its wearer, unless he has deliberately chosen it to contrast with his preferred outer clothing.

Normally, however, people wear overcoats that harmonize with their personal style and are also appropriate for the occasion. The overcoat then indicates the wearer's intention: whether he is going to the office, or hunting, or to the opera, or whether he is perhaps traveling. So the man who always wears his beloved Barbour jacket – lovely though it may be, suitable though it may be for many occasions – renounces a whole series of opportunities for stylistic self-expression. An overcoat appropriate for the occasion is always a true statement of style, as much as any other part of a true gentleman's wardrobe.

The overcoat always used to serve to highlight distinctions of social rank. The person who helped you on with your overcoat was your social inferior. No longer: today nobody is compelled to wait on other people in this way, though it is still a sign of respect toward a fellow human being who is older, or of whom you think highly. If this small, helpful gesture is unfortunately growing less and less common, this is due not only to the decline of politeness but also to the loss of overcoat culture.

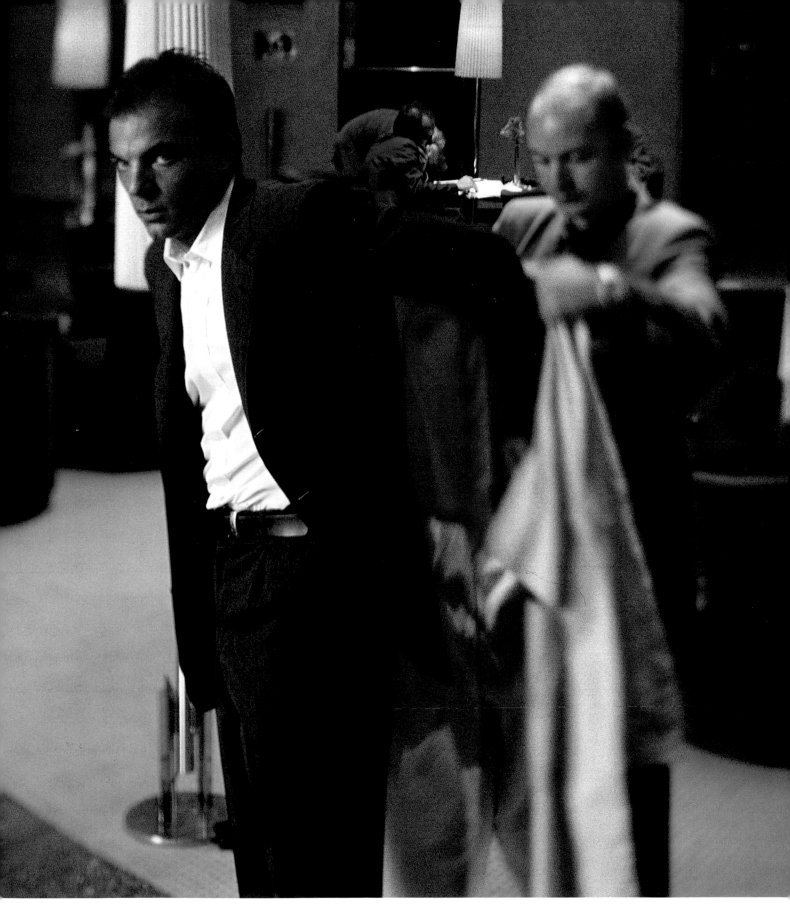

Essential Overcoats

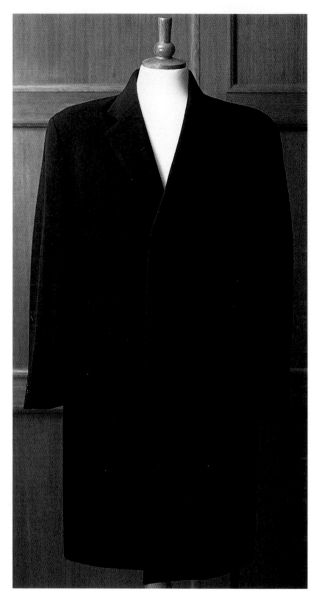

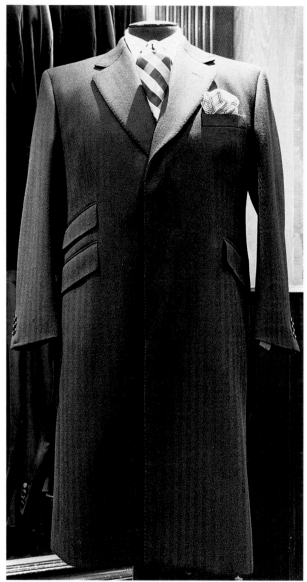

The dark-blue Crombie is the classic English town overcoat. Tailored from thick woolen cloth, the Crombie is especially suitable for cheerless autumn and winter days. Almost all makers of classic off-the-rack clothing include it in their basic collections in more or less modified forms. It often originates from the workshops of the traditional firm of Tibbett, whose roots go back to the year 1898.

The Chesterfield came into fashion in the nineteenth century. Its first devotee is said to have been a member of one of the many branches of the family of the Earls of Chesterfield, but whether the aristocrat in question actually invented this overcoat, that is to say was the first to order one from his tailor, is not recorded. There are both single-breasted and double-breasted Chesterfields, in beige, blue, and black – though most people think of it as the single-breasted version, made of woolen cloth in a gray herringbone pattern, with fly front and a black velvet collar attached.

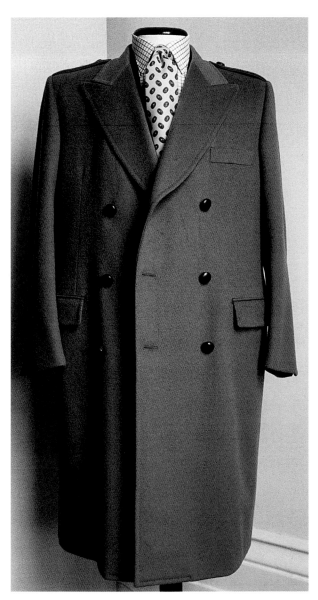

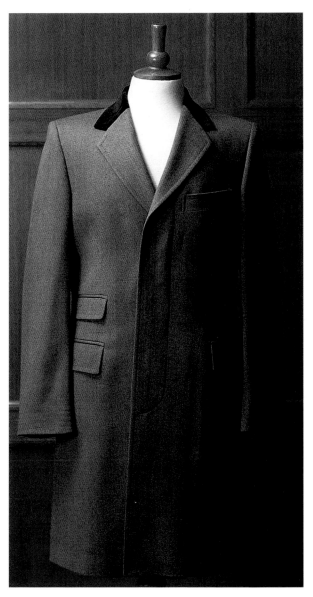

The British Warm, as they call it in England, was originally a military overcoat – as can be seen from the shoulder tabs. It really is warm: it is made from thick Melton wool, or sometimes from heavy cavalry twill. There is also a superior variant in cashmere. The long version shows how closely related it is to the trench coat, an ample military overcoat which has achieved great success in civilian life. Connoisseurs buy theirs at Gieves & Hawkes, unless they have their own tailors make them.

Slim and short: that is the covert coat. At first sight it greatly resembles the single-breasted Chesterfield. But the difference lies in the cloth from which the covert coat is made and derives its name, a light twill that can be worn practically all the year round. Also the covert coat has four parallel decorative seams – called "railroading" – at the cuffs and hem. The typical color is a pale, slightly mottled brown, and the covert coat usually has a contrasting collar in dark-brown velvet. It was originally conceived as a riding and hunting coat, and this is recalled by the large inside pocket at the level of the left thigh for provisions or ammunition.

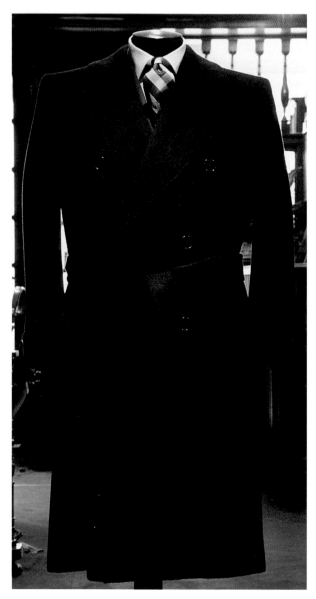

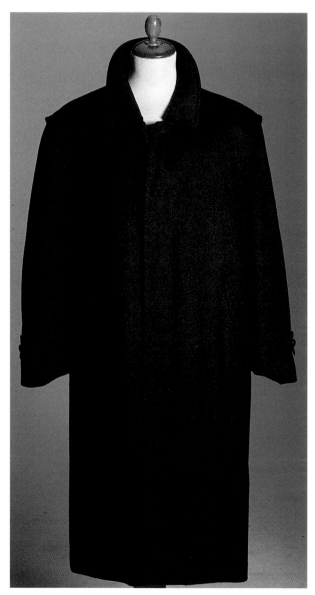

The polo coat is an American classic, though it is closely related to such traditional, more elegant styles of overcoat as the paletot, the Ulster, and the Guards coat. Brooks Brothers imported the style from England in 1910. The large patch pockets give it a casual air. The polo coat typically comes in beige, perhaps because at first it used to be made in camelhair cloth – though today it is generally made in new wool. London outfitters Turnbull & Asser recommend this coat in blue.

The green loden overcoat has long been a pan-European classic. We may initially associate the characteristic loden fabric with the alpine regions, but this overcoat is no less popular in England, France, and Belgium. When worn as a city overcoat, that is to say for other than folkloric reasons, it can be combined with tweed and cord. Loden is a wool weave that has been first fulled and then napped. It is comparatively waterproof and wind-proof, but above all it is highly resistant to damage by undergrowth, branches, and thorns. If a loden overcoat ever gets soiled, the dirt is simply removed by vigorous brushing. The classic design is cut wide and long, with a turndown collar and a long, vertical box pleat at the rear.

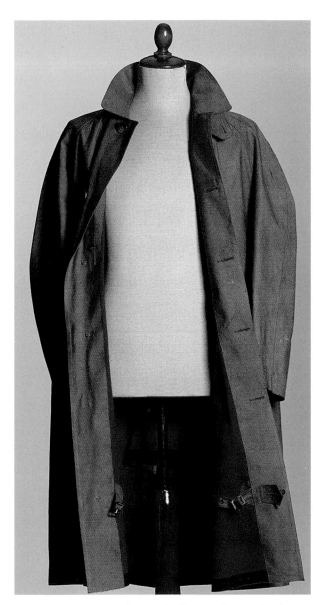

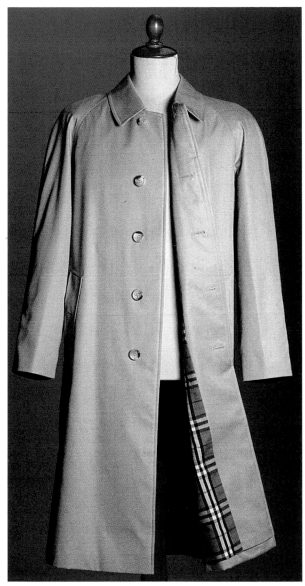

The macintosh – mac or riding mac for short – strikes us today almost as a fossil from the prehistory of the raincoat. Its construction, two layers of cotton fabric with a layer of rubber in between, wasn't originally intended for overcoats at all. In 1822 Scottish chemist Charles Macintosh patented his "India-rubber cloth" as a fabric for waterproof tarpaulins and the like, but soon the tailors pounced on the new material and used it to make raincoats. Disillusionment was not long in coming, however: water got in through the needle-holes in the seams. Macintosh had to do something to rescue the reputation of his "rubber cloth": he developed a process to seal the seams, and thereafter marketed the only really waterproof raincoat.

The slip-on or "raincoat" is closely related to the riding mac in cut and color, but it is made with a different fabric. The slip-on is not rubberized; like the classic trench coat it is tailored in gabardine. The raglan sleeves are typical of this comfortable raincoat; unlike the shoulder sleeves of the British Warm, for example, they give much freedom of movement. Enthusiasts for a sloping shoulder line should choose the one-piece raglan sleeve, though this is less common than the two-piece version. The slip-on has a fly front and flapped pocket-vents to reach through. There is a large inside pocket at the level of the left thigh, the perfect place for your morning paper.

For the Officer in the Gentleman

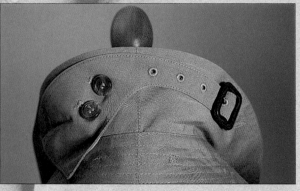

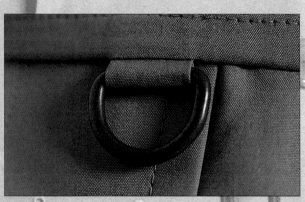

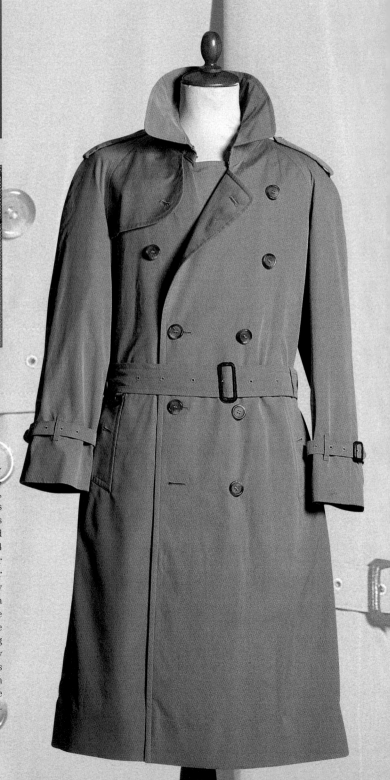

The classic authentic trench coat is made by the firm of Burberrys. Thomas Burberry may not, in fact, have been the inventor of gabardine, although he was enough of a businessman to patent this cotton weave, resistant to water and wind, in rain-swept England in 1879. Burberrys retained exclusive manufacturing rights to the material until 1917. This hard-wearing cloth soon came to the attention of the armed forces, and English officers first wore Burberry coats during the Boer War. In 1914 one version received official approval from the War Ministry, and over 500,000 of these "trench coats" were worn during the First World War (hence the name). The trench coat's military past is recalled today by its shoulder tabs, the storm flap at the collar, and the D-shaped rings on the belt, which were used to attach items of equipment. If you dislike these associations, avoid the classic Burberry in favor of a gabardine coat of a different design. Some people may also be put off by the lining in the Burberrys house check, a pattern which has become extremely well known. They can buy an Aquascutum trench coat, a make which is also of very high repute but still somewhat less exclusive. Or they can forget trench coats and wear Barbours, which in any case are waterproof and are much better protection from the rain.

The Duffel Coat

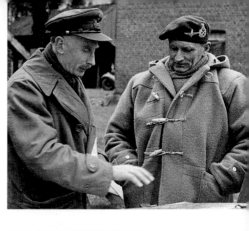

The duffel coat is the only classic overcoat to have a hood. This form of head protection has a long history, for gowns with hoods were known as long ago as the Bronze Age. The English word *duffle*, denoting a coarse woolen cloth and thought to be derived from the town of Duffel in the Belgian province of Brabant, hasn't been around for quite that long: only since the eighteenth century. The origin of the name is thus more or less clear. The origin of the design is thought to be the so-called "Polish coat," an overcoat with a toggle fastening that was popular in the first half of the nineteenth century. Some think the monk's habit was the forerunner of the duffel coat, and that would explain the hood. In common with many other overcoats the duffel coat made its entrance into menswear via the military, when the Royal Navy began to issue it to sailors: the hood and the thick woolen cloth protected them from wind and weather. In the Second World War Field-Marshall Montgomery wore a beige duffel coat, thus giving the design a new surge of popularity. And in the 1950s large quantities of army-surplus duffel coats came onto the market, which conclusively established them as hot favorites for cold winter days. In France the duffel coat quickly achieved great popularity among high-school and college students and intellectuals. Today it exists not only in the classic colors of dark blue and beige, but also in dark green, dark brown, burgundy, and yellow. The boxy cut and the hood, and not least the characteristic toggle fastenings, make this a very casual overcoat. If your wardrobe tends towards the elegant, you will certainly have trouble finding other items to combine it with. But if you favor casual outfits, you would still be well-advised to wear a duffel coat.

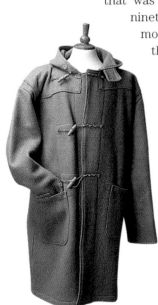

The original duffel coat is manufactured by the English firm of Tibbett. This one was made in 1941.

Even today the duffel coat still recalls Montgomery, the British Field-Marshall whose nickname was "Monty." The duffel coat is often called the "monty coat" in his honor.

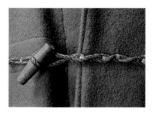

The duffel coat has traditional toggle fastenings made of buffalo horn. They have no real advantage over buttons; it is often said that they are easier to do up and undo with gloves on, but actually quite the opposite is the case.

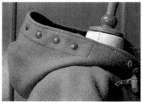

The duffel coat's hood is quite small, but it should be big enough to wear a beret or flat cap underneath it. It provides excellent protection from cold and wind, but cyclists should be warned that it severely restricts vision and hearing.

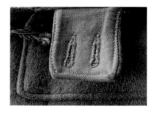

As the toggle fastenings mean that the duffel coat is not particularly wind-proof, the sensitive neck region can be protected from the cold with a buttoned tab. At moderate temperatures this makes a scarf unnecessary.

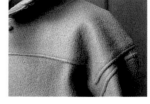

The extra layer of cloth forming the cape-collar provides additional upper-body warmth. In the rain it is intended to stop the water from soaking through the cloth too quickly, and it also protects the shoulders of the coat from premature wear.

A duffel coat always has two big patch pockets, with or without flaps. Pockets without flaps have the advantage of easier access, but things are also more likely to fall out of them. A breast pocket is not normal, but sometimes a larger inside pocket will be found at thigh level.

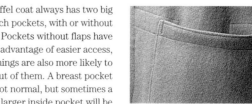

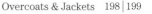

The Barbour Phenomenon

When you purchase a Barbour you are not only acquiring a rainproof jacket: above all you are buying your share of an international lifestyle. As soon as you put it on you're part of it – the world of those who have style, money, and success. This jacket protects you from bad weather, but it also protects you from the risk of being improperly dressed. And it's true: if you are not sure what to put on you can always fall back on the Barbour – as long as it's not too warm, that is. Absurd though it may seem, it is better to appear at an evening social event in sweater, jeans, and a Barbour than wearing the wrong shoes or a badly cut tuxedo. Throughout Europe the Barbour is something like an entrance ticket to high society, and if the other details – the wristwatch for example – are also right, then the wearer of the famous waxed jacket will be treated courteously in even the most exclusive stores. The Barbour is neither excessively costly nor especially difficult to get hold of. But it conveys taste, a sense of style, and an attachment to tradition – particularly if it is old and extensively patched.

It is hard to say what makes the Barbour stand out from other classic English garments, what makes it so successful in so many European countries in spite of all their actual or supposed differences of mentality; it can be found today, after all, in every large town in Europe from Helsinki to Madrid, and no gossip column anywhere lets a week go by without printing pictures of celebrities in Barbours. Perhaps it is the feeling that a piece of that glamorous world comes with a Barbour, which in contrast to most trendy items of clothing is a really long-term and worthwhile investment; the older it looks, after all, the higher its value. A worn and battered Barbour provides unspoken confirmation of the wearer's "membership since ... ," the same idea that a well-known credit-card company used in one of its recent advertising campaigns. The older the Barbour, the longer its owner has been a member.

Yet in spite of its fame the Barbour has remained a highly individual garment. It offers a multitude of stylistic, esthetic, ideological, and ethical associations, being equally popular with both the pro- and anti-hunting lobbies. The patent waxed jacket is at the same time English, practical, hard-wearing, sporting, in tune with nature, accepted, high-quality, casual, snobbish, classic – and so on, and so forth. But perhaps one of the things that fascinate us about the Barbour is simply the fact that it is part of the scenery. It is hard to imagine that there was ever a time when it did not yet exist, it seems to have been around for ever. Though the design of the various styles can be described as well-nigh perfect, nobody knows the name of the person who first thought up this brilliant garment. Perhaps that is a further reason why so many people can identify with the Barbour brand: there is no designer behind it, no specific individual to like or dislike. Barbour is simply an old English firm that makes jackets, very modestly and without a great deal of fuss – and there is absolutely no reason for not buying one.

The lining of each Barbour is graced by the Royal Warrants of not one but three blue-blooded customers of this legendary supplier of waterproofs.

The Story of the Waxed Jacket

The Barbour firm was founded by John Barbour, probably in about 1894 – but nobody is exactly sure. The relative uncertainty about the date testifies to a degree of modesty, which is also reflected in the firm's exiguous history. Why, when, and how the first Barbour jackets were made is shrouded in mystery. Evidently it never occurred to John Barbour that the foundation of his firm might one day become a memorable event in the history of costume. Presumably he simply decided one day to make waterproof overcoats and jackets, and all the rest somehow just happened. The oldest surviving Barbour catalogue dates back to 1908. On the back cover there is a prominent advertisement showing a man in a long coat with a rainhat on his head. The text describes the "special light-weight coat" on offer as "ideal… for yachting, fishing, driving, boating, walking, and shooting." A lighthouse, at the time the Barbour trademark ("the famed beacon brand oilskins"), can be seen in the background. It was not until the 1920s that it was replaced as the trademark by the family name. In fact the family – which still owns the company today – has always stayed well in the background, though many Barbour customers would undoubtedly love to glance through the family album. But the Barbour family is probably not that different from other English families, except that in their case the Barbour jacket which their great-great-grandfather used to wear was made to his own design.

Today Barbour is one of the few British clothing manufacturers with three of the prized royal warrants: from the Queen, the Duke of Edinburgh, and the Prince of Wales. We can hardly fail to be aware of the royal predilection towards the brand; there is no member of the Royal Family who has not at some time or other been photographed wearing a Barbour. These pictures, which go all over the world, relieve Barbour of the need to engage in expensive advertising campaigns. The Barbour phenomenon is an excellent example of the fact that a product can be sold without advertising – all that is required is a few decades' patience and confidence in the quality of one's product. Today there are a number of styles of Barbour available and these are described on the next two pages.

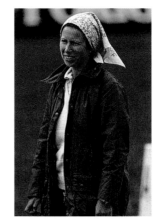

Princess Anne, like all the other members of the English Royal Family, is often seen in a Barbour. She also wears other makes, however, like Musto and Puffa. As the sister of the future king of all British citizens, perhaps she has to support all British makes.

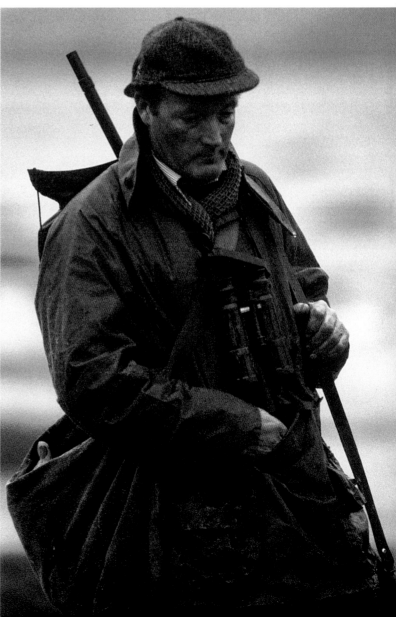

Shooting is one of the occasions when the Barbour proves its superior quality and useful design. The big pocket at the back is perfect for small game, the large bellows pockets have plenty of room for cartridges, and the fabric, proof against water and wind, protects the wearer from the rain and cold.

The Barbour in Detail

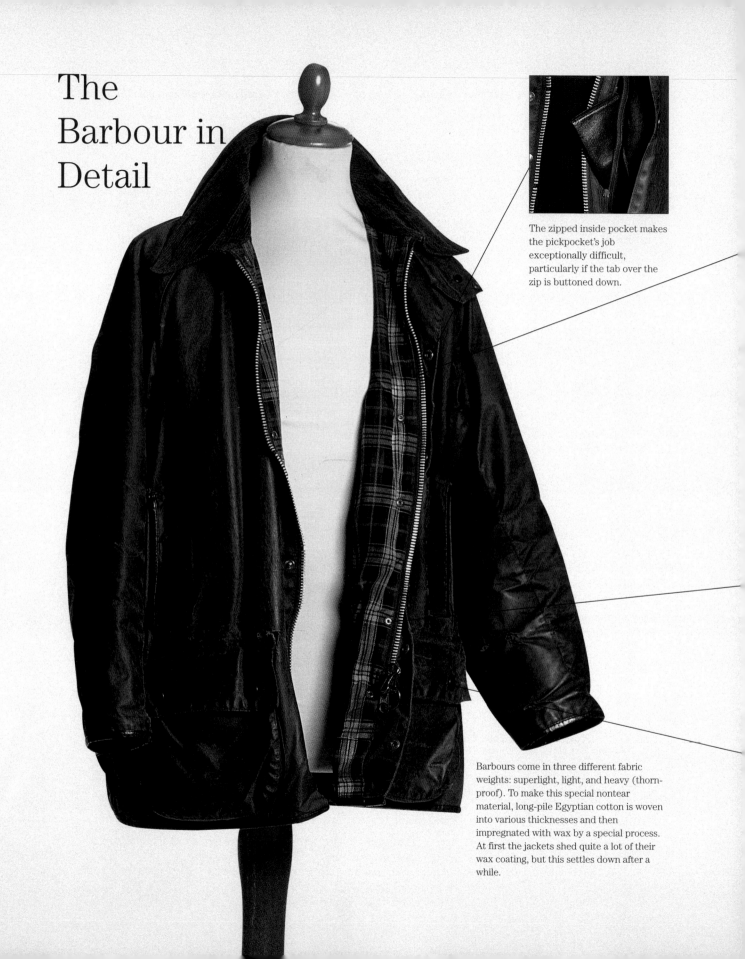

The zipped inside pocket makes the pickpocket's job exceptionally difficult, particularly if the tab over the zip is buttoned down.

Barbours come in three different fabric weights: superlight, light, and heavy (thornproof). To make this special nontear material, long-pile Egyptian cotton is woven into various thicknesses and then impregnated with wax by a special process. At first the jackets shed quite a lot of their wax coating, but this settles down after a while.

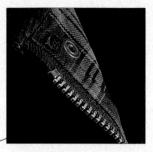

The press-studs are made of noncorroding brass so that they do not wear out even after years of use, closing just as firmly as on day one. The zip has large brass teeth and a big ringpull, both of which make it easy to undo and do up, even with gloves on.

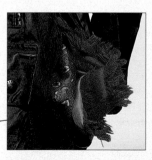

Depending on the model there are inside pockets with room for everything you could possibly need, both in town and in the country: sugar lumps for the pony, the dog's lead, your newspaper, your sunglasses, the obligatory chewing gum, or insect repellent.

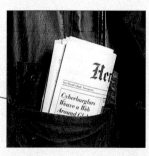

The capacious outside pockets, the size of which varies with the model, can be filled with all sorts of useful things: shotgun cartridges and the keys to the Range Rover in the country, mobile phone, cigarettes, and lighter in town.

The Top Six

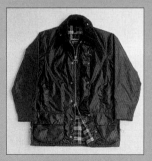

The green Beaufort is the most widespread Barbour, beloved of high-school students, young ladies, and society ladies who throw it on to go shopping.

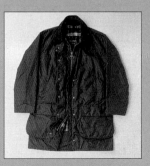

The Border, slightly longer, is almost a substitute for the trench coat. It comes in green and blue. Its big pockets inside and out endear it to people who carry lots of paraphernalia around with them.

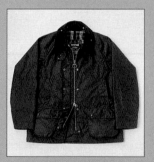

The Bedale is a particular favorite of ladies who ride, and also of Barbour-wearing parents and their children, as it is the only model which is made in small sizes.

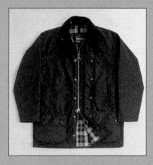

The heavy Moorland is only available in olive. It is bought by those who wish to set themselves somewhat apart from the Beaufort-wearing majority.

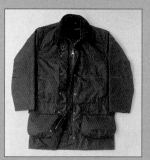

Instead of the characteristic Barbour "house check" the long, heavy Northumbria is lined with a warmer wool and polyester blend in a pattern known by the attractive name of "hunting McKinnon."

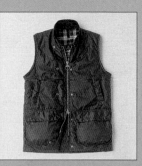

A sleeveless rain jacket? An odd idea, perhaps, but this vest really does protect the upper body from dirt if, for example, you have to pick the dog up.

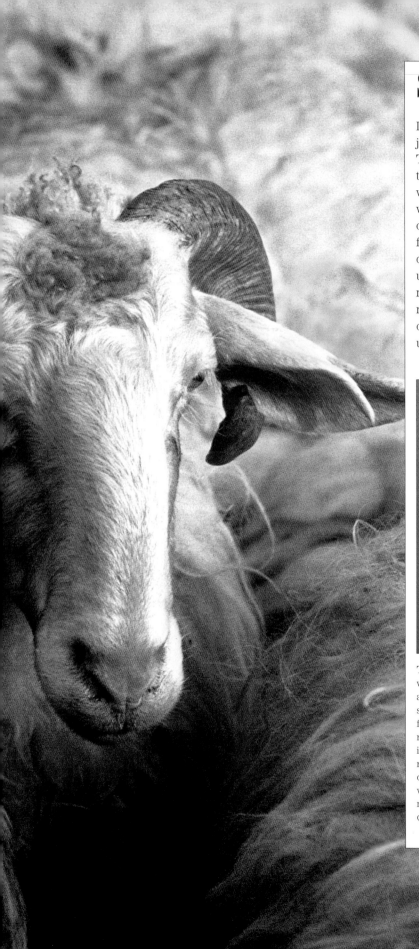

Short is All Right

Italy is the source of the modern preference for light jackets only marginally longer than the jacket of a suit. The Italians are mad about automobiles, and the trend toward short, light jackets may have something to do with the fact that these are much more practical at the wheel than long overcoats. These jackets, which are often quilted, may not necessarily be elegant, but they form an interesting casual contrast to the rather staid dark suits in wool or cashmere that are normally worn underneath them. In southern Europe they tend to be more courageous about contrast than in the neighboring countries to the north, and bright-orange or luminous-yellow quilted jackets are by no means an uncommon sight on the "piazza."

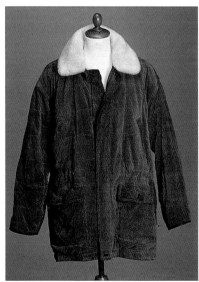

The lambskin jacket is always slightly reminiscent of the getup in which pilots protected themselves from the cold in the early days of aviation. It looks good in a convertible, and indeed for all other sporting activities. To many people it is the only acceptable form of fur (though fur was never really out; these days it is simply worn rather more discreetly). The drawback of the lambskin jacket is that it is not always of the highest quality, not to mention that it is redolent of *aprés-ski*. But this association can be avoided by combining the lambskin jacket with a classic wardrobe rather than with white broadcord or waist-pleat jeans. With a tweed suit or a navy-blue blazer and flannel pants the lambskin jacket is a true classic, both in the country and in town.

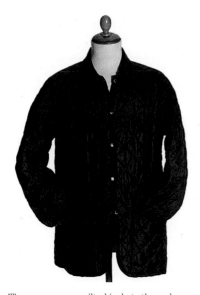

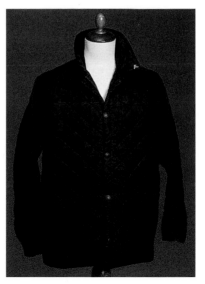

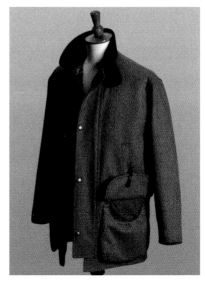

There are many quilted jackets these days, but only one original: the genuine Husky. It was invented by Stephen Guylas, an American colonel of Hungarian extraction who settled in Tostock, in the English county of Suffolk, on retiring from active service. When he was in the army Col. Guylas was involved in the development of special clothing for the US Air Force, and he was not entirely finished with this assignment even after he retired. He had always been a keen marksman, and in the early 1960s he designed his own clothing for the shooting range. First came a quilted and waterproof shooting vest, then a jacket in similar style. Col. Guylas' friends at the shooting range were fired with enthusiasm for these practical items. Their fame spread, creating a growing demand – which the colonel and his wife were soon spending all their time satisfying. The Husky jacket, as well as its numerous imitations, can now be seen all over England. In the 1980s this padded English cult item was launched on the continent as an in-product. With increasing success the range of colors also grew, and the Husky jacket is now available in almost all the colors of the rainbow as well as the original pale green and blue.

The original Husky can be recognized by its slightly boxy cut and the side vents fastening with press-studs. The Husky jacket's great success stimulated the appearance of numerous imitators. As the original – apart from its cord collar – is made of prosaic synthetics, and is amazingly expensive at that, most of its imitators have specialized in upgrading the quilted jacket by using better materials. For devotees of natural fibers there are highly superior quilted jackets from John Partridge in cotton, lined with decorative tartans or with soft leather collars. But these often costly variants of the quilted jacket are no longer what the original was, that is to say very light, virtually indestructible, and above all machine washable.

Those who like the cut and length of the Barbour – which reaches almost to the knees – are recommended to consider the tweed field coat from Cordings of Piccadilly, which is of a similar cut. The weave is not waterproof, admittedly, but it is treated against moisture. It is also much warmer than the Barbour, which can sometimes be pretty cold and damp. In England these field coats have long been known and loved as a casual half-way house between the Barbour and the traditional tweed overcoat. On the continent they still have insider status, and as they are a little too expensive to be espoused by the masses this will probably remain the case for some time.

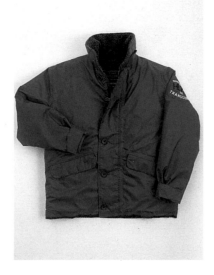

Henri Lloyd is one of the great in-brands of the 1980s, when the so-called yuppies were setting the trend. It is said to have originated when chic young Milanese wore Henri Lloyd's warm, waterproof sailing jackets to ride their motor scooters – which was a good idea, because jackets that could stand up to storms and seawater could be expected to defy rain and slipstream with ease. Soon a veritable tidal wave of Henri Lloyd swept through the clothes closets of youths and young adults. Today Henri Lloyd is simply a chic and expensive sportswear brand to most people, with its popularity concentrated on the shores of the Mediterranean. Only those who sail as well as drive motor scooters are aware that Henri Lloyd started in 1963 as a small specialist outfitter for yachtsmen.

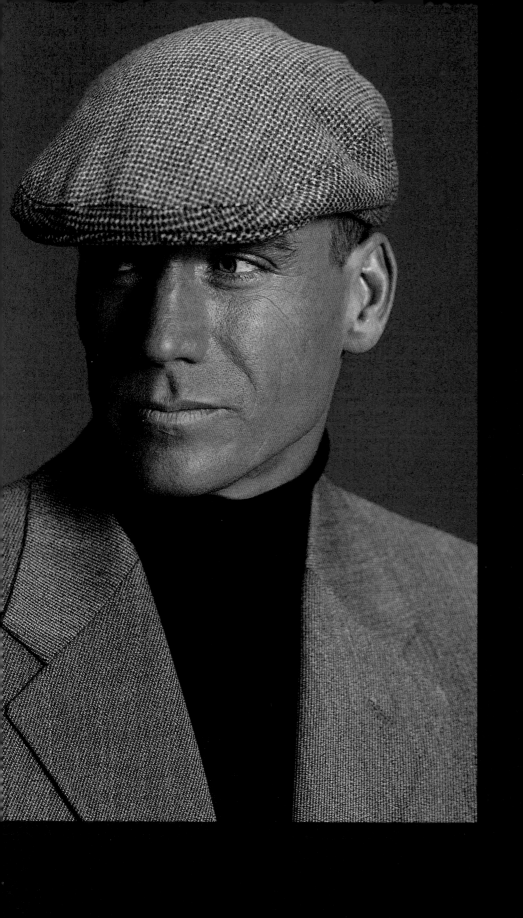

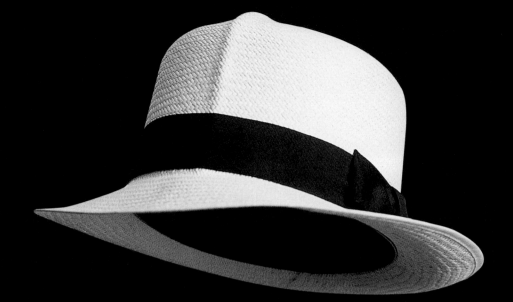

The Hat

The Hat Past and Present

Fifty years ago the hat was still just as important a part of the gentleman's everyday wardrobe as the necktie, shoes, and shirt are today. Until well into the 1960s wearing a hat fulfilled a dress code which was questioned by very few, and any rebellion against it involved wearing some other form of headgear rather than putting nothing on one's head at all. Anybody who went around without a hat was sending out a clear signal that he did not consider himself bound by social norms. In Thomas Mann's *The Magic Mountain* Hans Castorp admonishes his cousin Joachim Ziemssen that "one should always have a hat on… so that one can take it off on occasions when it is appropriate to do so." The hat is a good example of the fact that nearly every fashion springs from a practical need; in the case of the hat, protection from rain, dust, cold, and sun. But if the original need no longer exists, the article of clothing meeting it is sooner or later felt to be superfluous. Anybody who travels to work by car instead of covering long distances on foot can easily do without a hat. And anybody who is in a position to wash his hair as soon as it needs it does not necessarily have to protect it from dust and dirt. The 1950s with their weekly hair-wash are long past. The elaborate hair fashions of the 1960s and 1970s also threatened the continued existence of the classic gentleman's hat, for what follower of style would be inclined to pull a felt hat down over his artistically blow-dried coiffure, inevitably flattening the hair against his head and thereby destroying its laboriously fabricated body?

The hatbox has become a rare item of equipment indeed. When the hat used to be taken for granted just as the overcoat and scarf are today, this rigid container for soft headgear was a familiar sight. It acted simultaneously as transport packaging, a way of protecting the hat from dust, and an advertising medium for the hat-maker.

CHRISTYS' London HATS

Nor does hair combed down over the forehead go with a hat, however, for to show off a hat to its best advantage the forehead must be bare. Hair sprouting down over the forehead from under the brim of a hat recalls a shirt hanging out under a suit vest. Most dedicated hat-wearers therefore choose a classic gentleman's haircut, trimmed short at the back of the neck. At any rate they are firmly of the opinion that the sight of a hat – on the street, at least – is preferable to that of the hair. But as it is precisely the hairstyle which we see today as the expression of our individuality, it occurs to few men to cover it up with a hat. These days, as a rule, anybody who wears a hat every day does so in the firm knowledge that he is doing something unusual, almost eccentric.

Every day, mind – for on special occasions a gentleman still wears a hat, or rather a top hat. If a formal occasion requires tails (morning or evening dress) to be worn, a man who otherwise makes a point of dressing with discreet elegance and timeless style may bring himself to drag his good old top hat out of the farthest corner of his wardrobe. Wearing a top hat with anything other than morning or evening dress would, however, be a *faux pas*. A man whose hairstyle makes wearing a top hat impossible, or would at least make it look very odd, holds the hat in his hand. These days the most frequent occasions at which to wear a top hat are weddings, where the morning coat is seen as the international standard. But the top hat is certainly not essential with either morning or evening dress.

At present, except on formal and decidedly official occasions, hats are only encountered at certain sporting events. At horse races, for example – true to the English model – the brown trilby, of which we shall have more to say later, is the preferred headgear. Other hats are simply no longer worn; they have become outmoded, they no longer fit into our current sense of style – no more, for example, than do the pocket watch or the full-length umbrella. The international style may strike some as conservative, but it has nothing to do with nostalgia. We stick to the traditional only as long as it really makes sense to do so. The hat has largely lost its function, we have nowhere to put a pocket watch because vests no longer exist – and as for the full-length umbrella, we have lost the habit of taking walks. Thus many items disappear from the international style canon, while others – if they have proved themselves over a decade or two – are readopted or sometimes simply rediscovered. Perhaps the hat has prospects of one day reappearing on every head. In that case the baseball cap may possibly pave the way for its comeback. Say what you like, this quintessentially American peaked cap has managed to creep up on classic sportswear. One day it may perhaps be a classic, just as acceptable as the penny loafer and the polo shirt are today. And anybody who has once learned to appreciate the advantages of having something on his head may perhaps one day turn once more to the felt hat as an expression of style.

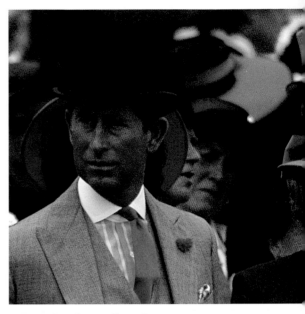

In England gentlemen still wear hats – a top hat, for example, if the occasion requires morning dress. Here the Prince of Wales is seen with a particularly elegant specimen in silk. Whether he holds this archaic headgear in high regard, however, we shall not inquire.

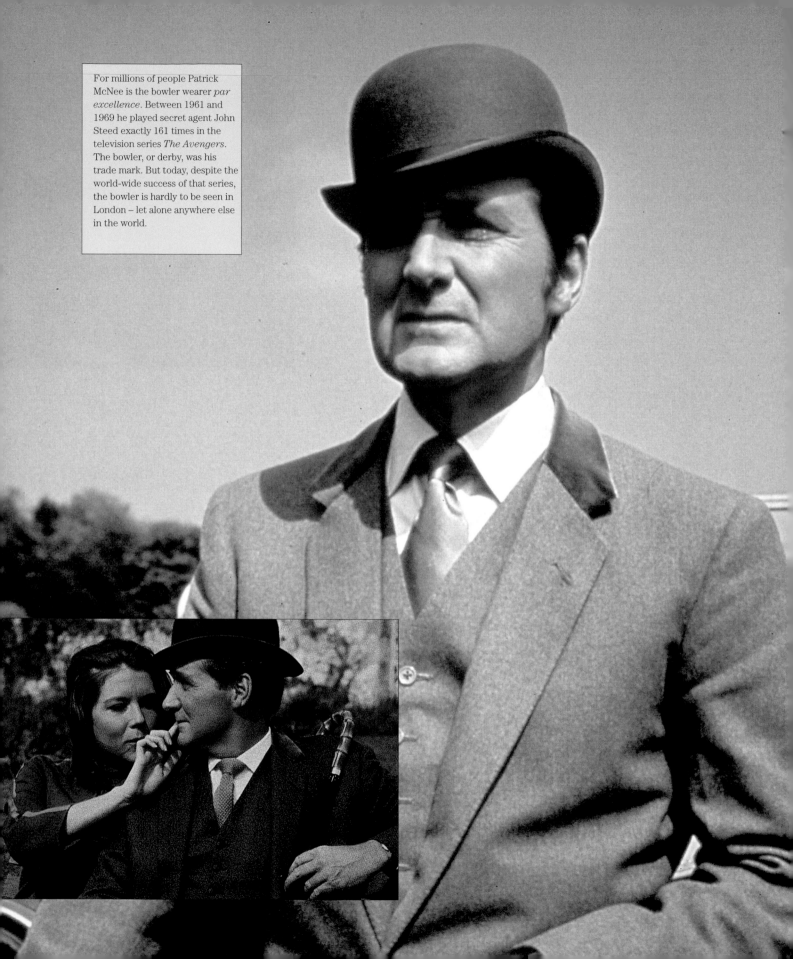

For millions of people Patrick McNee is the bowler wearer *par excellence*. Between 1961 and 1969 he played secret agent John Steed exactly 161 times in the television series *The Avengers*. The bowler, or derby, was his trade mark. But today, despite the world-wide success of that series, the bowler is hardly to be seen in London – let alone anywhere else in the world.

The Bowler

The bowler was designed in the workshop of Lock's, the legendary London hat-makers, on the instructions of a certain William Coke, who wanted to give his gamekeepers headgear that would not keep getting knocked off when they patrolled undergrowth and woodland. And indeed, this little, rigid, dome-shaped hat offers little purchase to obstructions. Initially the new hats were called "coke" in honor of that concerned landowner, not being given the name "bowler" until the firm of Bowler & Son began to make them in 1850 or thereabouts. In America it is known as a "derby." The French call the bowler "chapeau melon," while in German it is a "Melone." Until well into the 1960s the bowler was the unquestioned symbol of London stockbrokers and bankers, but today it is worn only by the Queen's Guards officers as part of their civilian dress. If you see a few men in pinstripe suits and bowlers carrying rolled umbrellas in the vicinity of Wellington Barracks in London, they are probably officers of the Coldstream Guards who have just come off duty. These days stockbrokers are hardly ever to be seen wearing bowlers.

The elegance of the bowler is not obvious at first glance – or, to many an observer, ever. Many people simply find this hat ridiculous, and it certainly does recall American comedians Stan Laurel and Oliver Hardy. But anybody with a feeling for the English style will sooner or later be fascinated by the bowler; it is still, after all, one of England's best-known national clichés – along with the bulldog, Big Ben, and afternoon tea. Should you feel the need to acquire this most English of all English articles of clothing, then do so – you will be buying a true myth. Of course, occasions to wear it outside your own four walls will be few and far between, but every now and then you can take it out of its hat box, put it on and feel like John Steed of *The Avengers* – childish, perhaps, but no less a pleasure for that.

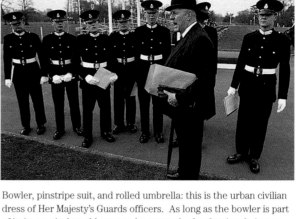

Bowler, pinstripe suit, and rolled umbrella: this is the urban civilian dress of Her Majesty's Guards officers. As long as the bowler is part of it, its survival would seem to be assured – for the time being, at least.

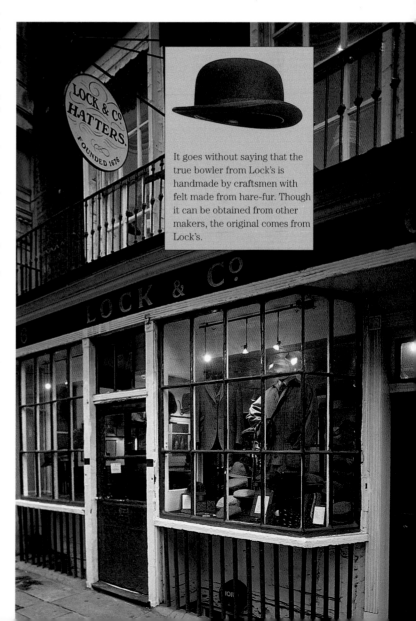

It goes without saying that the true bowler from Lock's is handmade by craftsmen with felt made from hare-fur. Though it can be obtained from other makers, the original comes from Lock's.

Besides the bowler, all the other classic hats are available at 6 St. James's Street, London – custom made, if required. Here the bowler used to be known as the "coke hat" in honor of William Coke, the first man to have one made.

Courage to Wear Hats

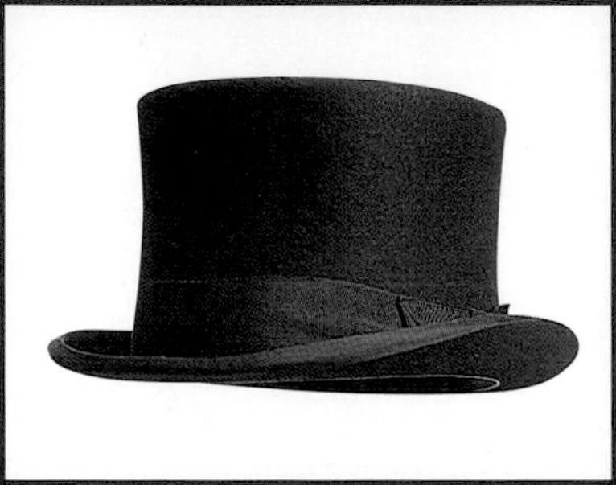

The black top hat is the most formal of all hats. Legend has it that it made its public debut on 15 January 1797 when English hatmaker John Hetherington first wore one in the street. Passersby reacted with horror to his new creation, and Hetherington had to pay a fine for his *démarche*. But this did not mark the end of the top hat's career. In the nineteenth century it was one of the most popular of all hats. Today it is worn only on specially ceremonial occasions, and even then only in combination with morning or evening dress. It takes a certain sense of style to wear to wear a top hat properly, even then.

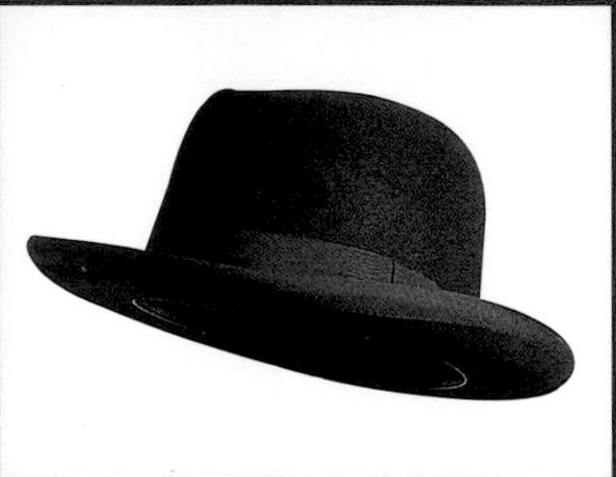

When King Edward VII, still Prince of Wales at the time, was once in the German spa town of Bad Homburg, he discovered a very special hat – the "Homburg" – which was traditionally made there. The style-conscious prince – who was subsequently to pass on his penchant for fashion to his grandson Edward VIII, who in matters of costume was far more famous and meritorious – liked this indigenous hat, and soon he had popularized it throughout Europe. Today the Homburg is second in formality only to the top hat, if we leave the bowler aside as an English specialty.

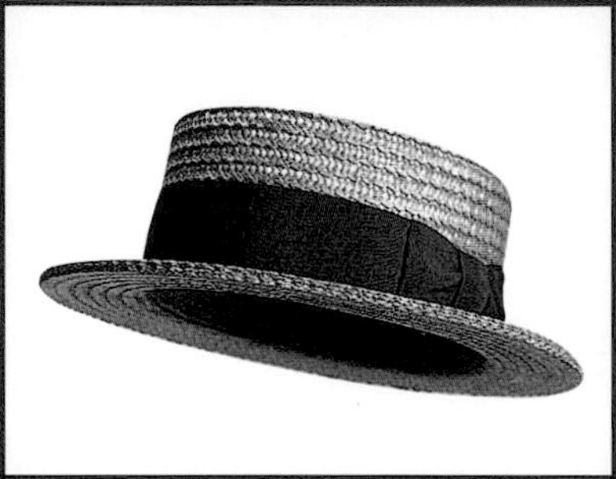

The round, rigid straw hat used to be common in France as the "matelot" or "canotier," in Germany as the "Butterblume" (buttercup) or, less flatteringly, "Kreissäge" (circular saw), and in England as the "boater." Originally the boater or "strat" (short for straw hat) was the favored headgear of English butchers. In the 1920s it began its worldwide progress as a universally popular summer hat. Today it is hardly ever seen except at the traditional English rowing regatta in Henley.

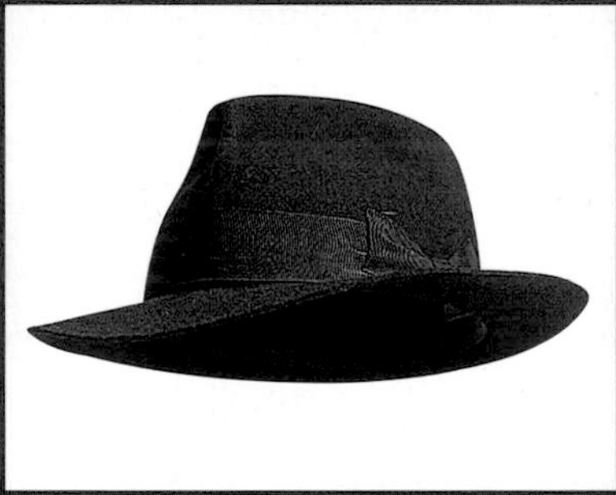

In England it is called the "fedora" or "snap brim," this classic gentleman's hat with the soft brim that can be worn turned up or down. It looks more elegant than the trilby thanks to its somewhat broader brim, but more casual than the bowler or Homburg. Though to most men this is the hat *par excellence*, it is perhaps at the greatest risk of falling into oblivion and extinction. For unlike the bowler, the Homburg, and the trilby, there is no niche in which a fedora can still be worn. The saying that [illegible] longer when [illegible] also applies here.

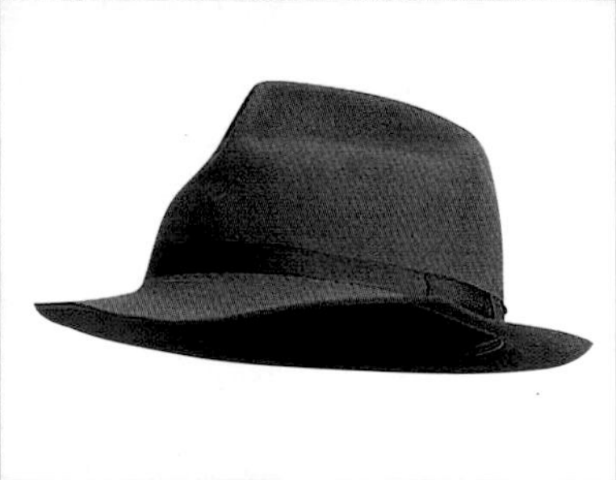

The brown trilby is known throughout the world as the insignia of the horse-racing fraternity. This crumpled brown hat is particularly beloved of the social and financial aristocracy. In England the racecourse would be unthinkable without the trilby, which is just as much a part of it as the tweed suit, the Barbour, and "hunter wellies," the typical green rubber boots of the English upper class. The trilby can be obtained from any English hatmaker who takes a pride in his work. The narrow hatband with the little bow on the left-hand side is typical. It also exists as a handy collapsible hat that will fit in a pocket.

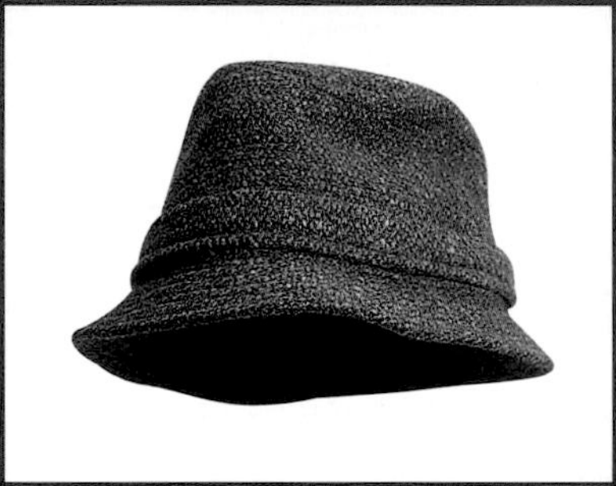

The soft tweed hat may be worn whenever a tweed jacket or suit is appropriate, that is to say at weekends and when traveling. And like all other tweed items, the tweed hat is favored by men of intellect and science, who would not wish either their heads or their thinking to be restricted by rigid hats. The tweed hat goes best with informal but traditional overcoats like the duffel coat, the British Warm, reversible coats with tweed on one side, and Barbours. In colder regions it is the ideal hat for winter wear, and it is popular with those gentlemen who enjoy country sports like shooting or fishing.

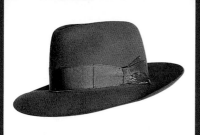

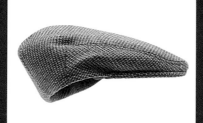

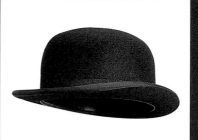

The Borsalino is a make of top-quality... with the reserved grace of those people. Borsalino is one of those... brims turned down even in... favourite styles.

The Homburg... a popular headgear throughout... UK days from Great Britain... the authentic nature... British hat makers... and Sardinia... in the country for shooting, riding or fishing.

The Bowler is now rarely ever worn by... and bankers... the heads of... the Second World War and a range of... regarded as a symbol of conservatism... in the world.

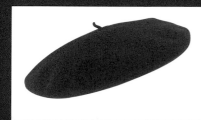

The Basque beret, or the Gauloise cigarette... Short and distinctive. It is favoured more in general use than for elegant gentlemen.

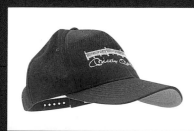

The Baseball cap comes into its own... sports with a brim...

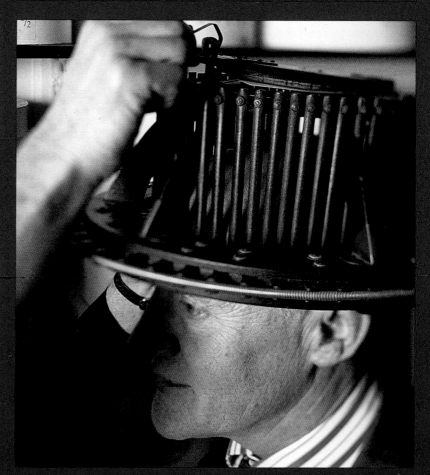

Who Wears Hats?

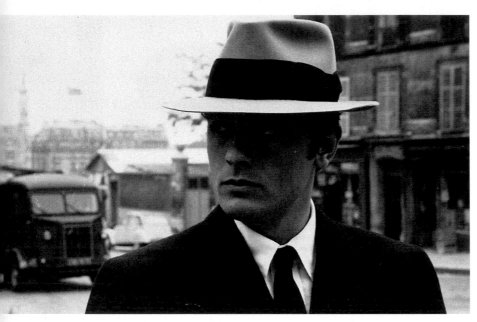

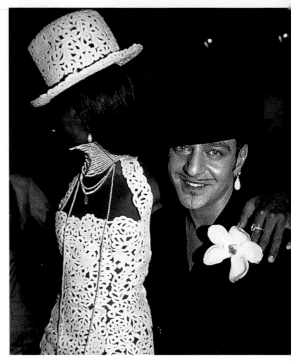

Alain Delon wore hats in many of his films. He is what we might call a professional hat-wearer. We have the cinema and television to thank for the hat's survival in our consciousness.

These days British designer John Galliano usually appears wearing a hat over a headscarf. But this is not taken amiss any more than the couturier's habit of wearing his hat indoors.

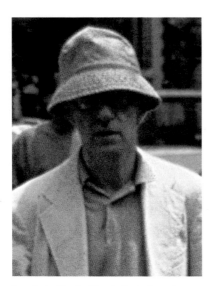

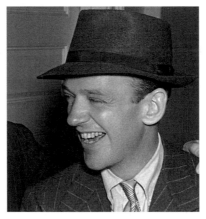

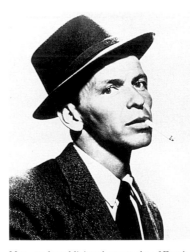

In private Woody Allen is fond of wearing a soft rainhat of the type sold by Brooks Brothers in his native New York, but whether this enables him to remain incognito is debatable.

Fred Astaire is associated with two famous types of hat, the top hat and the "pork-pie hat." The top hat was by way of being part of his working clothes, but he also wore the pork-pie in private. Like many other hat-wearers Fred Astaire had a massively receding hair-line, which in his films he always concealed under a toupee. In private life he often "went topless," preferring to cover his partial baldness with a hat.

Many early publicity photographs of Frank Sinatra show him wearing a hat. When he was starting out this was nothing unusual, for in the 1930s and 40s men wore hats as a matter of course, like overcoats and scarves. In the 1950s the hat more or less became the famous singer's trademark, to which the publicity photo for the film *Pal Joey* undoubtedly contributed.

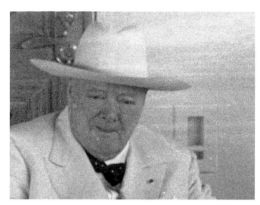

At first there may not be any obvious reason to pick out Winston Churchill as a particular hat-wearer: in his day, after all, hats were worn as a matter of course. But if you study the photographic archives attentively you will immediately be struck by Sir Winston's fondness for adventurous hats. At Chartwell, his country house in Kent, an extensive collection of the most diverse military, official and private headgear has been maintained. His favorites included a Homburg and a stetson, the second of which he mostly wore in private.

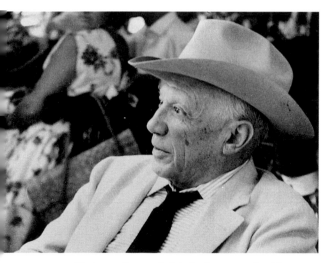

Most men who wear hats today have a penchant for disguise, for by putting something on his head a man can radically change his external appearance: by covering half of the head, after all, the hat masks its characteristic silhouette. As an artist Pablo Picasso stood outside social norms – nobody expected him to look conventional. When he wore a hat it was probably mainly for practical reasons, or perhaps for the fun of dissimulation.

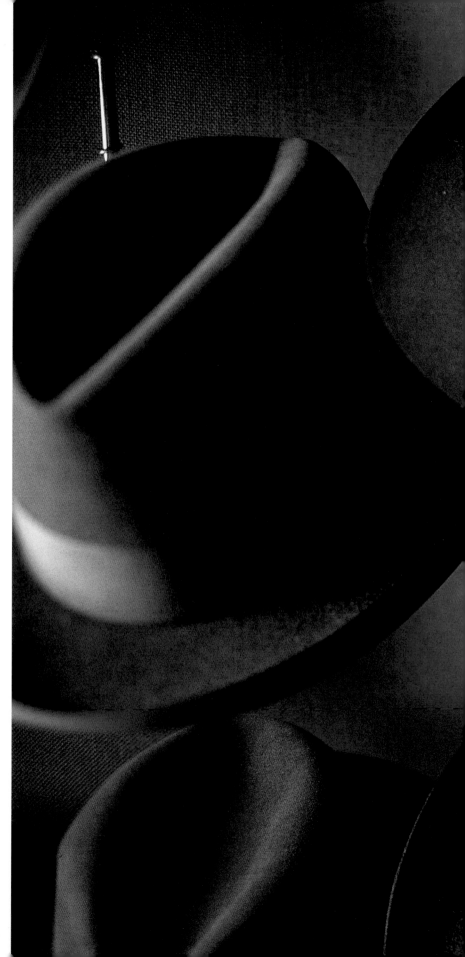

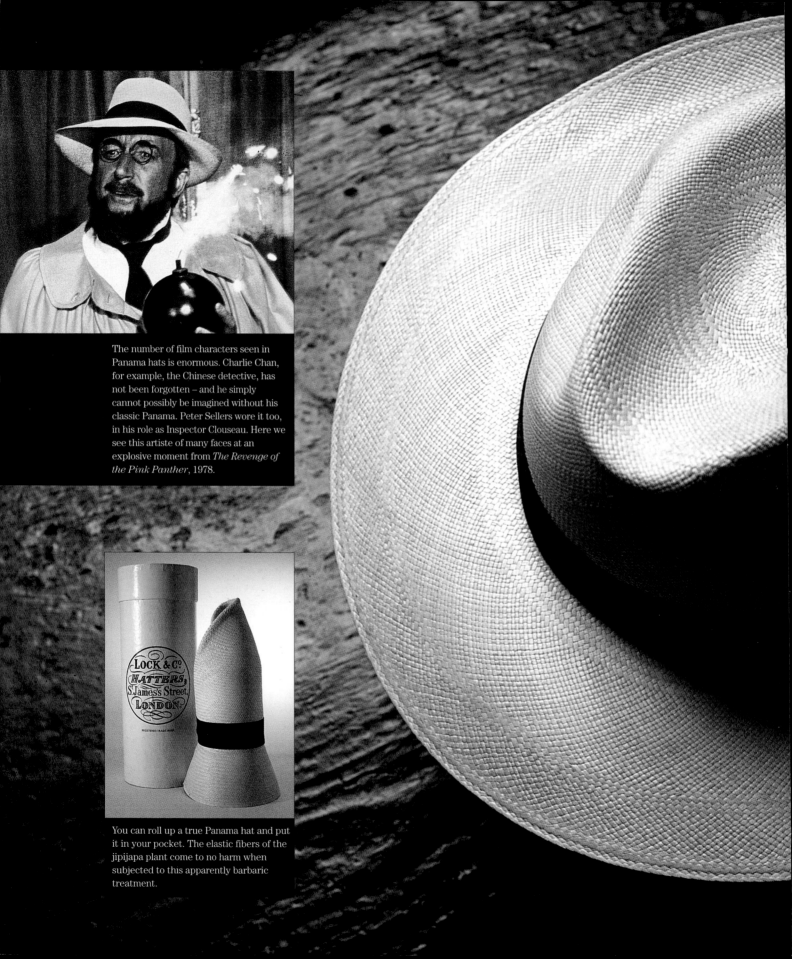

The number of film characters seen in Panama hats is enormous. Charlie Chan, for example, the Chinese detective, has not been forgotten – and he simply cannot possibly be imagined without his classic Panama. Peter Sellers wore it too, in his role as Inspector Clouseau. Here we see this artiste of many faces at an explosive moment from *The Revenge of the Pink Panther*, 1978.

You can roll up a true Panama hat and put it in your pocket. The elastic fibers of the jipijapa plant come to no harm when subjected to this apparently barbaric treatment.

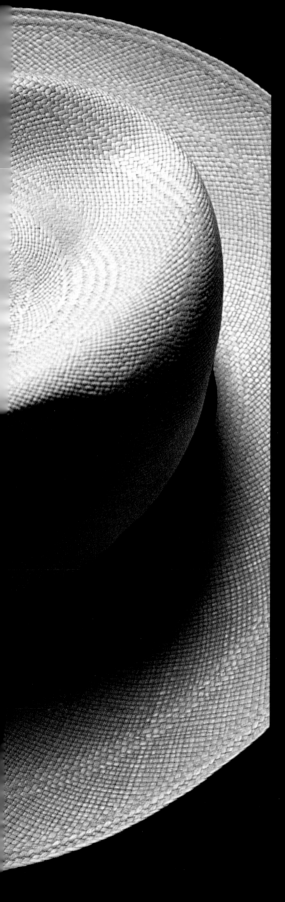

The Panama

One grand entrance is seen every year when the Wimbledon All England Tennis Championships are televised. We are not talking about this or that star in the tennis firmament, but about a hat, large numbers of which protect the spectators" heads from the sun – when it shines, which in England is admittedly not always the case. Perhaps this is why the English are so devoted to the Panama hat; they are not that accustomed to the sun, and they have particularly sensitive skin. It might be assumed from the name that the Panama hat comes from Panama, but actually Ecuador is the home and source of this hat, which is woven from the leaves of the Panama palm (Carludovica palmata, a cultivated plant known as the jipijapa). Still eminently wearable today, this hat presumably got its name when the waterway between the Atlantic and the Pacific was built, when North American engineers and workmen discovered for themselves that it was both light and lightproof. They took it back home with them, where it rapidly became a summer classic. The Europeans, too, quickly came to love the Panama hat. Since it was inseparable from the adventure of building the canal, in the early years it had associations of audacity, almost of frivolity, at any rate of excitement – which clearly set it apart from the European sunhats already in existence, like the traditional Florentine straw hat, for example. We might also describe the Panama hat by means of a metaphor: if headgear were compared with tobacco products, then the Basque beret would be something like a strong, plain cigarette made with black tobacco; the tweed hat, an agreeable pipe; and the Panama hat, a good cigar. And like cigars, the Panama hat is not everybody's cup of tea – but any man with a taste for the unusual will probably grow extremely fond of it. The Panama is also popular with umpires in that quintessentially English sport, cricket. Foreigners, except those from the British Commonwealth, find cricket incomprehensible in many ways and its rules esoteric. But it is certainly a sport for gentlemen, and the Panama hat will always have its place here.

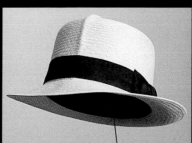

The really classic, original Panama hat has a so-called "optimo crown": this means that the top forms a sort of crest which makes the hat easier to fold up. Some Panama hats have a "flat crown," the shape of which is familiar to us from the "snap brim." Whether you decide in favor of the more traditional or the more conventional version is a matter of taste, but purists prefer the "optimo crown."

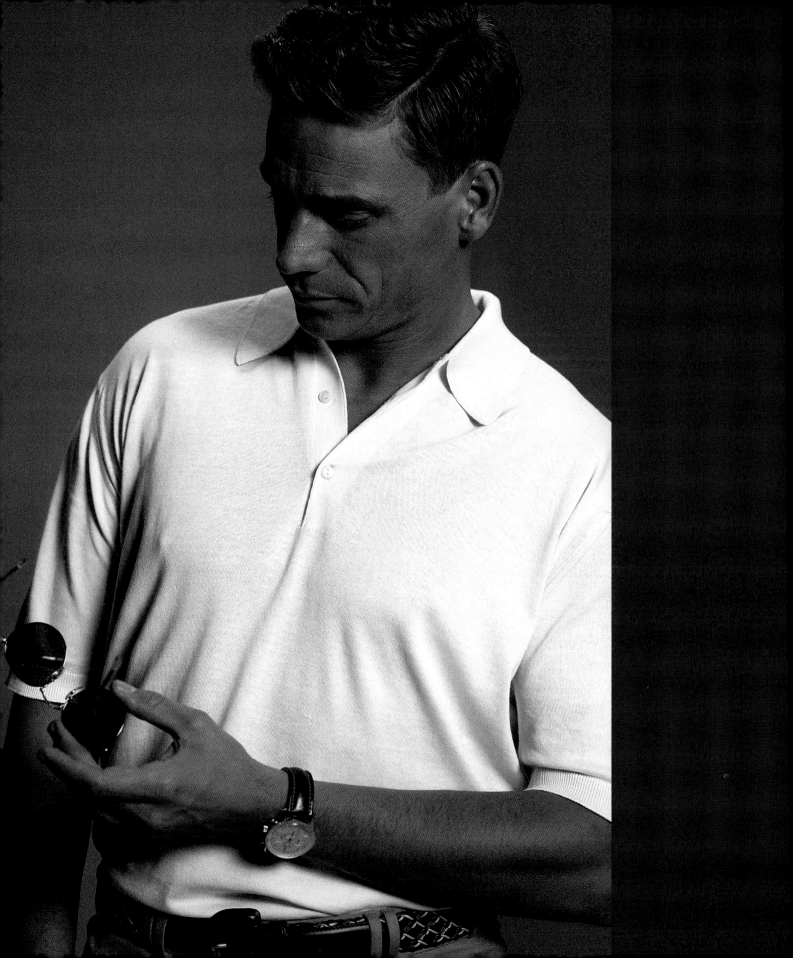

Accessories

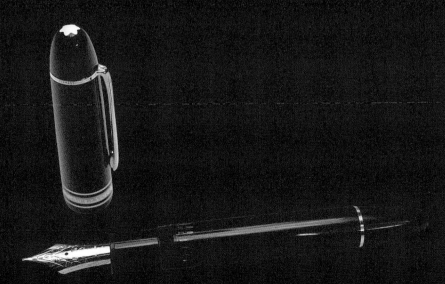

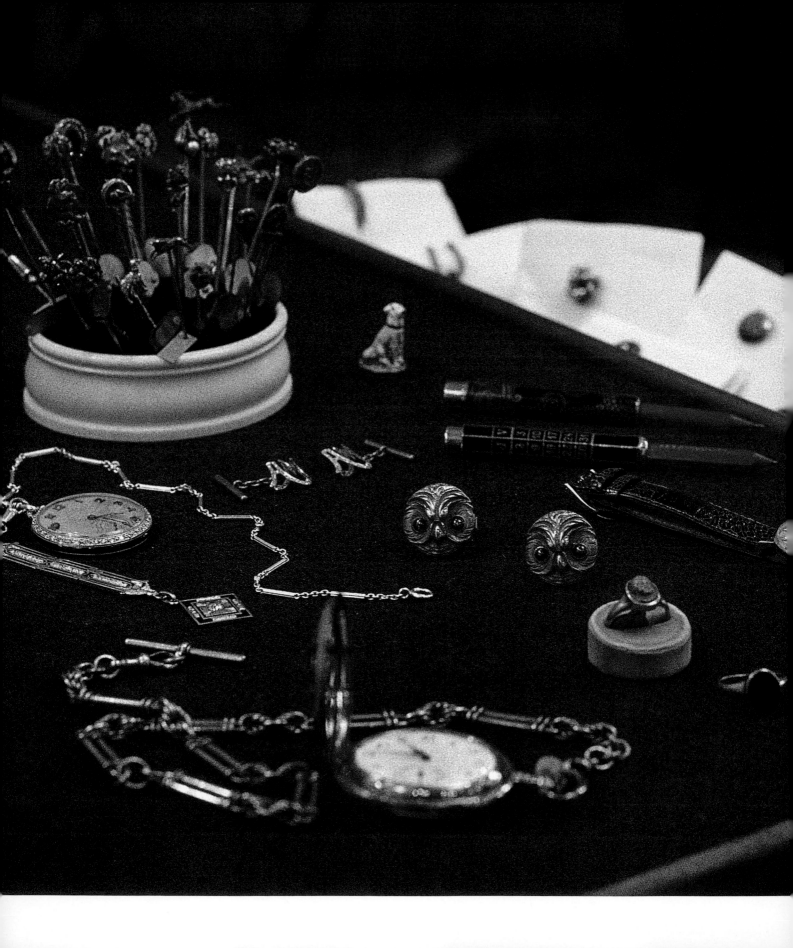

Those little differences

Man does not live from bread alone, and neither does style depend only on clothes. It is the small "minor details," the "accessories," that round off and refine the total look, sometimes even adding a very special and personal touch. We shall be concentrating in this chapter, therefore, on the subject matter of accessories, in other words, those items that are carried around with us, either in the pockets of clothes, directly on the skin, or as a small piece of luggage. They can be useful items like wallet or pocketknife, decorative items like a dress silk handkerchief, or appetizing items, like fine tobacco. These are objects with which we are associated and which enrich our daily lives. It is these very small and apparently minor details that reveal so much information about their owners. This is especially so if the meticulous care devoted to the selection of their clothes leads one to suppose that this same meticulous care went into the selection of their accessories.

In films and literature it is minor details that often serve to define the character of a hero, whether it be a certain cigarette brand that he prefers, the way he arranges his dress handkerchief, or his tendency to fold and clip his currency bills together. You may debate the importance of whether an accessory has been consciously or unconsciously selected, and whether the unconscious selection of an accessory makes a greater statement than a conscious selection does. Yet the total look incorporating the accessory without fail reveals whether it is a consciously planned accent, or more of a coincidence. If, for example, a Belgian living in Brussels smokes the Spanish cigarette brand Ducados, he thereby not only expresses his penchant for the aromatic taste of this type of cigarette, but also an obvious and probably somehow biographically well-founded fondness for the Iberian Peninsula. If a Spaniard smokes Ducados in Spain, he is simply smoking the popular strong cigarette. This is also making a statement, but one which is totally different. And it is not only cigarette brands that make such powerful statements. Small nondescript accessories are often also a focus of interest, because they convey unique regional traits. These can thus also be kept alive, whereas one's clothes are completely subordinate to international style. Irrespective of whether you are in New York, Tokyo, Hong Kong, London, Vienna, Cape Town, or Rio de Janeiro, you will find the same selection of clothes and shoes in expensive shops everywhere. Local specialties are practically of no importance. It is a different matter with the small items. They have stronger associations with our everyday lives, and from time to time express different regional and national preferences or dislikes that have been nurtured by innumerable historical connections.

Accessories are like local cuisine, which courageously holds its own everywhere against so-called international cuisine. It is thus the small minor details that constitute the genuine attraction of a journey – just like typical regional specialties. When we leave our familiar everyday surroundings, we want to experience change and variety in well-calculated measures. The current international style of clothes leaves very little room for national variations; in this connection, it is accessories that therefore often dictate the decisive accent. Those who are familiar with the language of accessories are not only capable of creating a more individual look to this style, but can also interpret more from the outward appearance of those they are confronted with. The attention we devote to the relevant detail will improve our feel for the total look.

Tiepin, watch, cuff links, ring, or writing equipment ought to be selected with the same meticulous care as clothes. This is because the things we use daily not only say a lot about us, but, over and above the fulfilling of their function, are also capable of bringing beauty into our daily lives. In this connection, accessories provide the opportunity for the biggest understatement, even more than suit, shoes, and shirt. After all, apart from you, only the jeweler knows that the tiepin perhaps cost a small fortune. The selection pictured comes from the firm of Peter Pütz in Cologne, the internationally renowned specialist in antique jewelry.

The Everyday Ballast

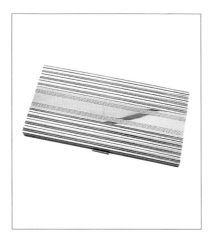

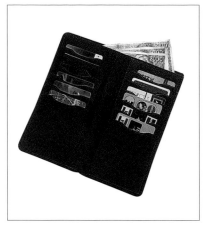

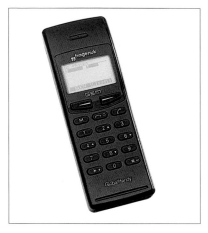

The cigarette case made of precious metal originated at a time when you did not yet buy an entire designer label world together with the associated lifestyle. The sales packaging was formerly considered too plain to carry cigarettes around in or even to proffer cigarettes from. It was preferable to fill the flat case with your daily requirement and leave the plain paper packet at home.

The square wallet is the best place to keep currency bills and credit cards. It is particularly recommended if you predominantly wear jackets with an inside pocket. By contrast, carrying a wallet in the back trouser pocket causes extreme bulkiness and looks comparatively unattractive. Those who do not like wearing jackets in summer or in their free time can make do with a small wallet.

The mobile phone is for many an automatic accessory. Depending on the size of the equipment, it can be carried in the trouser pocket, breast pocket, or, better still, the jacket pocket. A custom tailor will sew a special pocket for it in the jacket. Special holders that you can attach to your belt mostly look rather odd, however, because a mobile phone is an item of practical use that belongs in one of the many pockets of your clothes – like other things too.

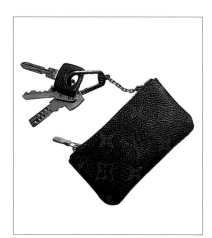

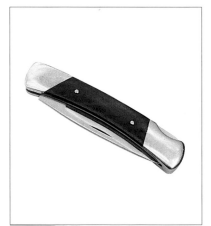

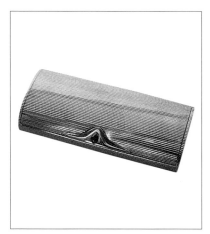

Keys belong in a holder, since otherwise their sharp edges and points can easily damage the lining of trouser or jacket pockets.

A small pocketknife can be put to good use in many situations in life. Depending on its facilities, you can uncork bottles of wine with it, use it as a screwdriver, peel fruit, open packages and letters, or slice salami.

If a large cigarette case is too bulky, you can also carry supplies of your favorite cigarette brand in smaller containers. The model illustrated here comfortably fits inside the trouser pocket due to its oval-shaped cross-section.

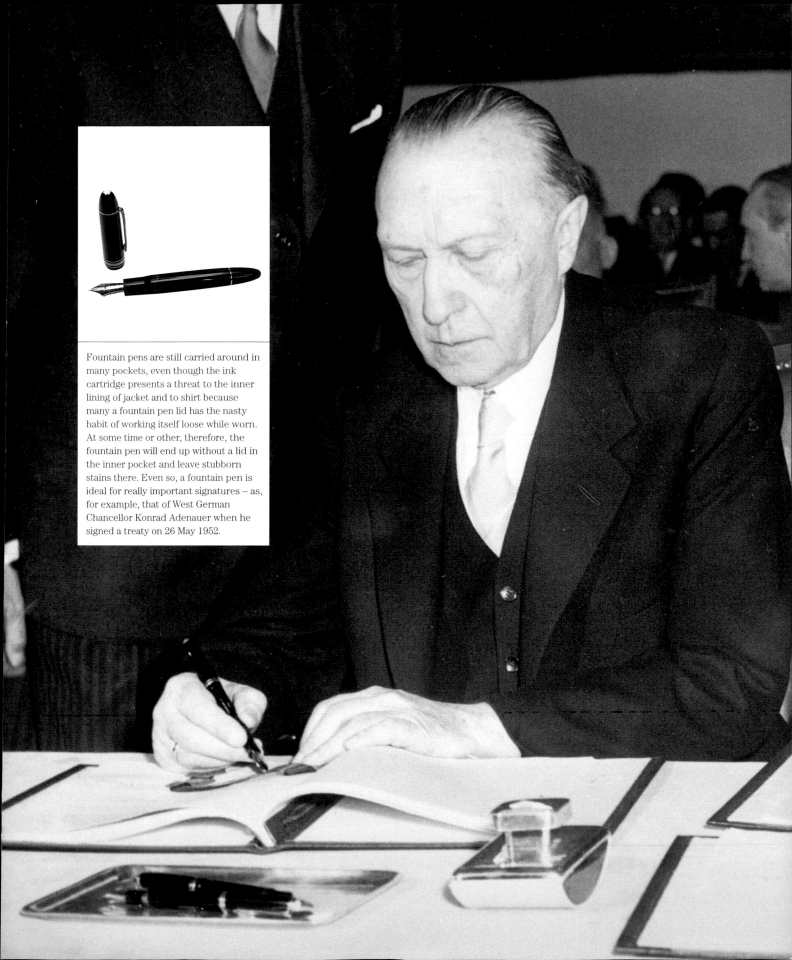

Fountain pens are still carried around in many pockets, even though the ink cartridge presents a threat to the inner lining of jacket and to shirt because many a fountain pen lid has the nasty habit of working itself loose while worn. At some time or other, therefore, the fountain pen will end up without a lid in the inner pocket and leave stubborn stains there. Even so, a fountain pen is ideal for really important signatures – as, for example, that of West German Chancellor Konrad Adenauer when he signed a treaty on 26 May 1952.

One has it – but where?

The way that people carry their ready cash around normally says a great deal about them and their attitude to money. Some arrange their currency bills neatly in a wallet, others tuck them in an unprepossessing bundle in the pocket of their pants; some hide them in the leg of their boots, others reveal how much they have on them with a bill clip. Legend has it that the Rothschilds fold each individual bill twice lengthways. The advantage of this is apparently that it makes you more thrifty with your money. Which branch of the family adopted this quirky idea is not mentioned.

Those who travel a lot often prefer to use a credit card, because it saves the bother of changing money and also provides a certain amount of safety. Nevertheless, despite the benefits, many men reject the card and instead choose the supposedly more substantial feel of ready cash.

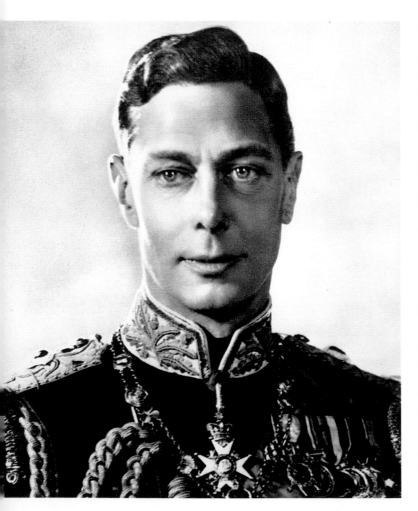

Once upon a time, problems with payment terms and conditions were largely unknown, because gentlemen did not have to settle their bills immediately anyway, but bought on account. For centuries, tailors, shirt-makers, shoemakers, gunsmiths, and saddlers were forced to tolerate this, despite often having to wait a long time for the unpaid invoices to be settled. In addition, being mere craftsmen, they were not in a position to issue reminders to their high-born clientele for payments that were due. Naturally, even today, there are still privileged clients whose invoices are sent discreetly to their home addresses, but the majority of high-born people nowadays have to pay on the spot in terms of the retail trade, before they are allowed to take the goods with them. Similarly, in the case of the ordering of custom-made clothes of any kind, it is usual to pay a deposit at the time the order is accepted – and with justification. It can take half a year or more to complete a suit or custom-made pair of shoes, whereupon payment is due. Nevertheless there are still clients who would be dumbfounded by the request for a small deposit, as though it were an absurd and unreasonable request. This is the situation in which tailor and shoemaker must weigh up the odds of losing a new customer or material. Anyway, in the era of the credit card, the advantage of ready cash is that you can often negotiate price reductions with it, because many business people still prefer the jingling of coins and the rustle of currency bills to plastic. It will therefore always be worth taking some ready cash with you. At the very least, you will need ready cash for possible tips. Apropos tips; it is now common worldwide to tip in dollar bills. Experienced globetrotters always carry a certain amount of American currency with them, so as not to have to fob porters, taxi drivers, head-waiters, or bellboys off with the somewhat lame excuse that they have not yet changed any money. Thus you will not be able to avoid taking a more or less large number of currency bills and coins around with you, whatever their proportions happen to be. There are various possibilities for how to do this, depending on your taste and need for ready cash.

The English monarch traditionally does not carry money around on his (or her) person. This applied to George VI, and it is equally applicable to his daughter, Queen Elizabeth II.

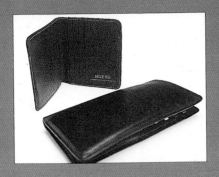

The narrow, rectangular wallet is a classic in terms of money receptacles. Apart from currency bills, you can also keep your credit cards and personal papers in it. It leaves no room for coins, but these you can carry loose in your pocket. If you dislike doing that, you can carry them around in a small coin receptacle.

A currency bill clip can be a very safe way of carrying bills around, depending on the pocket you tuck it in to. It is fairly well protected from the prying fingers of pickpockets in the front pocket of jeans or in other pairs of pants with horizontally cut pockets.

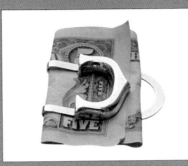

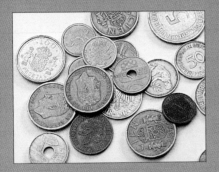

Englishmen love carrying coins around loose in their pockets. This habit is also common in southern Europe, but in northern regions men prefer to carry coins around in a coin receptacle. In the United States a coin really is "small change," since there is already a bill for as little as one dollar.

Small coin and credit card receptacles can be carried around perfectly well in the pockets of pants, and are then fairly safe from the prying fingers of pickpockets.

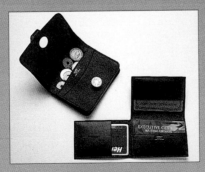

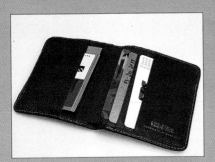

A credit-card holder is useful if the wallet is not provided with compartments for "plastic money." In addition it is advisable to distribute the individual means of payment around the body for safety reasons, in order to prevent total loss of everything in one go in the event of theft.

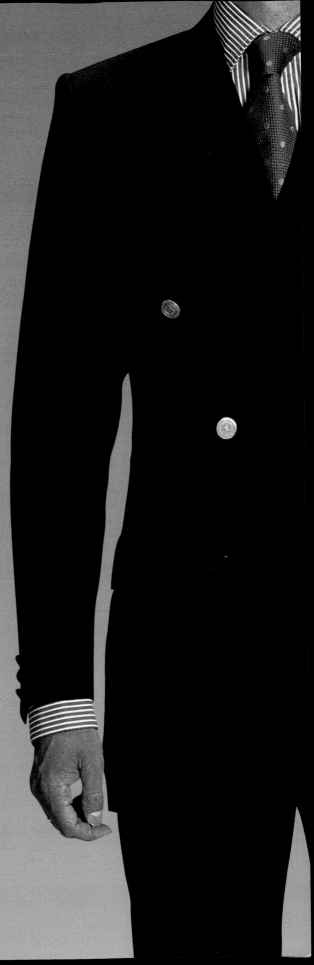

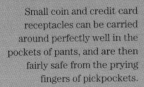

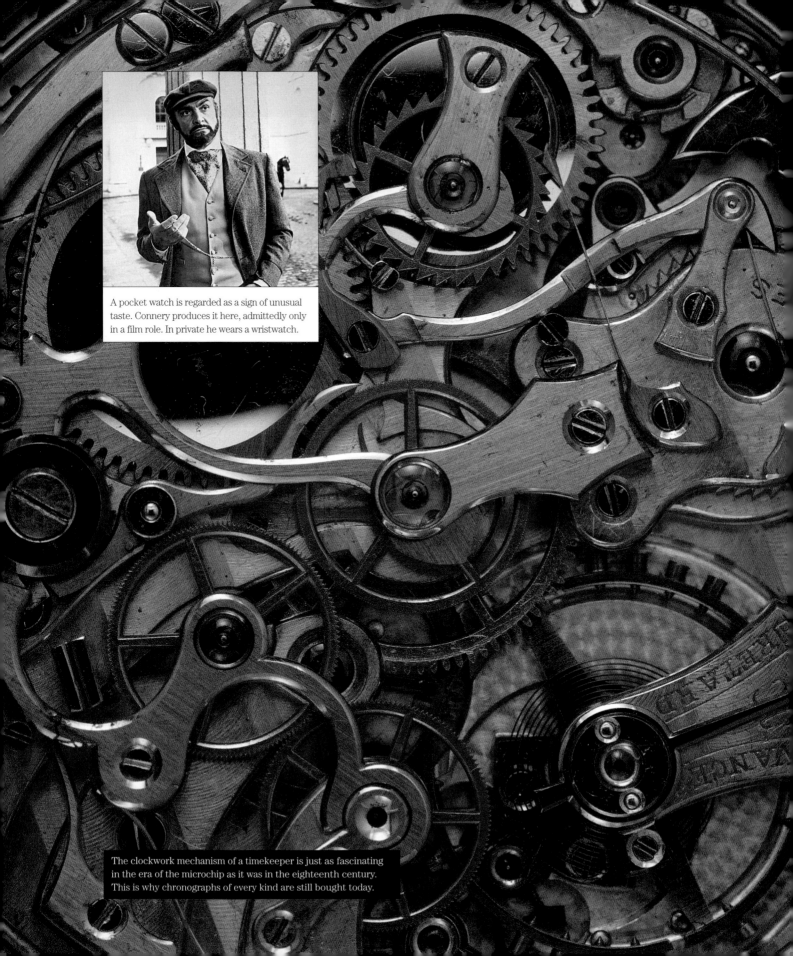

A pocket watch is regarded as a sign of unusual taste. Connery produces it here, admittedly only in a film role. In private he wears a wristwatch.

The clockwork mechanism of a timekeeper is just as fascinating in the era of the microchip as it was in the eighteenth century. This is why chronographs of every kind are still bought today.

What does it tell us?

Anyone wishing to analyze the style of the person opposite should not forget to glance at that person's watch. Like their clothes, it allows you to draw interesting conclusions on that person, provided of course you have a knowledge of current watch models. If not, you can acquire this knowledge within a few months in an extremely enjoyable way by looking in the windows of jewelers' shops, reading one or other book on watches, and talking as often as possible with watch experts and watchmakers. Involvement in this subject mostly ends with the purchase of a corresponding model, because hardly anybody can resist the fascination of a mechanical watch. In this respect it need not cost a small fortune. A few hundred dollars will buy you a good quality mechanical watch, even if it is not a famous make. The choice always depends, though, on what you expect from a watch. Do you prefer a reliable timekeeper that does not depend on a battery and can still be repaired even after decades? Or do you value prestigious items? In the latter case you must decide whom you are wishing to impress with this marvelous mechanism – the broad mass of the populace or the real expert?

The decision for or against a particular watch is often determined by quite personal needs and expectations. Those who need a waterproof sports watch with all kinds of additional features, or at least find it beautiful, will probably end up at the popular well-known models. Those who on no account want to wear their watches in the water, and merely wish to know the time and possibly a date, will primarily veer towards less conspicuous watches. A watch should, of course, also match the owner's style of dress. A very typical sports watch can definitely be worn with predominantly casual clothing. On the other hand, flat, dainty watches look better worn with a dark suit, although many men put on big sports watches in order to create a deliberate contrast to the suit. Owning several watches opens up a whole series of interesting combination possibilities, depending on the clothes and the occasion. Those who wear an elegant but somewhat sensitive watch as their main watch will quite happily fall back on a second robust sports watch for surfing, parachute jumping, or romping around (with the children, the dog, or all together). Whatever watch you choose, it should also suit your build. People with small hands and delicate wrists are not necessarily doing themselves any favors by wearing big professional diver's watches. Furthermore you should consider your own individual skin tone. Some look fantastic wearing stainless steel, white gold, and platinum; yet on others the light-colored metal can look rather pale and insignificant. Yellow and red gold do not look equally attractive on everyone either. The question of which metal should, therefore, not be decided in terms of the price alone. Before you purchase a watch, think also about what other jewelry you wear in the vicinity of the watch – that is, your rings and cuff links. If you are the proud owner of an extensive collection of gold cuff links, you ought perhaps to buy a gold watch too. The more you know about watches, the more you will consciously register what watches your fellow human beings are or are not wearing, whether the motive for buying a watch was the urge to show off, or expertise – or simply even watch collecting. No motive is better or worse

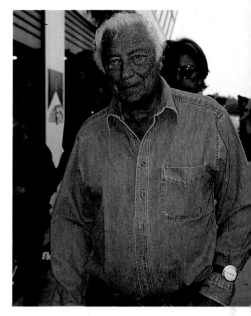

Like many Italians, Gianni Agnelli wears his watch over the cuff of his shirt, presumably to be able to see the watch face comfortably at all times. It would certainly not be to show off his watch. Anyone as rich as he is has no need of demonstrating the extent of his wealth with the aid of a watch.

than any other, and every good watch is still a product of great expertise. Yet it is equally a symbol of style that can be read and interpreted like all other style symbols. Therefore, the purchase of a watch should not necessarily be dependent on fashions or trends, because you will have it around you and on you too long for this purpose. What is crucial is whether the watch suits you and your style – and whether you are in love with the watch. Finally, it must not be forgotten that a watch is a functional object, that ensures that you are not late for important appointments or meetings. It should therefore have a clear face, so that it is easy to tell the time.

The best watches in the world

In 1790 *Abraham-Louis Breguet* invented the shockproof safety device for the storing of watches, and the tourbillon, a device that eliminates the influence of gravity on the accuracy of the watch, in 1795. The latter are merely the most famous of his numerous inventions. Breguet's clientele list reads like a who's who in world history. It included Marie Antoinette, Napoleon Bonaparte, the Duke of Wellington, Arthur Rubinstein, and Sir Winston Churchill, who all owned watches from the famous factory. Even today you can still recognize Breguet watches by the typical "pomme" hands (Breguet hands).

Audemars Piguet is famous for luxury watches with numerous complicated bits – that is, additional mechanisms like stopwatch features, supplementary time zone displays, chiming mechanism, and date or moon phase displays. Since 1972 the flagship model of the firm has been Royal Oak, a characteristic octagonal design that is available in many different variations.

William Baume, already a very successful watchmaker, joined forces with *Paul Mercier* after the First World War. At the start of the 1960s they were joined by Piaget, who brought fresh momentum to the traditional company. Today *Baume & Mercier* are particularly renowned for elegant bejeweled watches.

A pilot's watch by *Breitling* is a well-known prestigious item. The popularity of the label often makes people overlook the fact that Breitling originally became famous through watches that met the high professional standards of aviation. Anyone who is not a pilot is for the most part totally unaware of the possibilities of his Breitling pilot's watch. The famous Navitimer that came onto the market in 1952, apart from displaying the time and date, also displays ascending and descending gradients, and enables determination of fuel consumption and average speed.

The International Watch Co., *IWC* for short, was founded by an American and a Swiss in Schaffhausen in 1868. The American, however, pulled out of the business in 1876. The most famous watch by IWC is without doubt Il Destriero Scafusiae from 1993, the "war-horse of Schaffhausen," a mechanical watch with 750 wheels and a total of 21 features, including chronograph with "Rattrapante" (see page 231), moon phase display, perpetual calendar, and details of year, decade, and century. Only 1,625 copies of this watch have ever been produced.

Watch collectors treasure above all the old mechanical watches with the American make of *Hamilton*. The firm was founded in Lancaster, Pennsylvania, in 1892. Military watches from the Second World War are particularly popular. At that time Hamilton was supplying the armed forces of the United States with pilot's chronographs, marine chronographs, and watches.

If there is a make of watch particularly identifiable with one single model, then it is *Jaeger-LeCoultre*, which is always named in the same breath as the Reverso. The Reverso is a reversible watch; the case is mounted on the base plate in such a way that it can be folded down 180 degrees, thereby protecting the sensitive watch face from shock damage. Thus the Reverso was originally a sports watch that has since become the term for a classically elegant watch.

Apart from the Reverso Jaeger-LeCoultre have other legendary watches in their range, like Memovox, the wristwatch alarm clock, and many different highly complex chronographs.

Longines rank with Breitling as the second biggest label in terms of pilot chronographs. In 1927, flight pioneer Charles Lindbergh had the duration of his flight over the Atlantic timed by a watch from Longines. In the same year, Lindbergh himself designed a special pilot's watch for the Swiss company – the hour angle chronograph.

Cartier have been making watches since 1898. Thus this make, that is synonymous with jewelry, also has a long watch tradition. The Santos was launched in 1908, the Tank in 1919, and the first Pasha was designed in 1932 for the Pasha of Marrakech. The most famous Cartier watch is probably the Panthère, in gold and steel. Many men, however, find Cartier's style too feminine, although if you examine the Santos design closely you will notice it has a somewhat warlike appearance with its screwed on, angular casing, and the modern Tank in steel or gold can be regarded as quite a sports watch.

The *Omega* make of watch has so far not achieved the reputation of the *Rolex* make. Nevertheless, it would be unthinkable to omit Omega from the list of prestigious legendary watches, because when the American Neil Armstrong took his first step on the moon on 21 June 1969, he was wearing a Speedmaster Professional. Since that time, Omega watches have participated in all NASA's space programs.

Besides this, Omega has particularly made a name for itself with diver's watches.

Germany too has contributed in a modest way to the fame of watchmaker craftsmanship through Ferdinand Adolph Lange, for example, son-in-law of the Dresden court watchmaker Gutkaes, who in 1844 set himself up in business in the Saxon glassworks along with 15 journeymen. From this there emerged an extremely successful watch factory that had acquired an excellent reputation by the Second World War. Since the reunification of Germany the firm of *A. Lange & Söhne* has been able to start up again, producing top-quality watches. A typical Lange watch is the patented large-date display.

Patek Philippe has produced no more than approximately 600,000 watches since the founding of the make in 1851. Nevertheless Patek Philippe is synonymous worldwide with supreme craftsmanship. Calatrava, Ellipse, Gondolo, and Nautilus are names that express the entire broad range of the make, and can be elegant, luxurious, and casual.

There is probably no other watch make that is as controversial as *Rolex*, being simultaneously adored and despised. Some reject it because, as every child knows, Rolex is expensive and therefore is an unmistakable object of prestige. Others love this make because of this tag. Rolex has indisputably produced timeless classics, particularly including the first ever waterproof watch in 1926, the Oyster. Its design broke new ground and is still an absolute classic today. The worldwide enduring success of Rolex proves that watch connoisseurs also look beyond the image and see the quality.

Anyone wearing a watch by *TAG Heuer* is mostly also interested in fast two or four wheelers. There is hardly another manufacturer today that has such close links with motor sports. The make was founded in 1840 by Edouard Heuer and acquired by the TAG (Techniques D'Avant-garde) Group in 1985. TAG Heuer does not have the same prestige as Rolex and is not as well known as Omega or Breitling, yet the design of these watches is unmistakable.

Zenith became famous particularly as a result of their chronograph El Primero, although the watch factory had already collected hundreds of awards by the time of the launch of El Primero in 1969. The watch mechanism of El Primero is an absolute pièce de résistance of Swiss watchmaker craftsmanship and is an established classic.

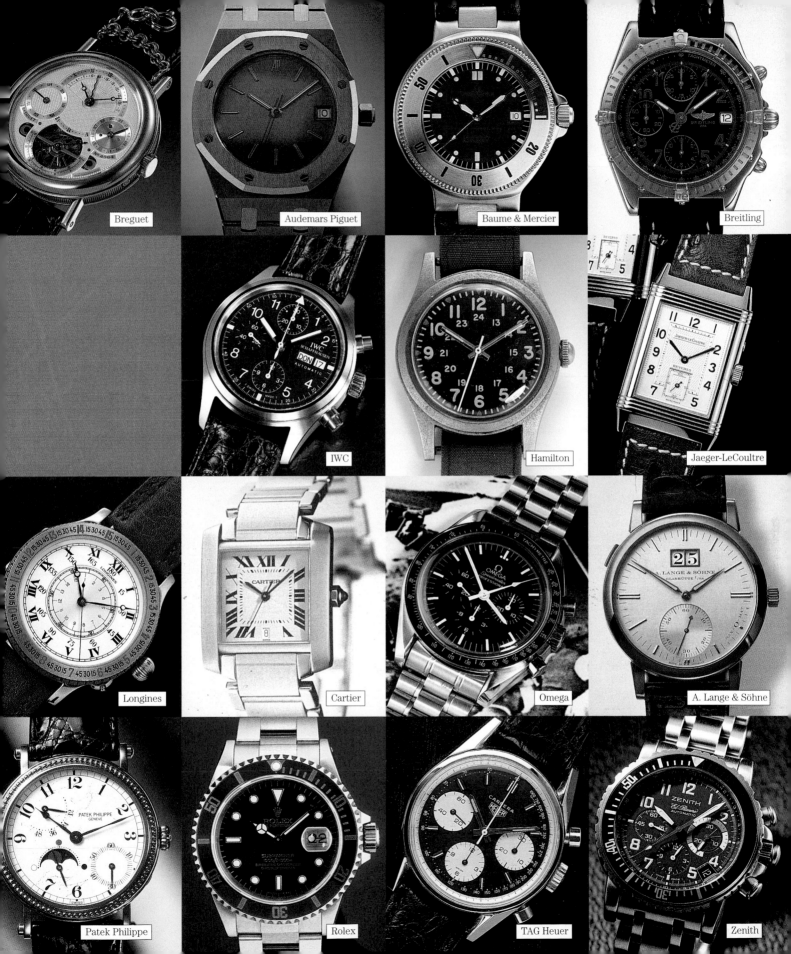

Breguet

Audemars Piguet

Baume & Mercier

Breitling

IWC

Hamilton

Jaeger-LeCoultre

Longines

Cartier

Omega

A. Lange & Söhne

Patek Philippe

Rolex

TAG Heuer

Zenith

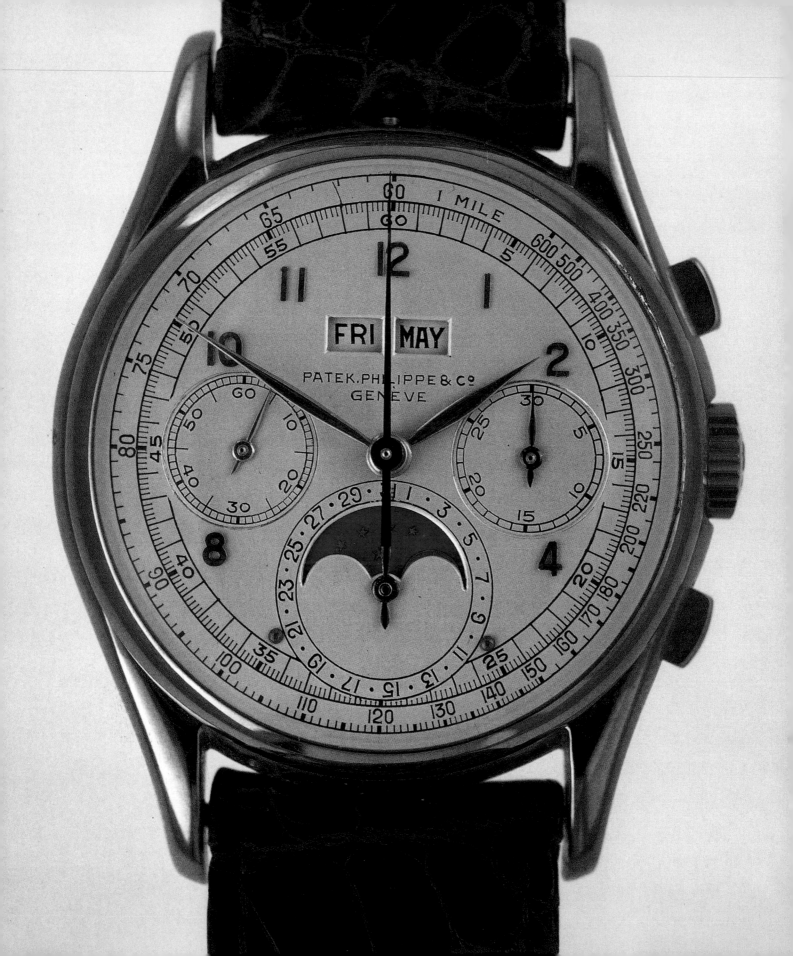

All About the Watch

Automatic movement
A watch with automatic rewind. Arm movements cause a rotating part that rewinds the mainspring of the watch to rotate. An automatic movement watch is also called a self-winding watch.

Barrel
The barrel contains the mainspring that is curled in it like an endless screw. The mainspring stores the energy that is necessary for the operation of the mechanical watch. The mainspring is wound manually or indirectly by a rotating part (see **Automatic movement**).

Cabochon
A highly polished, unfaceted gem for decorating the dial or winder button.

Chronograph
A wristwatch or pocket watch with an additional stopwatch mechanism.

Chronometer
An extremely precise watch that is finely attuned to different locations and temperatures and for which an official watch certificate has been issued.

Complication
Additional features to the watch mechanism like chronograph, second time zone display, chiming mechanism, or calendars. Also the term for a watch with one or several of these additional features. A watch with several complications is also termed "Grande Complication."

Diver's watch
Diver's watches must not only be absolutely waterproof, but also withstand water pressure. Casing, winder button, glass, and base must therefore be particularly stable. The revolving ring for measurement of the diving time can only be adjusted in one direction, so that the diving sequence can never turn out to be too long, or if necessary too short, if the ring is inadvertently altered.

ETA
Biggest Swiss manufacturer of watch mechanisms. ETA mechanisms are inserted in many Swiss makes of watches. The very famous and very expensive manufacturers, however, use their own mechanisms.

Jewel
A jewel in a watch is a synthetically produced gem that is used in the watch mechanism as a pallet jewel and wheel bearing to minimize friction and wear. The more jewels there are used in a watch mechanism, the better the quality.

Lunette
Circular glass covering or decorative ring, sometimes revolving, that fits on top of the casing.

Manual rewind
A watch whose spring is tightened by using the rewinder button.

Mechanical watch
Watch in which the working mechanism is stored by means of a mainspring. Rewinding is manual or occurs automatically by means of a rotating part.

Mineral glass
Mineral, mostly flat watch glass, that is harder and more scratchproof than plastic glass.

Minute repetition
The most complex complication. A system whereby the alarm can be triggered by a push button or lever. Famous manufacturers of these watches are Audemars Piguet and Patek Philippe.

Moon phase display
Display of the moon cycle by means of a usually dark blue disk that is turned by the hand mechanism under the dial.

Perpetual calendar
Calendar that takes into account the length of month, and leap years.

Power reserve
Running time of the clock after it has been rewound. The power reserve can be as much as 50 hours, which preserves automatic movement watches from undesirable stoppages and loss of time in the event of long, motionless intervals by the wearer.

Rattrapante – perpetual equation of time
An additional second-hand or trailing "delayed" hand that moves independently from the first. Chronographs with Rattrapante enable simultaneous measurement of two different times for one and the same event.

Sapphire glass
Watch glass made of synthetic sapphire. Due to its hardness it is extremely scratchproof, but it can shatter.

Screw base
Base fitted with a screw thread is screwed into the watch casing.

Screw button
Button that is screwed in to make the watch more airtight in terms of dirt and above all more watertight. Before you can set the watch, you have to unscrew the button. This is typical of diver's watches and sports watches.

Sealing ring
Waterproof watches are mostly fitted with sealing rings on the casing base, glass, and button.

Small second-hand
Second-hand display that does not stem from the center of the dial.

Waterproof
In terms of diver's watches, the diving depth to which the watch is waterproof is indicated on the dial, often in feet and meters. This detail is unique in that it is really reliable, even if there are no operating instructions for the watch. Always comply with the manufacturer's details and have the waterproof aspect regularly checked. You must be especially careful with second-hand watches. Incidentally, Rolex applied for the first patent for a waterproof watch in 1926.

Winder
A shaft with a button at its outer end, with which we wind up or set the watch. The winder is the link to the watch mechanism.

Less is More

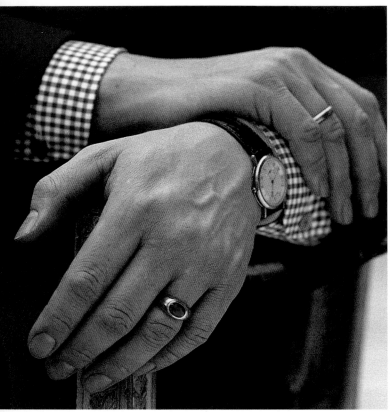

Watch and cuff links are simultaneously jewelry and a necessity. Furthermore, a gentleman will wear at most two types of ring in addition to his wedding ring – one with his family coat of arms and one with a beautiful stone.

The times are long gone when men wore rich jewelry. Some regret this – others do not! On the other hand, anyone who feels the need for the fairly visible wearing of precious metal or valuable stones on his fingers, around his neck, or on his arm, only has a few possibilities for doing this. In this connection, we are going to start by mentioning pieces of jewelry that are worn directly on the body. Cuff links are not included among these, since they are attached to the shirt.

The list of precious objects that can be worn by a gentleman is short. On the one hand there is the gold neck-chain that very many men wear. It can be seen predominantly in southern climes, though this is not necessarily attributable to the fact that gold neck-chains are actually more popular with Italians or Spaniards than they are with British, Austrian, or Hungarian men. The reason is partly that those who live on the Mediterranean simply have more opportunity to

be seen in casual clothes, or even swimwear, thus revealing the jewelry around their necks. With northern Europeans, the jewelry around their necks tends to remain concealed beneath their shirt collars. There is really little more to say about the gold chain. It is an extremely personal item, that goes beyond a matter of taste, yet mostly no one sees it except for the wearer himself, apart from companions, doctors, or fellow users of saunas, steam baths, or swimming pools. Openly displaying a gold neck-chain undoubtedly is somewhat dubious. This depends of course on whether we are talking about a chain that is mostly worn concealed and that makes short appearances – for example, when swimming on holiday – or whether it is one that is always worn in a deliberately open way. The former is acceptable, but beware of the latter, because the only items of jewelry that a man can wear, if he wants to be on the safe side stylewise, are his rings and watch. In this connection, the latter does not necessarily have to be regarded as an item of jewelry.

There is a manageable number and type of wearable rings intended for gentlemen. The most common is the gold wedding ring that is made in either red gold or yellow gold, depending on regional taste. It is worn on the ring finger of either the left or the right hand, again depending on the country and the custom. Avoid any ring with an eccentric design; the plain shape with a semicircular cross section is still the most timeless and best choice always. Anyone who is married and also wears a wedding ring has already used up one-third of the possibilities, because then a gentleman should only wear two other rings at the most. Those who own or have inherited a ring with the family coat of arms either wear this on the ring finger without the wedding ring, or on the little finger of the hand without the wedding ring. Rings with the family coat of arms always make a very aristocratic impact, though imaginative family coat of arms or initials are no real substitute for the ring of an ancient noble family. Be a proud citizen and do not attempt to add an aristocratic touch with the aid of signet or family coat of arms rings that you have bought. Either you are or you are not of noble lineage; it is not commendable if you are; it is no disgrace if you are not. To pretend to be noble shows very little taste, but if you own a family coat of arms ring, this is then a beautiful and very wearable piece of jewelry for a man, just like the wedding ring. In this way your hands are complete in terms of jewelry; it is hardly likely that you will want to wear any other rings. If you do, then choose one or two plain classic rings at the most. Anyone wearing a reasonably sized family coat of arms ring may possibly wear another ring below it. Those who generally like wearing a ring on the small finger will perhaps, at some time, want to add a second one. At any rate, it is advisable to concentrate jewelry on one finger rather than adorning two or three fingers of one hand with rings, since this often looks overloaded.

A timeless supplementary ring is the three-in-one "Trinity" ring by Cartier. It consists of three intertwined rings fused together in white gold, yellow gold, and red gold, symbolizing friendship (white gold), faithfulness (yellow gold), and love (red gold). This absolute classic is also preferably worn on the little finger. Also by Cartier is the "Bague love" (love ring) that looks good worn below the "Trinity" ring on the little finger. Its design is inspired by a bracelet that was launched in 1970; a design with small screws that we are already familiar with from the "Santos," one of the most famous Cartier watches. The "Bracelet love" (love bracelet) can only be opened and closed with the aid of a small screwdriver. Both bracelet and ring are worn as symbols of eternal love. Many a man also wears a diamond ring on his little finger. Wedding rings or rings with family coat of arms are not really worn for aesthetic reasons, they are primarily symbols or emblems. Therefore, anyone who wants consciously to wear jewelry needs additional rings, like a diamond ring, though rings for men should always be selected with great care; a man's hand adorned with rings can very quickly look very feminine. Anyone who likes buying jewelry should do this for the woman in his life.

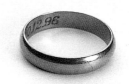

The wedding ring should be of the plainest possible design. A bejeweled ring is worn for preference as proof of unusual taste.

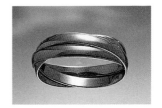

The "Trinity" is an original design by Cartier; its three types of gold symbolize friendship, faithfulness, and love. Connoisseurs choose it as an engagement ring.

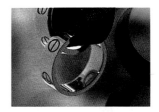

The "Bague love" (love ring) by Cartier is the lovers' ring. Its design is inspired by the classic "Santos" watch. There is also a matching bracelet in the same style.

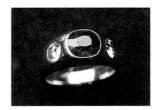

A diamond ring is a gain for both the wearer and his opposite number. After all, hands are almost permanently on view. A ring with a stone is thus a good choice.

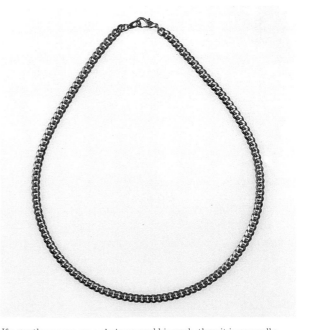

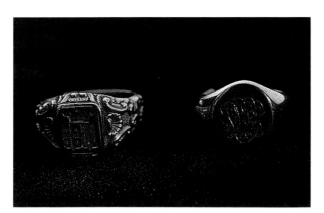

The family coat of arms ring is mostly worn by members of the aristocracy. The signet ring is distinct from the simple ring with initials in that the letters appear as a mirror image.

If a gentleman wears a chain around his neck, then it is normally under his collar and invisible. In southern climes it is sometimes adorned with a cross and perhaps a memento like a lucky charm.

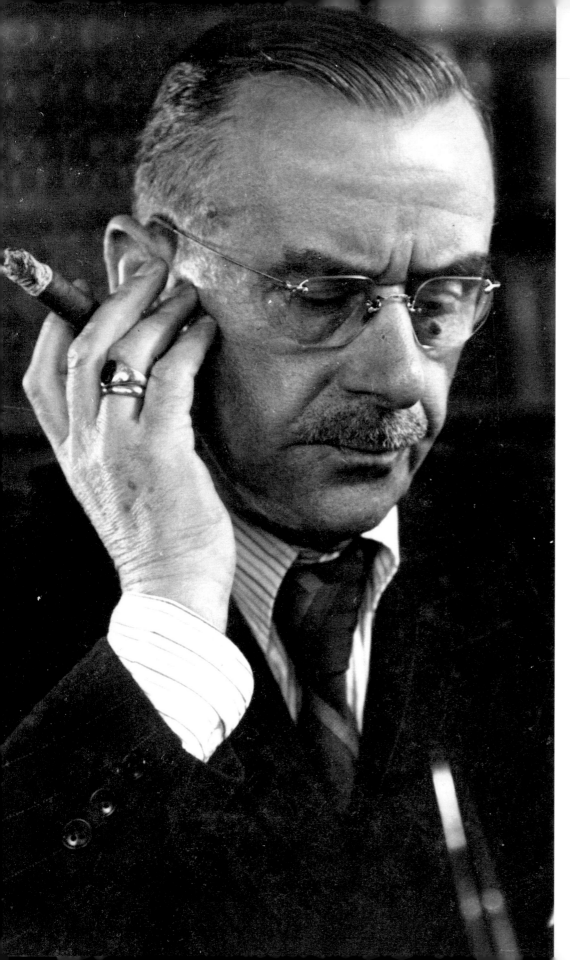

Thomas Mann describes the pure bliss of dabbling in tobacco at many points in his works. Here is a sample quote from *The Magic Mountain*, where he has the hero, Hans Castorp, saying: "I can't understand how some people don't smoke. They are rejecting, as it were, one of life's best parts, and certainly something that gives utmost pleasure." In this way the Nobel prizewinner also revealed his own opinion, because Thomas Mann himself had smoked cigars and cigarettes since his early youth.

Preface to Tobacco

Very few people can resist the fascination associated with cigarettes, cigars or pipes, and practically everyone has, at some time or other, made an attempt to savor and enjoy tobacco to the full. Who can forget the first surreptitious cigarette, the first tentative drags, and the disappointment of only minor enjoyment? Who can forget the excitement of the purchase of the first packet of your own cigarettes – for many the first step towards many years or a lifetime of this habit and passion? Smoking usually starts with accepting cigarettes from other smokers, until you reach the point where you are overcome with a feeling of decency about not unduly exploiting the generosity of your fellow human being. It is then that you buy your own first packet of cigarettes. Opening the packet, you enjoy the first view of the wonderfully white and pure tobacco roll that seems to have been untouched by human hand. Carefully you draw out a cigarette, place it clumsily between your lips, and light it in a fairly deft way. It takes years before your movements acquire that sureness with which long-serving smokers handle their cigarettes. However, when the beginner smokes his first own cigarette, he looks furtively around to see whether his "skilled" tobacco friends have noticed that he is not smoking "correctly." They would presumably notice if it were worthy of attention; however, it does not interest them. They smoke in peace and do not want to be disturbed. These feelings on the part of the newcomer to tobacco resemble those you feel when wearing a pair of really good shoes for the first time, or at the moment you step out into the street for the first time in a custom-made suit. You are afraid of somehow betraying the fact that you have only "belonged" since a short while ago, yet simultaneously you would like to share the feeling with others and be admired.

There are, of course, people who can gain absolutely nothing from tobacco. They are either envied or pitied by smokers, though doubtless their inherited sobriety will protect these fellow men from the disadvantages and ridicule that may be attached to tobacco enjoyment. But perhaps those who are immune to tobacco, and are oblivious to its appeal, may be missing a certain amount of enjoyment. What has driven millions of people for centuries to light up the dried and fermented leaves of the tobacco plant, and take pleasure in smoking them, must involve some kind of pleasure. Sir Walter Raleigh, the English explorer and admiral, and his crew introduced tobacco smoking into Europe in 1587. The plant acquired its Latin name of *Nicotiana* from Jean Nicot de Villemin, the French Ambassador at the Portuguese court, who takes the credit for having brought the first tobacco plant seeds to the French court. Whereas tobacco was initially used in France as a medicinal plant, and appropriate experiments were carried out to determine its healing effects, the English, thanks to Sir Walter, used it right from the start as a stimulant and smoked it in their pipes. Those who are interested can find out more details about the origin, content, and cultivation of tobacco elsewhere; we are concentrating here on the processing of the plant. The harvested leaves are dried in different ways. Before they can be smoked with relish, however, they have to be fermented. For this purpose, every element of the tobacco that would smell unpleasant and taste bitter when smoked is destroyed. The dried and fermented raw tobacco product is cut and roasted to remove surplus moisture. The consumer cigarette or pipe tobacco finally emerges during the last stage of blending of different sorts and adding of aromatic tobaccos. The skill of blending is a matter for tobacco manufacturers who have managed to maintain the constant taste of the tobacco brand over many years and despite changeable harvests – a difficult task, similar to producing a constant-tasting wine.

What is it that produces the very special effect of the tobacco? It is primarily nicotine. Pure nicotine is a dangerous poison, but in the diluted form in which the smoker encounters it, it acts as a stimulant. Nevertheless, people who are not used to tobacco can experience the sensation of feeling unwell, even with a comparatively small dose. They can and must get rid of this sensation if they want to become smokers. Most succeed in this and are drawn into a world devoted to tobacco consumption. Like other pleasures, enjoyment of smoking is relative, and assessed in highly different ways. It is left to the individual to decide how essential he regards this consumption for himself and his life. Perhaps one of the greatest pleasures of smoking is its social aspect. There is nothing better than enjoying a smoke with amiable companions.

The Cigarette

The cigarette was originally nothing more than a by-product. Left-over tobacco remains from cigar production were rolled in paper and smoked. This presumably first happened in Spain, where the first cigarette factory was founded in 1784 in Seville. This early form of the present-day cigarette spread from Spain to Portugal and France, and then as far as Russia and Turkey. However, it was not until French, English, and Turkish soldiers joined forces and went into battle against the Russians in the Crimean War from 1853 to 1856 that the triumphant progress of the cigarette began. What soldiers had learnt from their Russian enemies and appreciated, they were not prepared to do without at home.

Therefore, merchants from London and Paris started to import cigarettes from St. Petersburg, Moscow, and Constantinople. Admittedly, they were at that time still real luxury goods, since they were handmade at the rate of only 120 to 150 cigarettes per hour. Not until the invention of the cigarette machine did mass distribution of the cigarette become 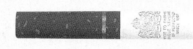 possible. Presented at the World Exhibition in Paris in 1867, this machine produced a minimum of 3,600 cigarettes per hour. This was enormous progress at that time, though compared with current machines this vintage machine is rather slow. Modern cigarette machines produce between 8,000 and 10,000 cigarettes per minute – that is, 480,000 to 600,000 cigarettes per hour. The history of many cigarette brands can be traced back to the early days of the cigarette. We have singled out just three examples here. In 1847, Philip Morris founded a business in Bond Street, London, for the

import and sale of cigarettes, and thus paved the way for a global operation. In 1890, the Ukraine-born Louis Rothman opened his first cigarette store at 55a Fleet Street, London, never suspecting that a cigarette bearing his name would today become one of the most famous brands of all times. Our third example goes by the name of José Joaquin Carreras. He was the son of a Spaniard living in exile in London. He moved into business premises in Leicester Square in 1852 and quickly earned a reputation as a tobacco blender. His special Earl of Craven blend later became the famous Craven A cigarette brand. These three gentlemen alone were responsible for numerous tobacco creations – whose names, such as Marlboro, Rothmans King Size, and Pall Mall – are music to the ears of passionate smokers. Even non-smokers can hardly resist the special fascination of these traditional brands. Perhaps that can be attributed to the fact that the cigarette packaging is often a masterpiece in terms of graphic design: small, colorful packets enticing and tempting you to touch and buy. Furthermore, it is without doubt the sound of these names that imparts a note of adventure, worldliness, or elegance, depending on the brand. Personal preference for a particular cigarette brand actually has very much to do with these brand names that are to some extent synonymous with a certain lifestyle. Rothmans promise classical English elegance; Gauloises promise an earthy enjoyment à la French farmhouse pâté or simple but good vin de pays. Lucky Strike, Camel, and Marlboro make us think of America, though, admittedly, an America that only exists in the imaginations of Europeans – a land of cowboys, Cadillacs, and rock 'n' roll. These associations have largely turned Marlboro into the most successful cigarette in the world, even though Marlboro is actually a totally English name, as proved by the original spelling of

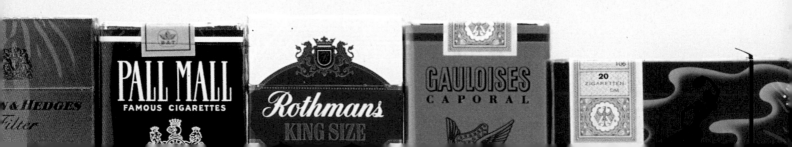

the brand. At Philip Morris in Bond Street they were still referred to as Marlborough in 1885 and the spelling was not Americanized until as late as 1924.

Apart from the name, the type of tobacco also determines one's preference for a particular brand. Cigarette fans can accordingly be divided up into those who prefer dark tobacco and those who prefer light tobacco. Examples of dark tobacco brands are Gauloises Caporal, Gitanes, Ducados, Bastos, and Roth-Händle. Examples of light or blond tobacco are most other brands, like Camel, Lucky Strike, or Chesterfield. The only exceptions are oriental cigarettes that have their own type of taste. Their popularity has sharply declined, although until the Second World War they were extremely popular. One of the best oriental brands is Finas by the Kyriazi Company. For smokers, the question of dark or light tobacco is basically similar to that of car drivers deciding between a diesel or petrol engine. Fans of dark tobacco cigarettes find light brands insipid and limp; on the other hand, smokers of blond tobacco can hardly bear the smell of dark tobacco Gauloises or Ducados cigarettes.

There is a similar basic difference of opinions in terms of filter cigarettes and light cigarettes. The only guide here is personal preference. Beginners should simply try both, but here is a word of warning about experimenting with non-filter cigarettes. You can familiarize yourself with the taste of dark tobacco by trying Gauloises Caporal filtre or the Spanish Ducados. Try out the pure taste very cautiously later – you may find you actually enjoy it better than the filter cigarette. However, as already mentioned, it is a matter of taste.

The many internationally known brands mentioned here are not, of course, the only brands available. Many countries produce their own popular cigarettes, of varying quality.

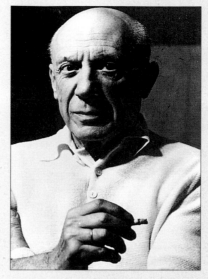

Pablo Picasso smoked throughout his whole adult life – his choice included Gauloises.

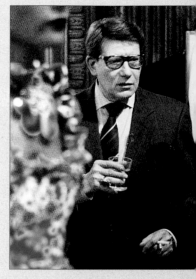

Yves Saint Laurent is a famous and elegant smoker.

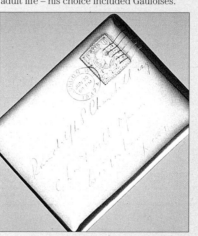

Sir Winston Churchill had a solid gold cigarette case made for his son Randolph by Cartier in 1932. In case his absent-minded son left it anywhere, the lid was designed like an addressed envelope. Anyone finding it would, therefore, have no trouble in handing back the valuable item.

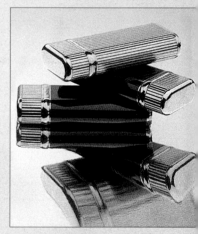

Dunhill, Dupont, and Cartier lighters are welcome presents for smokers, but can be repeated, so the proud owner may come across one exactly like his own.

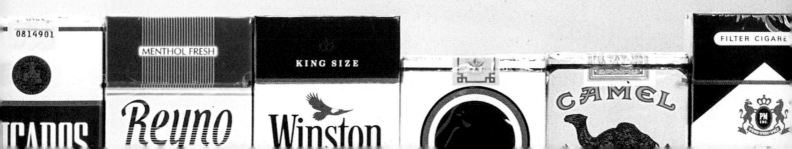

The Pipe

Pipe smoking is regarded as very English, and many people actually believe that the male population of the British Isles consists predominantly of pipe-smoking gentlemen in check tweed suits. Even if this image only partly corresponds to the reality, the Old World nevertheless attributes the introduction of the pipe to an Englishman, Sir Walter Raleigh, who taught mankind tobacco consumption. After the death of his patron, Queen Elizabeth I, Sir Walter fell from grace and was finally sentenced to death. According to legend, he was still smoking his pipe on his way to the scaffold, and presumably died with tobacco smoke in his mouth. "Death, where is thy sting?" a pipe smoker may think, whereas a non-smoker will shake his head and dismiss such anecdotes. The fascination of the pipe smoker for his smoking instrument, and the enjoyment of a well-smoked pipe, seem strange and incomprehensible to him. Unfortunately, only very few people actually smoke pipes, although nearly every male makes an attempt at some time in his life to become acquainted with a pipe. Many give up again prematurely in disappointment. No

one seems to know why that is. Perhaps it can be attributed to a special gene that decides who will be a pipe smoker and who will not. At any rate, pipe smoking must have something going for it, otherwise countless males would not be paying substantial sums of money for pipes, tobacco, and accessories, and would not be walking around in public with a pipe in their mouths – something which does not suit everybody. Presumably, apart from the pure enjoyment of the tobacco, the seemingly long-winded procedure must also contribute to the enjoyment. The choice of pipe alone requires a great amount of basic consideration, and frequent visits to homely and very well-equipped specialist stores, and also permits the purchase of interesting pipe literature. In short, it is an accepted pastime that many people elevate almost to a kind of science. Compared with real science, a pipe is highly accessible – to anyone with the capacity to enjoy tobacco.

As already mentioned, pipe smoking makes an impact and is very English. Therefore, as a rule, very good pipes come from England. The most famous brands doubtless include Dunhill, a name that to most non-smokers conjures up an exclusive label for clothes and equally beautiful useful accessories. Pipe smokers covet Dunhill in the same way that photographers covet a Leica. It also has an equally comparable value as a visual statement. The white dot on the mouthpiece makes it immediately recognizable. Dunhill supply both pipes and fine tobacco to smokers. Even today in the famous store at 30 Duke Street in London's West End, smokers can still have their personal tobacco blend made up, the ingredients can be noted and repeat blends made up upon request. Other good English pipe makes are Charatan, Loewe, GBD, and Parker & Barling, to name but a few.

Apparently the best-selling English pipe is the Falcon, a patented pipe. Only the bowl is made of wood;

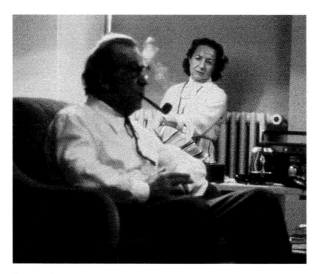

Georges Simenon smoked a pipe – like his famous hero Maigret.

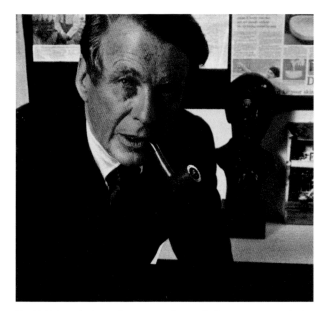

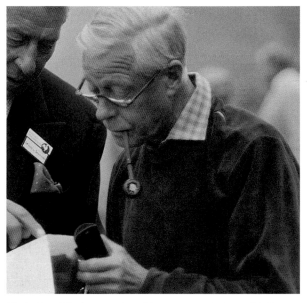

David Ogilvy, the legendary copy-writer and advertising expert looks like a picturebook Englishman. Tread warily – he is a Scotsman!

The Duke of Windsor was also a big supporter of tobacco like his brother.

the stem of the pipe screwed to the bowl is, instead, made of aluminum. This structure is very practical, because it facilitates changing the pipe by exchanging the bowl, which obviously saves a lot of space, especially when travelling. In addition the smoke cools down well in the exposed metal smoke canal, and the pipe is overall lighter. Nevertheless, opinions on the Falcon are very divided.

Naturally, outstanding pipes can also be found outside England. In Italy, for example, the Savinelli label provides excellent quality, and good pipes are also produced in France, Germany, and Denmark. Apart from involving the entertaining devotion to the smoking utensils, pipe smoking also has the advantage that this is the one form of tobacco enjoyment generally tolerated best of all. The smell of pipe tobacco is pleasant to most people, and any anxiety about the

dangers of passive smoking seldom occurs in its presence. Since pipe smokers are moreover regarded as calm and collected, sociable, and thereby largely trustworthy people, let the pipe be recommended to all those smokers who are really fed up with continuous well-meaning, and even hostile, remarks about their love of tobacco.

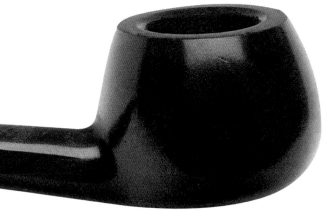

Classic Pipe Squad

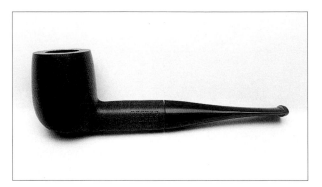

The *Billiard* is the pipe shape most frequently encountered. It is available in numerous sizes and wood types. Every pipe smoker should have at least one of them.

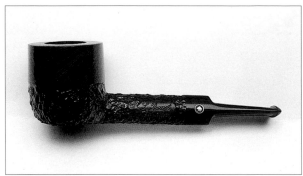

The *Pot* is particularly recommended if the pipe is hand-held sometimes. It is somewhat heavy and not best held longterm between the teeth.

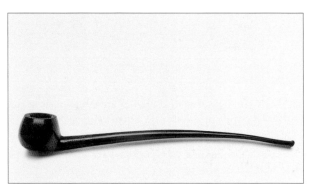

The *Churchwarden* is particularly suitable for home use. It is too long and unwieldy to walk around with in your mouth. Ideally, the cool smoke of this pipe should be enjoyed in a sitting position.

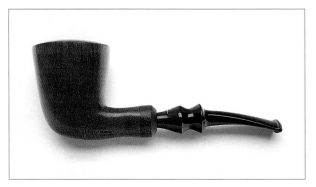

The shape of this bowl is called *Dublin*. The Dublin is just as classic as the Billiard, and like the latter it is also available in numerous variations. Here it is seen with a mouthpiece that slots in.

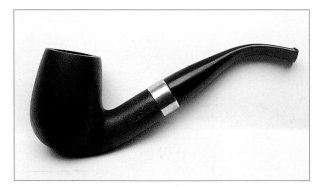

The mouthpiece of the *Bent Army* is not screwed in, but slotted in. The metal ring serves to reinforce the stem. There are also Army pipes in the Billiard shape.

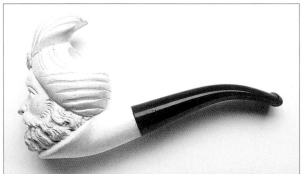

The *Meerschaum* gives an extremely cool and dry smoke. Nevertheless, the material is very sensitive, which makes this style unsuitable for use while on the move.

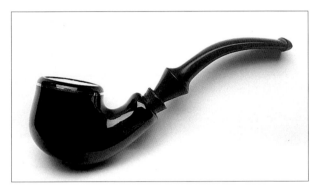

The *Prince* is a somewhat more robust edition of the Billiard. Short and squat, it sits well in your hand and does not become hot too quickly when you smoke it.

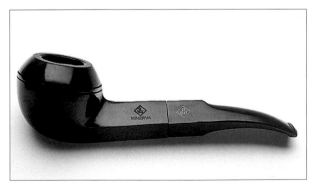

The pipe with the bend is called *Bent*. The low, heavy point of the hanging bowl means it is ideal for when your hands are otherwise occupied – for example, when you are driving the car.

The *Bent-Rhodesian* is as robust as the Prince, but the slight bend in the shape means you obtain a better balance in your mouth. It is an ideal everyday pipe that can stand anything.

The Manufacture

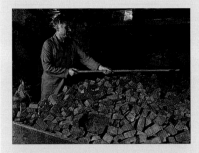

Before being processed to make pipes, the wood is baked and then dried for half a year.

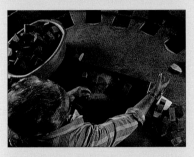

The pieces of wood – *ébauchons* in French – are sorted in such a way that, depending on the eventual shape, as little waste as possible occurs.

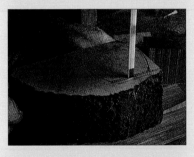

The pipe bowl is first of all roughly hewn out of the *ébauchon*. The shape of the pipe is already recognizable.

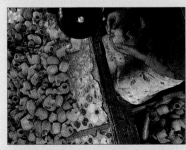

Pipes are still made by hand. This explains the high price of good pipes, also accounted for by the cost of the material.

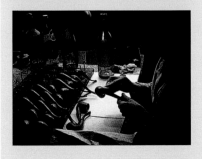

The mouthpiece is fitted, so now the pipe only needs to be stained, polished, or decorated.

The Cigar

If you look carefully at the goods on display in a cigar store, you will, as a rule, discover cigars in three different colors: dark brown to black, beige, and beige olive types. The dark ones are Brazilian cigars, the beige-colored ones are Sumatra cigars, and the beige olive ones are Havana cigars. This is, of course, only a very rough classification, and we could certainly have a discussion on the exact color definitions. However, the main purpose here is to mention the three classic areas of origin.

The most popular and simultaneously best cigar is without doubt the third one mentioned, the Havana. Thanks to a transformation of the image in the 1990s, it can nowadays be seen literally "between everyone's lips," even between the lips of actual non-smokers who enjoy being offered a cigar after meals. What was previously reserved for staid gentlemen, whom you would occasionally mockingly and pityingly smile about, is suddenly in vogue – even for the fairer sex. How long the present trend is likely to last remains to be seen. The fashion for cigars has doubtless made life somewhat easier for the passionate cigar smoker. A few years ago, he had to assume that he would be inundated with shocked glances in public bars if he lit his cigar. Nevertheless, even though the number of occasional smokers may have risen, the core of habitual smokers will not have substantially increased. Depending on the country, it represents a more or less large proportion of tobacco consumers. In Spain, this proportion was traditionally certainly bigger than in northern Europe. In Barcelona, Madrid, or Seville there have always been many cigar smokers apparent; the smell of cigars hangs permanently in the air.

In America, too, the cigar was always around, and therefore smokers there perhaps fell back on them automatically when cigarette smoking in public began to have a detrimental effect on their own reputation. Like the pipe, the cigar is relatively immune to the hostility of those opposed to tobacco; their specific aim is to get rid of cigarettes.

If you now decide to try cigar smoking, you will quickly notice that it is not as simple as cigarette smoking. Naturally, you can go into a good cigar store, request the best cigar, and then light it at the first suitable occasion.

However, generally speaking, you do not obtain much real enjoyment from the first few attempts. The potential cigar smoker, therefore, initially needs a little patience, and naturally a little knowledge of cigars. Whether a cigar tastes good or not depends on whether it has the right degree of moisture – that is, it is not too dry – and whether it meets the expectations of the smoker in terms of taste. Since cigars can taste extremely different from one another, it is advisable to have a detailed consultation with the dealer before buying cigars. The dealer will put together a selection of half a dozen cigars from his vast range, that you can then try out like tasting wine. In this way you slowly develop your own personal preference.

Once you have found it, you are then faced with the question of how to store the stock of cigars being purchased. The best place is in a humidor, an air-conditioned box set at the correct temperature. They are available in all sizes, ranging from shoebox format right through to walk-in wardrobe format. This retains the moisture in the cigars, essential because a dried-out cigar is lost and cannot be salvaged. Experts recommend different storage facilities to anyone at the early phase of cigar smoking who does not yet want to invest in a humidor; for example, in the vegetable compartment of the icebox. Others advise storing cigars in their cedarwood boxes in the wine cellar. If you do not have a wine cellar, you can put the cigar box into an airtight bag with a moist sponge. Both must then, however, be stored in a cool place, because in moist and warm surroundings cigars can fall prey to pests. Particularly lucky people live in direct proximity to a good cigar store. They can buy their weekly supplies fresh, and need not store big amounts at home.

There are also cigar clubs that offer members storage facilities. Each person has his own personal humidor that is rented like the safe-deposit box of a bank. A cigar compartment also contains valuable treasure. The cigars can then be enjoyably consumed alone or in the company of other cigar fans.

These establishments also solve the problem of the smell. If you do not have a smoking lounge at your disposal, you will not enjoy smoking cigars at home – that is, unless you want to risk members of your household urgently imploring you to switch back to cigarettes again. The latter go up in smoke considerably quicker than a 7-inch (178 mm) long Cohiba Esplendido, making your own premises that much easier to ventilate.

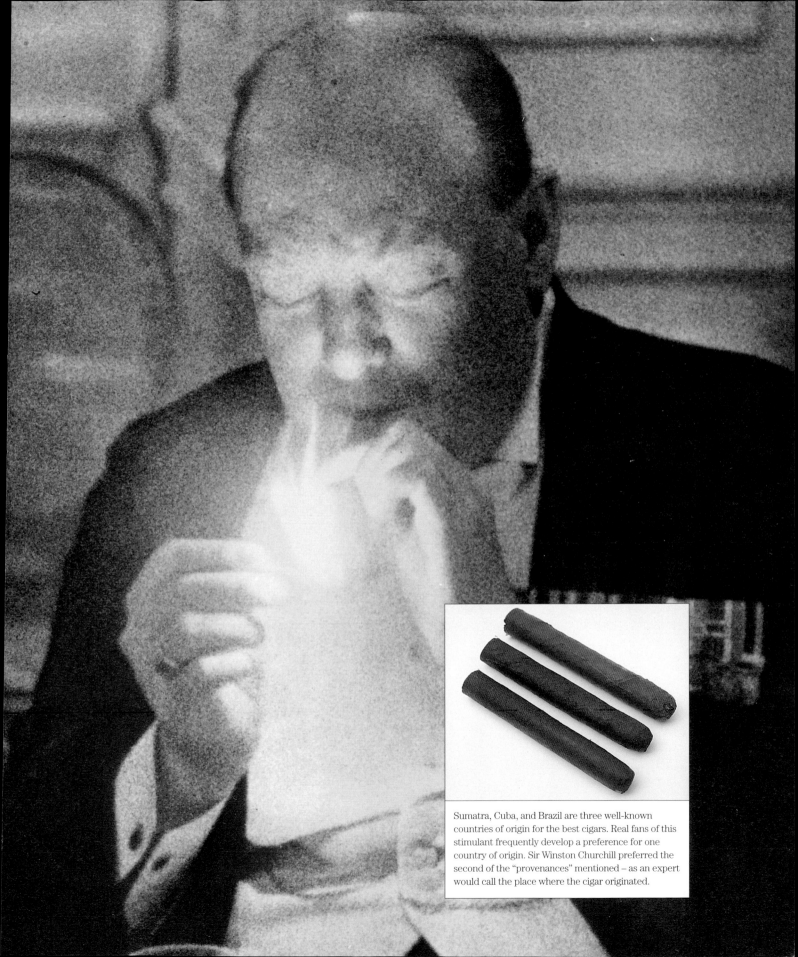

Sumatra, Cuba, and Brazil are three well-known countries of origin for the best cigars. Real fans of this stimulant frequently develop a preference for one country of origin. Sir Winston Churchill preferred the second of the "provenances" mentioned – as an expert would call the place where the cigar originated.

The Sizes

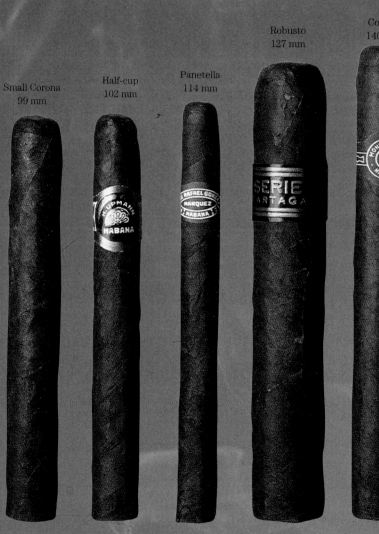
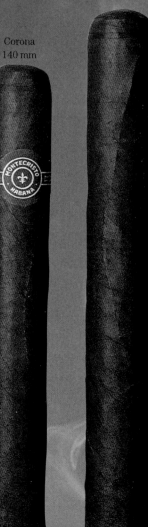
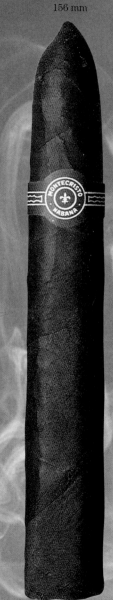

Small Corona
99 mm

Half-cup
102 mm

Panetella
114 mm

Robusto
127 mm

Corona
140 mm

Corona Grande
152 mm

Pyramide / Torpedo
156 mm

Double-Corona
200 mm

Especial
191 mm

Churchill
178 mm

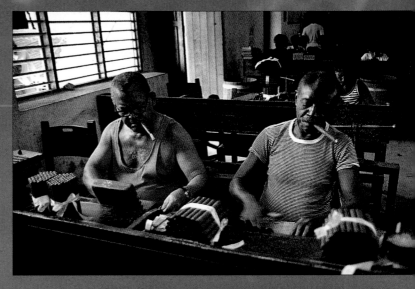

The best cigars are still made by hand even today in Cuba and the Dominican Republic. In this connection the cigar-maker fits together the three parts that go to make up the cigar: wrapper, rolled leaf, and filling. The filling consists of three sorts of leaves from the center, foot, and tip of the tobacco plant. Naturally, during this challenging work you are allowed to smoke – a cigar, of course.

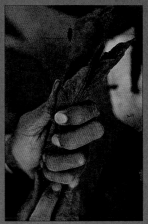

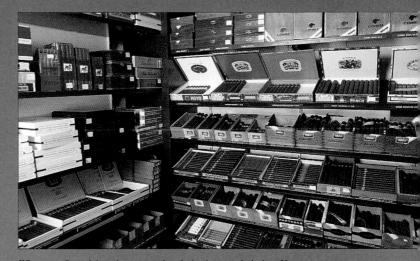

When you first visit a cigar store the choice is overwhelming. If you find out something about them beforehand, either from specialist literature or by talking to cigar enthusiasts, you will feel considerably more confident, and be in a better position to assess the advice of the seller.

The Bar in the Pocket

A person who does not drink alcohol certainly does not need a pocket flask, though you do not have to be a victim of the demon drink to appreciate one. However, their existence is under threat everywhere where travel is undertaken predominantly in your own car and you yourself are at the wheel. A sense of responsibility fortunately prevents most men from treating themselves to a sip from their flask during the day, and thus before the next car drive. Therefore, you are more likely to encounter it in surroundings where you are not responsible for your own locomotion, and simultaneously not automatically supplied with good-quality alcoholic beverages. This can be, for example, on public transport, on trains without a restaurant car, in taxis, and everywhere where men who enjoy the privilege of having a chauffeur at their disposal assemble – that is, in parliaments and ministries, and on the management floors of business conglomerates.

Many a boring ride on the train home to the suburbs is made a little more bearable by a sip of whisky from a flask, and the stupid chatter of fellow passengers can be ignored more easily if your gums are moistened with a little cognac. Also in emergency situations, in which the supply lines have been interrupted, it can be very comforting to know you have a quarter-liter of your favorite alcoholic beverage in your pocket. Anyone who has ever been stuck in winter at a train station because the Trans-Europe-Express has got stuck in snow can easily imagine that a full flask can be an extremely sensible accessory. It is comparable to a pocketknife; you do not miss it until you need it. A clever man, however, makes provision in advance, and he will have learnt to love his personal flask long before there is a shortage of supplies.

More precisely, there is also the question of hygiene when you are traveling: whether you should drink your cognac in a dubious restaurant car in a train, or out of your own flask in your own compartment. In addition the flask also guarantees the quality of what is being drunk. After all, its owner most likely filled it himself with his favorite tipple, or assigned this task to a person in his trust.

The flask should be handled in a self-confident and open manner, unless you find yourself among militant anti-alcohol supporters, or in a country whose laws prohibit alcohol. In addition, exaggerated secrecy gives the impression of a bad conscience, which is typical of people who have a less than perfect relationship to alcohol. The latter type of person can also be encountered among fans of the flask, but any worry we may have about being mistaken for one of them should not prevent us from availing ourselves of the undisputed benefits of the flask in a self-confident manner. A true gentleman is not afraid of taking a sip from his flask whenever he feels it will aid his enjoyment of life.

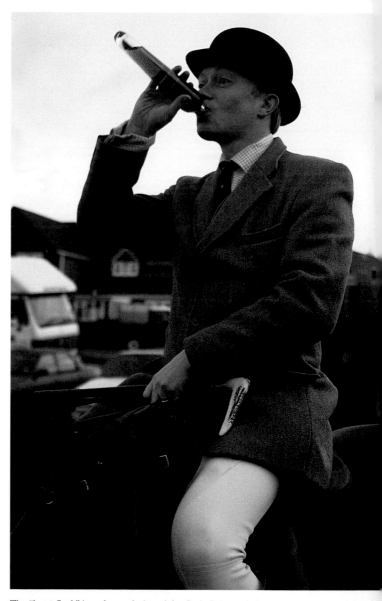

The "hunt flask" is a close relative of the flask. It is carried around in a leather case on the saddle, and helps to drive out the winter cold on a fox hunt.

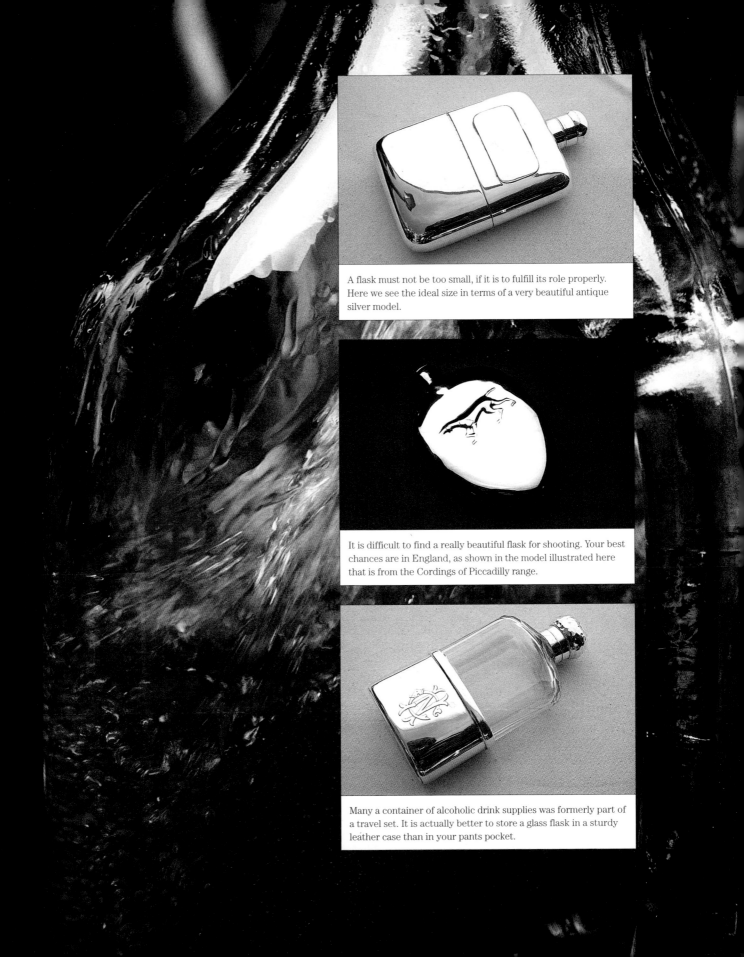

A flask must not be too small, if it is to fulfill its role properly. Here we see the ideal size in terms of a very beautiful antique silver model.

It is difficult to find a really beautiful flask for shooting. Your best chances are in England, as shown in the model illustrated here that is from the Cordings of Piccadilly range.

Many a container of alcoholic drink supplies was formerly part of a travel set. It is actually better to store a glass flask in a sturdy leather case than in your pants pocket.

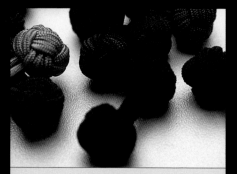

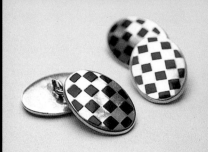

If you want a little additional color in your cuff links, you should try these small fabric knots that are on display in large sweet jars and offered for sale in gentlemen's outfitters and by shirtmakers. If you like wearing one-color ties, you can coordinate its color with the fabric knots.

Blue and silver are a good color combination for cuff links, if you predominantly wear light blue or blue-patterned shirts. There are, of course, other color combinations that also include silver.

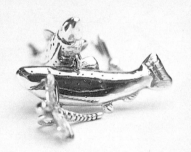

You can also choose cuff links that match your hobby – as an angler, for example, with trout and fly. This kind of cuff link with motif is available in innumerable variations, but requires careful selection. If you are not absolutely sure of your feeling for style, you should stick to the classic oval shape in silver or gold. An over-exaggerated "witty" cuff link is almost as big a *faux pas* as the tie clip with the New-York skyline. The most famous address for interesting cuff links can be found in the London district of St. James. At Longmire's, 12 Bury Street, the cuff link fan will be proffered a gigantic selection of these small jewels. Those who were fortunate enough to inherit beautiful cufflinks may best avoid buying these important accessories.

What never fails to astound are the potential variations that can be produced with combinations of silver, gold, and the classic colors of the gentleman such as dark blue, red, wine red, and bottle green. Anyone not wishing to buy new cuff links for practically every shirt and tie should ideally acquire one pair of gold oval cuff links. Cuff links are available in two different price categories: a very high one for samples in gold or precious stones, and a lower one for costume jewelry. Good shirtmakers also have a stock of the latter, because not everyone wants to wear a small fortune on their cuffs. Many gentlemen, however, do just that.

Cuff links can add a further important note, in a distinctly rich variety of ways, to the combination of suit, shirt, and tie, so they are also an expression of taste.

The Cuff Link

Cuff links belong to the group of accessories whose impact is inversely proportional to their size, because although they are minute, and are often not even visible, they make a very big contribution to the overall look. The right cuff links at the right moment can give the crucial note to an outfit. The wrong cuff links, or even good cuff links on the wrong occasion, can spoil a whole suit. Cuff links are worn exclusively on shirts with a double cuff, and also on a dress shirt, that although it does not have double cuffs, nevertheless does not have buttons. This rule may sound banal, but it is sadly justified. There are shirts with single-buttoned cuffs that apart from the button also have a hole for the cuff link. This so-called combination cuff is neither one thing nor the other, because cuff links belong on double cuffs, with the exception of the dress shirt (more on this subject on page 326). Anyone who does not like cuff links should wear shirts with single-buttoned cuffs for preference. However, cuff links not only show the wish to produce more in terms of style than the required minimum, but also a certain readiness to spend money on appearance, in spite of the fact that they are rather awkward to handle. Those who are seriously interested in and enthusiastic about style will not be put off by these factors, especially since the financial aspect can be estimated as being quite low. Beautiful costume jewelry cuff links can be purchased very cheaply, but if you develop a liking for these small pieces of jewelry, you can spend a lot of money on them, as in the case of all other beautiful things.

A cuff link consists of two identical objects, made in such a way that they can pass through the buttonholes in the cuff, and these objects are joined together by a bridge, a chain, or a length of elastic. These can also be connected via press studs, snap fasteners or screw devices; but as a rule, a small chain links the two objects. The objects are mostly flat, oval shapes and made of gold or silver, and can also be set with precious stones. Colorful enamel cuff links are also available. Apart from the flat, oval shape, replicas of objects are also for sale, like tiny gold teddy bears, dogs, dice, and horses – in short, anything that can be pushed through a buttonhole. Many people have inherited jewelry adapted to make cuff links. Earrings are particularly suitable for this, since they occur in pairs. The fabric knots already mentioned are also very popular, and look like tiny plaited balls. They are available in one color or are multicolored. Their low price means you can have a matching color in your wardrobe for every potential combination of jacket, pants, shirt, and tie. Originally they were a kind of substitute that the customer would replace with his own more valuable cuff links after buying a shirt. Nowadays they are both a popular accessory that can be a perfect color match in terms of the rest of the outfit, and a good interim solution for anyone who does not own any other cuff links.

When can you wear cuff links? Always when you wear a shirt with double cuffs. A shirt with double cuffs goes with almost anything, whether it be a suit, a sports jacket, or a blazer. Although it is rather unusual to see double cuffs with casual suits and jackets, it would definitely not be considered a *faux pas*. As a rule of thumb, double cuffs would be inappropriate if you were not wearing a tie with the shirt under the selected suit, sports jacket, or blazer. Yet even that is left to individual interpretation, stylistically speaking. Those who only wear button-down shirts with a soft roll collar have to do without cuff links, because this American classic is only available with buttoned cuffs. Whether cuff links should be worn with a casual outfit depends on whether they would make you look "overdressed" or not. That is, unless you are aiming for a contrast and quite deliberately wear gold cuff links as well as jeans and loafers. In terms of the choice of cuff links, you should consider whether and what jewelry you are wearing with them. Naturally, you cannot make sweeping decisions about whether or not you wear gold cuff links with a stainless steel watch. However, you should consider the impact generated by the joint tone of watch, rings, and cuff links. Every detail counts – even minute cuff links.

Our Daily Companion

"Form follows function" – this somewhat overworked phrase certainly still has a meaning when attached to the selection of a briefcase, because the case really does take its shape from its function. Those of you who take work home with you need a different model from those who earn their living exclusively at their place of work. The quantities of paper being transported range from a motorsport magazine to a bulging file, from a filofax to a statute book. Work tools that must be packed in can be a pile of technical books, one to two laptop computers, or also just a slim dictating machine.

Depending on our profession, we carry the most diverse things around with us. They give rise to certain forms of cases. Some carry a slim briefcase, which holds at the most newspaper, banana, and mobile phone; others need a flexible and roomy case that can hold a file, if necessary. The goods being transported, however, should not alone determine their form of transport. Almost equally as important is the matter of the route that the case, including its contents, will be taking each day to the place of work and back home again (in the company of its owner). Anyone using public transport should choose an upright briefcase that is case-shaped, or a briefcase that is stiffbacked and has a broad base. Then the faithful companion can be put down when it becomes too heavy. Or you might choose a type with a shoulder strap, leaving your hands free so you can read the newspaper standing up. For car drivers, the stability

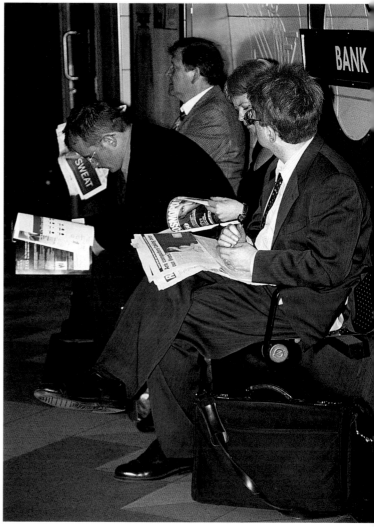

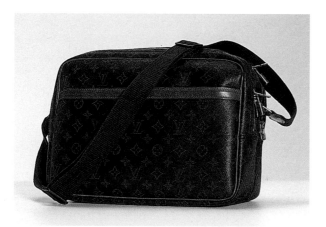

The *Reporter* from Vuitton recalls the canvas bags that airline passengers used to be given by airlines as a present. In the 1990s they were rediscovered by the young and acquired cult status. The upmarket Vuitton version enables all age groups to benefit from the advantages of a bag with shoulder strap, without looking suspiciously as though they are trying too hard to look young.

of the case is unimportant, since the precious thing will be laid or stood on the seat or in the trunk. Cyclists should ensure that nothing could fall out of the case if it is wedged horizontally on the carrier. Furthermore, the case should as far as possible be rainproof. Those not particularly interested in traffic safety can hang a traditional type of briefcase by its stiff handle on the handlebars. Pedestrians are also well-advised to choose a sufficiently weatherproof model.

Commuters are traditionally among the most intensive users of all sorts of briefcases. So the London Underground, for example, is a good place to admire the variety of bags and cases.

Despite all these sensible considerations concerning a functional choice, we often make the most impractical or nonsensical choice, whether it be for esthetic reasons, or because we feel obliged to maintain a supposed status. Some people cannot help going to work with an elegant briefcase, because they believe they owe it to their position. Others cling for their whole lives to a bag they learnt to love as a student or when they entered their profession.

As already mentioned, the principle of "form follows function" has a certain significance, but it is by no means the only consideration, because we could all carry our papers around just as well either in a plastic shopping bag or in a gaudily colored nylon backpack. Instead of this, considerable sums of money are now and then invested in calfskin briefcases and brass-studded cases. They are perhaps not the most practical items in terms of transportation, but they are definitely the most beautiful.

When buying a briefcase you should always consider the fact that this accessory will be accompanying its owner for many years on a daily basis to his place(s) of work, and rising up many rungs of the career ladder with him. This is reason enough to decide on a model that is worthy of being your daily companion. For a few dollars more, you can buy a case that you really like, and that is perfect for you. You will never want to relinquish it! Perhaps the battered leather briefcase that has done many years service has certain prestige value, showing that its owner has an important job.

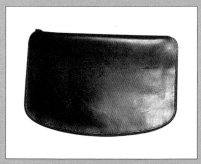

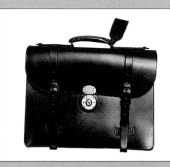

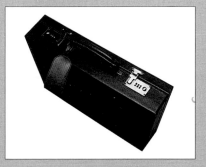

The classic briefcase, being a real workhorse, will often last the entire duration of a career, even if it has been constantly stuffed full with files or thick statute books. The broad base and low center of gravity means it is popular with commuters all over the world, because it rests firmly in an upright position.

This is the second big classic in terms of briefcases. It is available in numerous variations, but the basic principle is always the same: the back panel of the case extends to form a wide flap that folds over the body of the case and closes either with a buckle or lock. Space is limited here.

With more modern case shapes there is a concise closing of lid and body that gives the case rather a box-like appearance. Its stiff construction is both an advantage and a disadvantage. Fragile contents are safely protected, but it is not possible to expand it if it is likely to become overloaded.

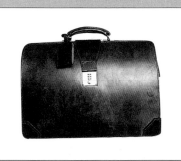

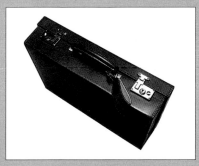

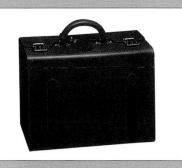

Compared with the very businessman-type effect of the other briefcases, there is something artistic or intellectual about the portfolio. Connoisseurs choose typical brown tones like chestnut or Havana.

The prototype of the briefcase that is still made in England today. Here the lid closes properly over the body of the case. The best place to buy these cases is at Swaine, Adeney, Brigg & Sons in England.

The pilot's case does not make much of an elegant impression, and its origin from the world of aviation can lend it only a certain amount of charisma. Despite all this, if you swear by pilot cases, you should perhaps go for the high-quality Vuitton version.

The Original

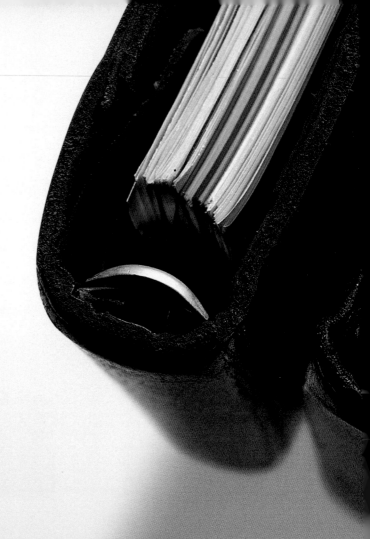

The heyday of the Filofax ought really to be long past. In an era when the size of computers, and of mobile phones that send and receive faxes, is ever diminishing, and the data network is of global magnitude, it seems like a contradiction in terms to carry your personal data around with you in a collection of notes. Yet maybe it is that contradiction that many people still find so attractive. The fairly large ring binder gives them security. It cannot crash like a computer; therefore, you cannot end up in a "black hole." In short, nothing can go wrong, provided you do not mislay your handy "personal organizer." In this respect, the Filofax is nowadays still just as trendy as the good old printed book that, despite all competition from CD ROM and other data carriers, stubbornly holds its own. The Filofax, self-confidently labeled "The Original," has

been in existence since 1921. The word "Filofax" is a newly coined word made up of "file" and "fax" (like "facts"). Its name also denotes its agenda; all the facts you need are collected and stored in a small ring binder – for example phone numbers, street maps, hotel addresses, and statistical sales graphs – in other words, all the data that make life easier, but are only useful if you have them at your fingertips at the crucial moment, or better still, in your small ring binder.

You would think that it was just what the world had been waiting for, yet it took a while before the Filofax became popular outside Great Britain. Not until Margaret Thatcher was prime minister of Great Britain did the world sit up and take note of the Filofax. During that decade, the 1980s, the Filofax became established worldwide as symbolic of "Yuppies" (Young Urban Professionals). In this connection, early P.R. campaigns were deliberately aimed at avoiding this image. It was stressed that in England, even schoolchildren and poor students used a Filofax. To reinforce this message, the range always contains an economical version of the "wallet" made of plastic alongside the expensive

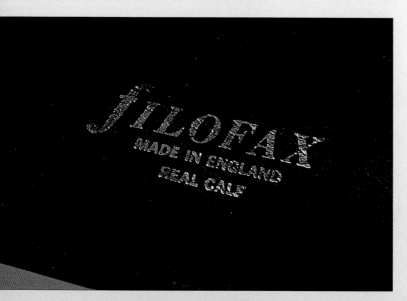

What counts with the Filofax is what is inside, though it must be assumed that the international success of the attractive ring binder would be far less, if the profound inner thoughts and feelings were wrapped in unattractive plastic or cheap cardboard. It was an army officer whom we have to thank for coming up with the idea of the Filofax, although when in 1921 Col. Disney founded the company of Norman & Hill that began to produce the forerunner of the current "personal organizer," it did not have a name. It was first christened "Filofax" by Grace Scurr, initially a secretary at Norman & Hill, who later became president of the company. Her work paved the way for the international success of this practical collection of notes. However, the rich pickings were established by David and Lesley Collischon who acquired Norman & Hill in 1980 and renamed their new company "Filofax," synonymous with the product. They made Filofax what it is today – a product with an unmistakable brand identity – a true "original."

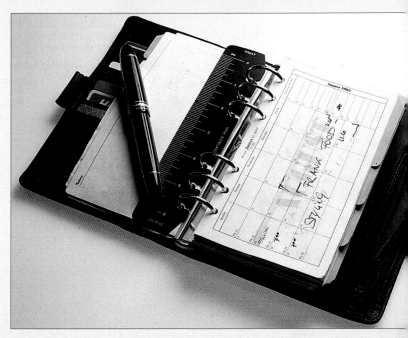

The "personal organizer" by Filofax is notebook, appointment book, address book, telephone list, yearbook of personal statistics, and much more – depending on the individual arrangement of the ring binder with lists, indexes, and collections of data. Fans of this English classic definitely swear they could not live without their Filofax.

"wallets" made of fine leather, though it is the leather cover that lends the Filofax its quaint and typical English charm. The more the "personal organizer" looks dog-eared and worn, the better it is, because the noble store of notes follows in the tradition of numerous English products where signs of wear and tear are known as "patina."

The secret of the success of the Filofax could also be defined thus: it is something like a pair of shoes by Church's in which you can enter your appointments, a walking-stick-length umbrella by Brigg complete with integrated telephone list, or a wax jacket by Barbour plus a list of good vintages of Bordeaux wines. In short, the Filofax is splendidly English and thus fascinates all those who were not lucky enough to be born in the United Kingdom. Anyone who is not prepared to spend so much on the original leather-cover version should try a different method of organization. After all, to be seen with a blatant copy of a real Filofax always implies more lack of style than jotting down notes on odd scraps of paper.

Traveling in Style

The history of the firm of Louis Vuitton officially starts with its founding in 1854. The suitcases that the "malletier" (suitcase-maker) Louis Vuitton was producing at the time were of particularly high quality and also lighter and flatter than those of the competition. Louis Vuitton did not cover his suitcases with leather, but instead with canvas fabric soaked in glue, so that they acquired a water-repellent surface. This invention was soon copied, and Louis Vuitton had no option but to replace the gray "toile Trianon" with a characteristic beige canvas with red stripes. A new stripe pattern was due again a few years later, in order to wreck the plans of plagiarists. However, because this design was also copied, the son of the founder, Georges Vuitton, designed a new cover in a check pattern, the "toile à damiers." Also, in order to prevent this pattern soon surfacing as a counterfeit, Vuitton junior provided it with the inscription "Louis Vuitton, marque déposée" (registered trademark). These suitcases from the firm of Vuitton were thus the first products that carried the brand name in a visible position (and still do today, of course). This firm step of self-assertion was a landmark event in the history of marketing and product design, because for the first time it was acknowledged that in terms of free competition, counterfeit goods can definitely do harm to an established make. Yet even the "toile à damiers" was not adequate protection for Vuitton from counterfeit, so Georges Vuitton went a step further. He created the "toile monogram," a suitcase cover that deliberately and stylistically uses a monogram of the firm of Louis Vuitton as the pattern. Apart from the staggered arrangement of the "LV," standing for Louis Vuitton, the pattern also contained a four-pointed star inside a rhombus, and a stylized flower inside a circle. These shapes recall the decoration in late Gothic cathedrals, and also the painting of the Nabis (Hebrew 'Prophets'), members of a post-Impressionist movement, into whose pictures symbolic and decorative elements were integrated. In a definitive way, all the products of the firm of Vuitton bear the signature of the firm's founder as a guarantee and protection against fakes. The fact that it is one of the signatures that is copied most frequently is ironical. Even though Vuitton meanwhile had a wide range of extremely varied leather goods and accessories, suitcases and bags of all kinds remained the actual specialty of the firm. It had started as a "malletier" (suitcase-maker), and still kept this title very proudly in the company name that had in the meantime become famous and treasured worldwide. For those who need to travel extensively, Vuitton's range of products is invaluable in ensuring that clothes can be transported without being harmed.

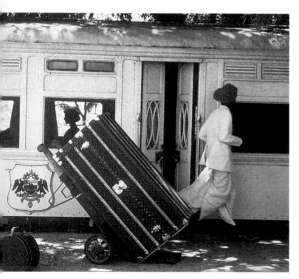

Traveling with an enormous piece of luggage only seems like a contradiction in terms to those who feel properly dressed for every occasion in T-shirt, jeans, and trainers.

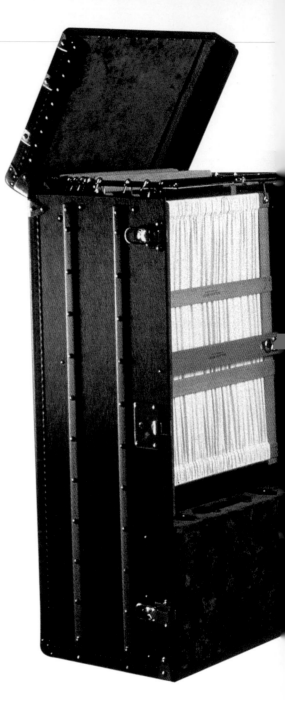

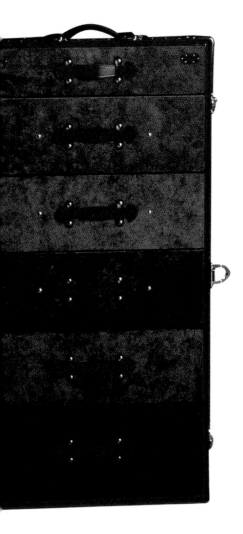

The wardrobe trunk is symbolic of traveling in style, but not necessarily because of its price. It is more to do with the fact that it can only be moved with the help of willing service staff – something only found in the best hotels nowadays.

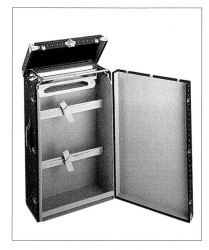

A smaller wardrobe trunk is adequate for shorter trips. It is, however, big enough to cater for the right clothes for different occasions.

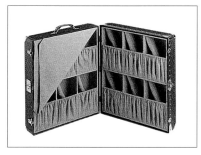

Vuitton will make a special shoe trunk upon request, in which there is room for eight or twelve pairs of men's shoes, depending on the model; that is, enough shoes for a trip lasting several weeks. This is a very good acquisition, because shoes take up a lot of room in other suitcases, yet are absolutely vital.

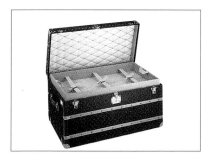

Cabin trunks are available in different sizes with removable horizontal subcompartments. They are a good alternative to the wardrobe trunk, since the clothes lie tidily folded as in a chest.

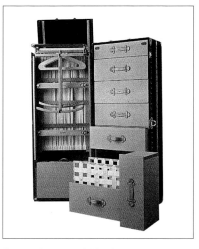

In a wardrobe trunk like this you can even transport a large wardrobe of clothes without any risk of them creasing, and they can be stored in it at journey's destination. Depending on the design and layout, the trunk can contain more wardrobe space or more space for a chest of drawers. There are versions with numerous drawers, while others provide more room for hanging clothes. Trunks of this kind are quickly and easily packed, because everything is simply transferred from wardrobe or chest of drawers into the relevant compartments – then off you go on your journey.

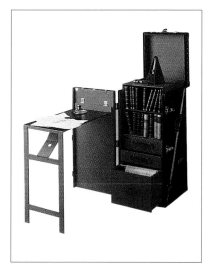

This "Stokowski" travel secretaire is highly recommended for travelers who like having their own desk with them. It was designed for the conductor Leopold Stokowski in 1936, but has now become a fixed item in the range.

For the Short Trip

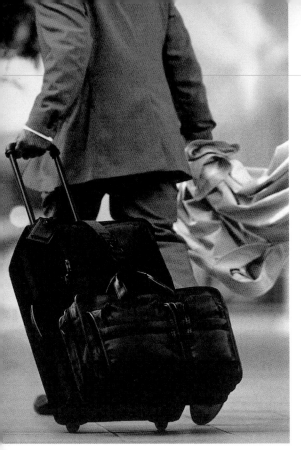

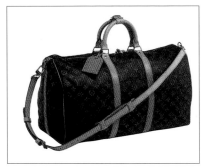

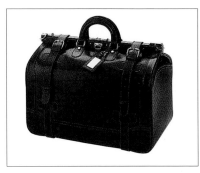

The Vuitton Keepall epitomizes the holdall. This shape has been in existence since 1924. Depending on the model, you can take the Keepall as hand luggage on board an aircraft, or as an overnight bag over the weekend. The classic Keepall is made of the "toile Monogram" (monogrammed fabric), but it is also available in different leather versions.

Luggage made of leather – irrespective of whether it is a suitcase or holdall – is only practical on air trips if it can be taken on board. The same restrictions do not apply to auto passengers. Anyone who is away for the weekend and only needs the minimum amount of clothing will readily select the Gladstone bag. This classic leather holdall is offered by numerous manufacturers, like Asprey & Garrard of Bond Street, London.

Holdalls on wheels are ideal flight companions on internal American flights.

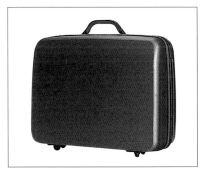

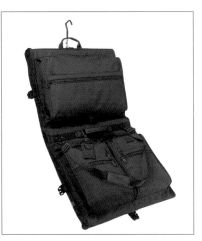

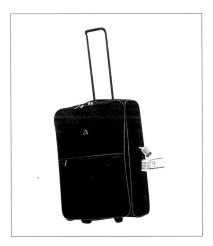

The roots of the Samsonite make stretch as far back as 1910. In that year, Jesse Shwayder founded a suitcase factory in Denver, Colorado. The family business was already mass producing particularly stable suitcases during the 1920s, by the name of "Samson." The hard-shell suitcase with aluminium frame emerged in 1958. The streamlined design of the 1950s still continues in existence today, and the Samsonite range always contains models that are unmistakably connected with this look. The robust nature of Samsonite means it is still the first choice for air trips.

The "kitbag" form is usually also allowed to be taken on board in Europe, if it is flat and really only fulfills its stated purpose. The basic kitbag style really only has room for a single suit. The hook of the hanger, on which the suit hangs, is often simultaneously the grip of the kitbag. If at all possible, you should put the suit in a hanging position inside the holder during the journey. Bigger kitbags that hold several articles of clothing often have the disadvantage that the contents – and particularly the suit – end up crumpled. A suitcase is usually the ideal solution here.

The American Tumi firm produce extremely heavy-duty luggage made of nylon fabric that was originally developed for bulletproof vests. The strength of Tumi is the ideally designed board case; the permissible size in the USA is much larger, but smaller-size board cases are available for pan-European flights. They are particularly suitable for those who fly a lot, and prefer practicality to elegance.

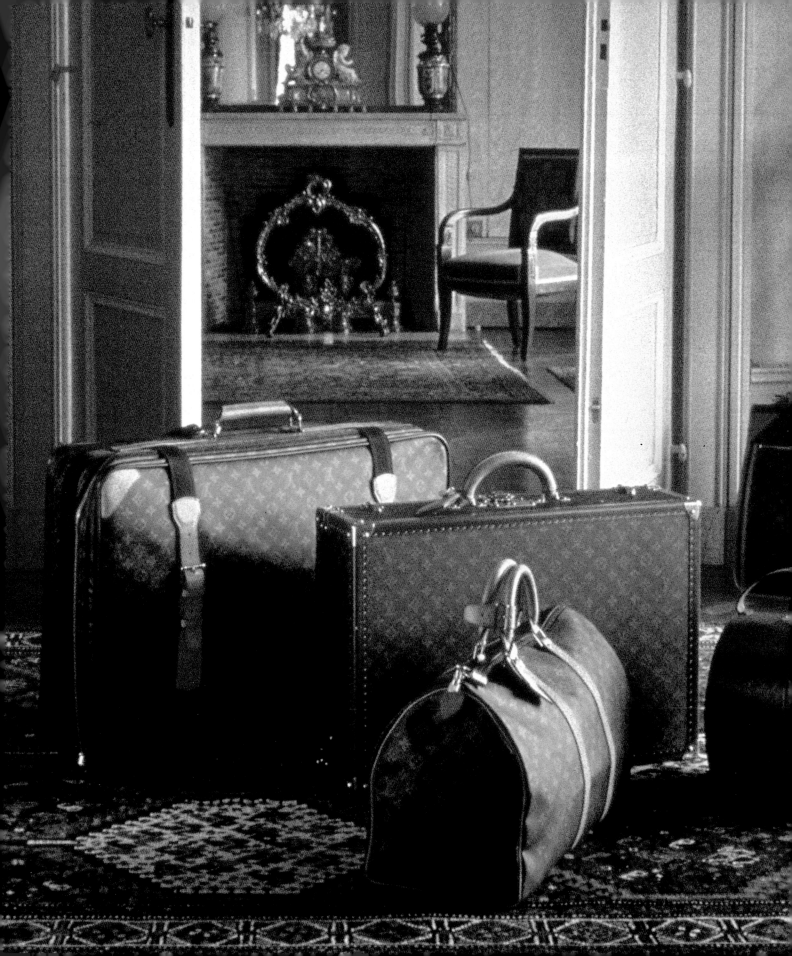

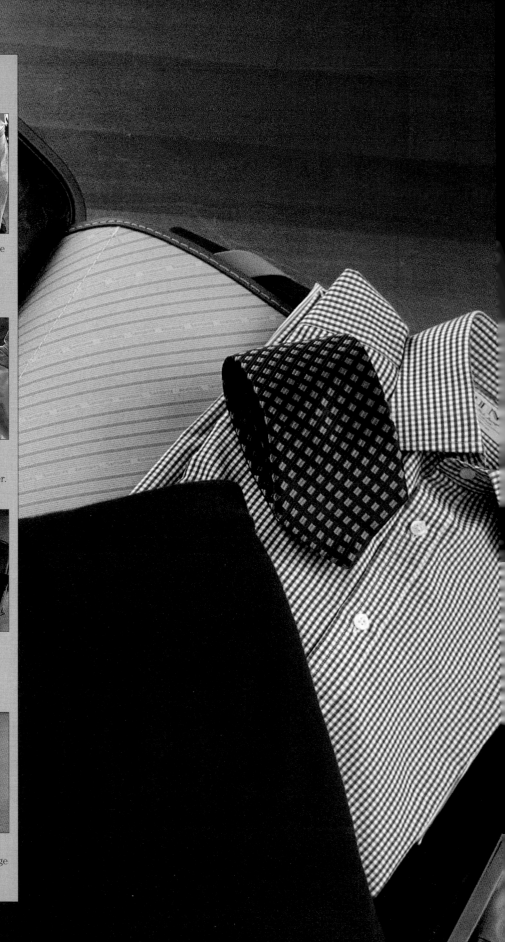

The Knack with the Jacket

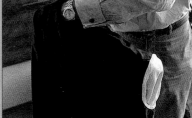

First of all, turn one half of the jacket inside out. For this purpose, turn the shoulder completely inside out, but do not pull the sleeve through.

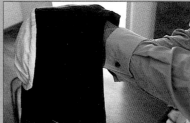

Place the jacket half that is not turned inside out carefully inside the other half, pushing it right into the inside-out shoulder.

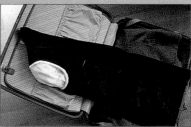

The invisible, nonsensitive lining of the jacket is now facing outward. Both shoulders, being one inside the other, are protected against pressure.

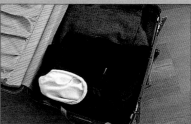

Folded once in the middle, a jacket now becomes a handy-size, nonsensitive package that fits into any holdall.

The Right Way to Pack a Suitcase

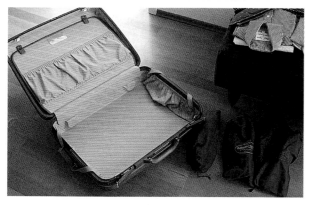

There are many different ways of packing a suitcase. Priority should always be given to sensitive suit jackets that should be protected from being crushed.

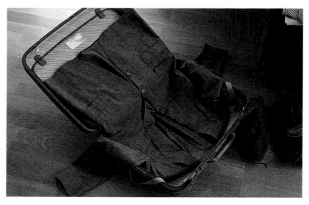

Now we fold the pants along the pants crease and place them underneath the front chest of the suit. This protects the jacket from being pressed together too tightly. After all, the chest of your jacket should retain the slight three-dimensional shape.

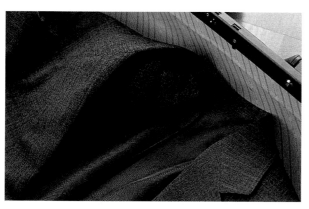

Let us assume we are taking two suits with us. Start by placing the first jacket on the bottom on the suitcase with the front facing upward. We fold the other one as demonstrated on the left and then place it on top of the first suit.

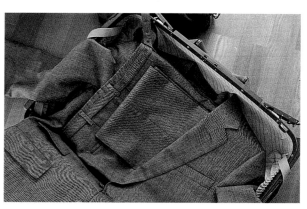

Now fold the sleeves and lower parts of the jacket over the chest. Collar and sleeves can also be stuffed. Tissue paper can also be used for this purpose.

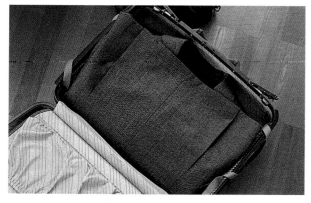

Stuff rolled-up socks or underpants in the shoulders so the latter cannot get pressed completely flat later. With the method on the left, we stuff one shoulder with the shoulder of the other jacket half.

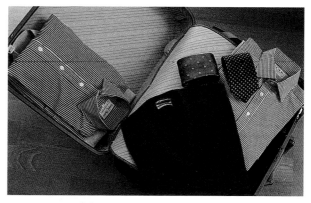

You can now pack a pullover (and shirts) in the upper half of the suitcase under the packing panel. Shoes that travel in your suitcase should be distributed around the bottom of the suitcase, so that they do not slip down when the suitcase is placed in an upright position.

The Walking Cane

Once upon a time, gentlemen never ventured out without a walking cane, hat, and gloves. Nowadays, it is the complete opposite. Hardly any man would dare to be seen on the sidewalk with a walking cane. Mark you, there are walking sticks and walking canes. We are not talking here about a walking stick that is used as a walking aid. Even though walking canes served originally to support the person holding them, and also as a weapon, since the start of the twentieth century the cane has merely been used as an accessory. Antique dealers usually keep a large selection of historic examples in stock, and the huge variety of decoration, material, and metal fittings reveals the former popularity of the stick or cane. Although it is totally superfluous today and has no bearing on fashion, a good old walking cane exerts a certain fascination. We enjoy picking it up and imagining how it would have been to stroll along with a walking stick and hat, in the manner of our forefathers. There is additionally something ceremonial about a walking cane; it imparts a certain formality to the appearance. In actual fact, a richly ornate cane is a sign of rank and authority in many cultures in our world. The joy of owning beautiful walking canes drives many a man to become a collector, yet even though he has several dozen at home, he is hardly likely to venture out onto the sidewalk with one. Only extreme eccentrics do this. Most men wait until old age or fragility finally supplies a reason or excuse to be seen parading with a beautiful walking stick.

❶ Those who need the support will select a corresponding walking stick. The handle is shaped in such a way that it provides sufficient hold and a supporting surface for the hand. There are many beautifully shaped and also elegant walking sticks that fulfill these requirements, and harmonize with a stylish appearance or even round it off.

❷ This classic is suitable as a walking stick and hiking staff. For long hikes it really does substantially take the weight off the leg joints. A stick with a pointed metal tip is recommended for soft ground underfoot, since it provides a good hold. The pointed tip can be covered in rubber to prevent slipping over on slippery floors.

❸ Country-style walking sticks are appropriate for the countryside. They are not only used as a support, but also to fend off over-friendly – or even aggressive – dogs, clear a way through undergrowth, or to test the firmness of a layer of ice. Hunters like using walking sticks the height of a man to rest their guns against, if there is no other surface within reach. Long walking sticks are also very useful in the mountains, especially during a descent into difficult terrain.

❹ Those who quickly work up a thirst on walks should purchase a walking cane with an integrated drinking flask from Brigg in London. The test-tube-shape container is concealed under the silver knob.

❺ The black walking cane with the silver knob is classically elegant. It goes exceedingly well with evening dress, and also looks good with a dark suit or morning coat. This kind of cane is often chosen if the person holding it does not want to give the impression of fragility, even though he perhaps rather needs a walking aid. This cane with the silver knob is too elegant to be mistaken at all for a walking stick; therefore whether the cane is of ornamental or practical value remains the secret of its owner.

❻ The human desire to embellish practical objects naturally also extends to the walking stick. There is an endless variety of designs and styles available. The carved heads of animals in wood, horn, bone, or semiprecious stones are very popular. These kinds of canes usually form parts of collections, and are seldom used for their real purpose.

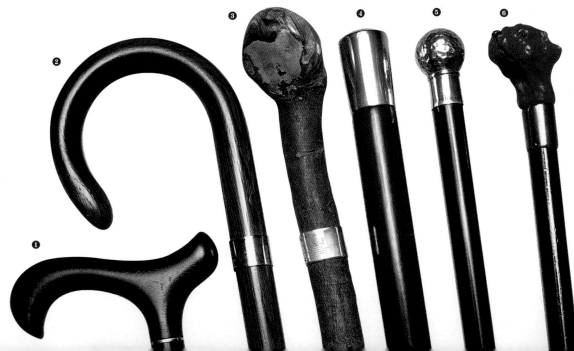

The Lap Robe

Although it stems originally from the times when travelers had to protect themselves from the cold in draughty horse-drawn coaches, the travel lap robe is still extremely useful even today. Not for nothing do we find it stocked by all big saddleries and luggage manufacturers – usually rolled up into a handy bundle and held together by a leather harness. You do not really have to be particularly sensitive to the cold to learn to appreciate the benefits of a warm blanket. In summer an air-conditioned train compartment can become like an icebox if you are sitting still for long periods. This is even more so in winter, when the compartment has to be shared with strict enemies of heating. Even in an aircraft, the lap robe can be of good service, since although airconditioning is a godsend, it quickly becomes a nightmare if you fall asleep on a long-haul flight and then wake up, frozen to the bone. Of course, you can ask the cabin personnel for a blanket, but who wants to wrap something round themselves without knowing when it was last cleaned, and who the last person was that used it? The travel lap robe is, therefore, above all recommended for those people who have a low threshold in terms of cleanliness. A personal lap robe can additionally lend a familiar note to the impersonal surroundings of a hotel room. It is a simply wonderful feeling to be able to wrap yourself up in your own blanket and lie on an unfamiliar sofa, breathe in the familiar smell of home, and to know that this blanket had been a throw on your comfortable armchair in the livingroom right up to your departure. However, a lap robe is not only something that travels well, but is also just as at home in the yard, or out in the countryside, where it is very practical for sitting on for a picnic, or for relaxing on the lawn. Spectators of leisure and sport activities often take a lap robe with them, because a blanket is ideal protection and warmth for the usually windy spectator galleries and hard benches. A lap robe is also extremely useful in the automobile; for journeys in the open convertible, for front-seat passengers taking a nap, or as a blessing in disguise to keep out the cold when you are stuck in a traffic jam in winter. On seeing this nondescript travel lap robe lying there on the holdall waiting to be used, it is hard to imagine all these potential situations. They will materialize, no doubt of it, because there are numerous occasions for proving the item to be worthy of investment.

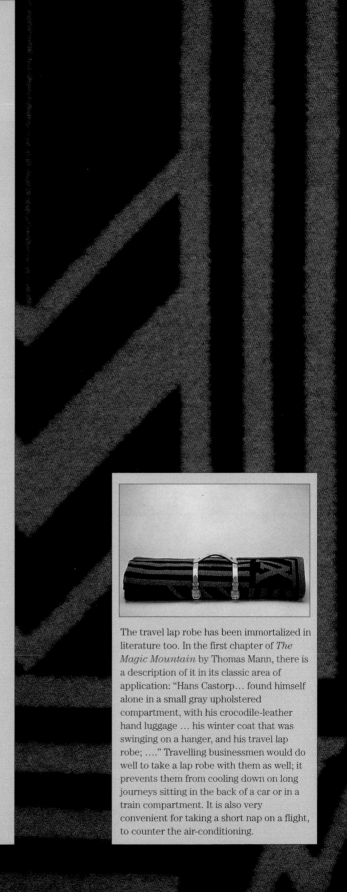

The travel lap robe has been immortalized in literature too. In the first chapter of *The Magic Mountain* by Thomas Mann, there is a description of it in its classic area of application: "Hans Castorp… found himself alone in a small gray upholstered compartment, with his crocodile-leather hand luggage … his winter coat that was swinging on a hanger, and his travel lap robe; …." Travelling businessmen would do well to take a lap robe with them as well; it prevents them from cooling down on long journeys sitting in the back of a car or in a train compartment. It is also very convenient for taking a short nap on a flight, to counter the air-conditioning.

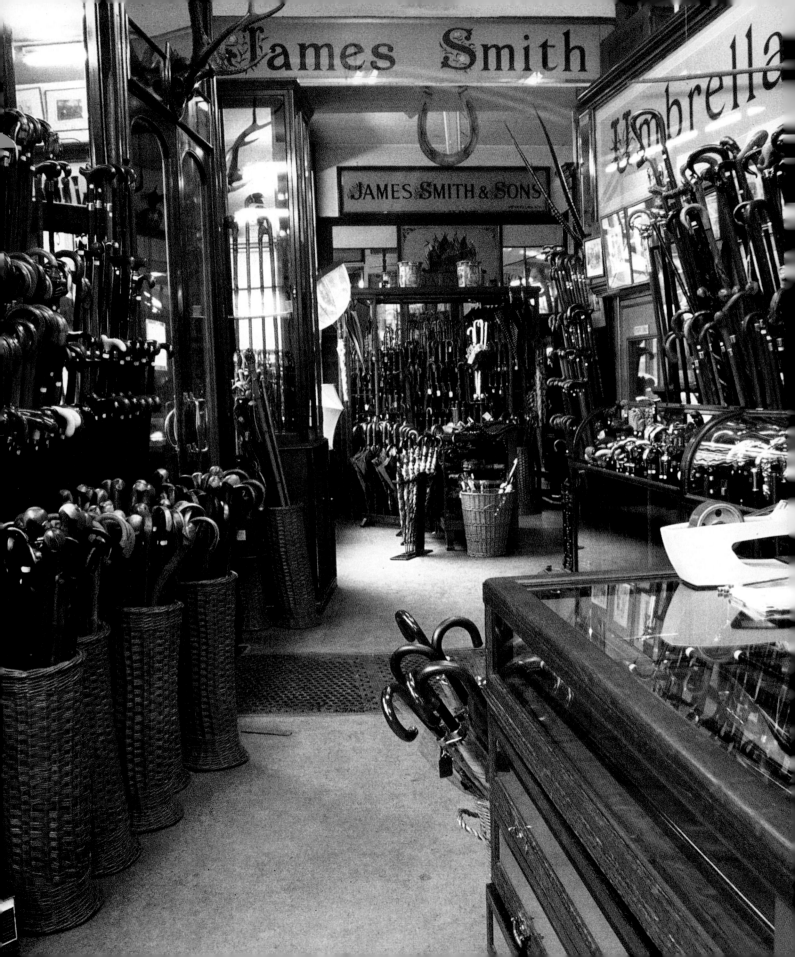

No Fear of Rain

The umbrella is by no means a recent invention; the portable roof over your head, protecting you against rain or excessive sunshine, has been known to mankind for thousands of years. It has been found in the art of the Greeks and Romans, as well as in the China of times long past. Nevertheless, it sank into oblivion for a very long time in Europe, for, according to legend, it was not introduced in London until 1756 by a certain Jonas Hanway. Reactions to the "expanding roof over your head" to combat the notorious London rain ranged from amusement on the one hand, to strict rejection on the other. Hackney coachmen, for example, regarded the umbrella as unwanted competition. Even polite society was initially skeptical, because being seen with an umbrella could lead people to the conclusion that you did not own a carriage. Even so, umbrellas gradually became a permanent feature, presumably due to the lack of anything more effective in the way of rainwear, and because a shower could surprise anyone, even someone that owned a carriage. However, the early models were still very cumbersome and heavy. The modern shape of umbrella is attributed to a certain Samuel Fox, who made a crucial improvement to the construction of the frame that ensured that the shape of the umbrella was narrow and even in a closed position. Despite its indisputably elegant shape, few gentlemen still carry a rolled walking-length umbrella around with them nowadays. Gentlemen with a form of transport, nowadays an automobile, have less need of an umbrella than the user of public transport. The latter will most likely tend to carry articulated rain protection around with him. Nevertheless, many of us regularly take a walking-length umbrella when going for a walk, because it is useful as a walking stick in dry weather, and it provides excellent protection in the rain. In the city you can always find a place to shelter from the rain; on the other hand, an umbrella is often the only salvation from the rain if you are walking across a field or a spacious park. Two's also company when you are sheltering under your umbrella waiting for the rain to stop...

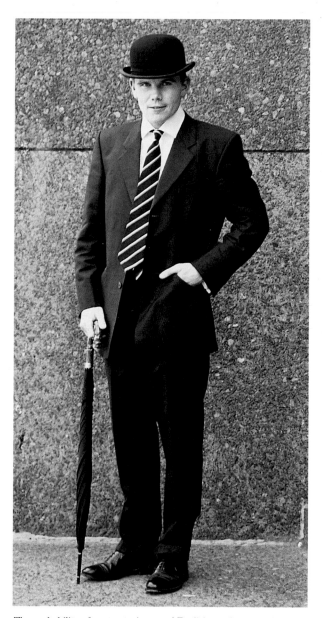

The probability of encountering a real English gentleman with rolled umbrella is greatest in the London district of St. James's. If he is also wearing a bowler hat, he is likely to be a soldier of one of the Guards regiments in civvies.

If you are not happy with the three umbrella lengths available from Brigg, then try your luck at James Smith & Son of 53 New Oxford Street, London. The handles of their umbrellas are not shortened to standard lengths at the outset; instead the length is customized to suit customers. In this way the customer can obtain intermediate sizes that often provide exactly what he had in mind.

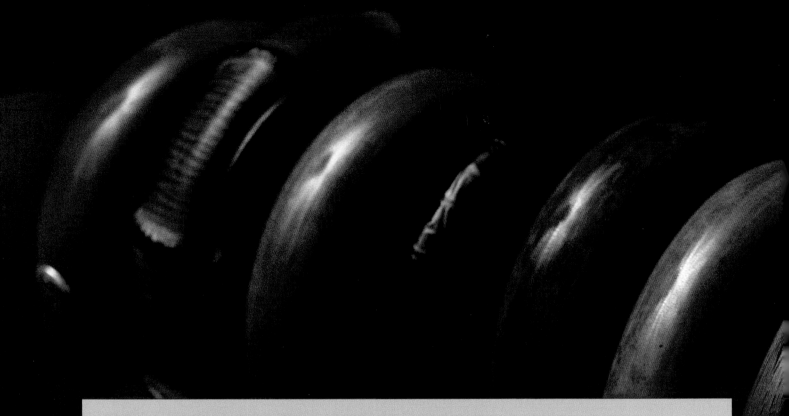

The Other Word in Umbrellas

Swaine, Adeney, Brigg & Sons were resident at 185 Piccadilly, London, for 250 years, and many shoppers still make a pilgrimage to this address, full of happy anticipation at the thought of a Brigg umbrella – "Brigg" being the shortened version of the company name. The disappointed tourist, however, only needs to make a short detour finally to reach his destination at St. James's Street, where the traditional firm has set up a new home at No. 54. What will come as a surprise to many is that you will find somewhat more than just umbrellas here. In this connection, the use of the word "just" is not to suggest that the umbrellas from this firm are wrongly regarded as the best in the world. Here you will find a big selection that are available in three different standard lengths. Especially enticing for the non-English anglophile is that the umbrellas all bear the Royal Warrant. After all, Swaine, Adeney, Brigg & Sons are suppliers to the members of the English Royal Family. Nevertheless, umbrellas form only a part of the range. Not as well known, but just as good, are the leather goods of the venerable firm, comprising valises, holdalls, and containers of all shapes and sizes and of outstanding quality, in which the trophies from a stroll through London's West End can be carried back home safely and in style.

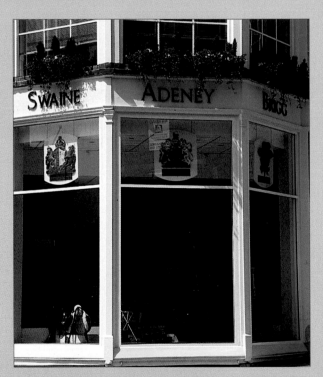

Swaine, Adeney, Brigg & Sons have a big selection of umbrellas in stock. Umbrellas purchased here are regarded as the best and, above all, the most famous in the world.

Top of the range models by Brigg are covered with real silk that is triple woven and slightly inflatable in wet weather, making the fabric absolutely waterproof. If silk umbrellas are too expensive, they are also available in synthetic and cotton fabric mixes.

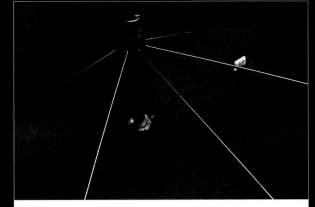

The frame is a "Fox Frame" made of oiled tubular steel, named after its inventor Samuel Fox, who applied for the patent of his construction in 1873. When open, the "roof" of this model measures over a yard [1m] in diameter.

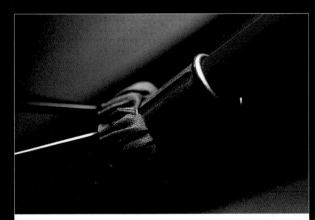

Every detail of a Brigg umbrella, like the retractable clasp of bronzed brass, is of high-quality workmanship. This guarantees the long lifespan of the object.

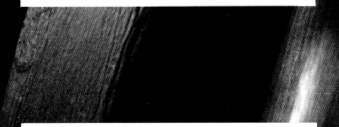

There are umbrellas made from extremely different types of wood, and for the most divergent applications, from the slick black city umbrella to the golfing umbrella with the straight handle, or the umbrella for horse racing. In the handle of the latter there is room for a pencil with which the racing enthusiast can fill out his betting slips. The core of a Brigg umbrella is a real stick, not a metal tube. Naturally, the wood is processed and polished by hand. The handle is bent into shape over hot steam, presumably because this way they can guarantee that it is a really good fit. Such details make the London firm a must for the real umbrella enthusiast.

Glasses

Over the last few decades, glasses have evolved from an unpopular necessity to become a fashionable accessory. In this connection, those who wear glasses are envied for the creations they wear on their noses, whereas previously they were used to being ridiculed by their fellow men.

Women especially were doubly hard hit if they suffered from poor vision, because in addition to the handicap, they had to spoil the look of their faces even more with unattractive spectacle frames. Everyone can recall the unfortunate role that Marilyn Monroe played in the film *Gentlemen Prefer Blondes*, that of a woman who suffered so much from wearing glasses that she preferred to go without them, and thereby landed in all sorts of amusing situations.

Men have it easier in this respect. In terms of the saying that a man does not need to be beautiful, glasses will not necessarily make him flawed. Quite the contrary, glasses still supposedly make him look intelligent, as they always did, yet make him touchingly helpless when he takes them off. Countless attempts have been made to try and establish a correlation between poor eyesight and intelligence. For a time, people who wore glasses were not regarded as more intelligent, but were thought to be more educated than other people, because they had read more and thereby ruined their eyesight. This theory, of course, collapses under closer scrutiny, because apart from the matter of whether bad eyesight is caused by too much reading, reading itself is not necessarily a sign of good education. Ultimately, it depends on what you read, yet in spite of this, prejudice in favor of the idea of the intellectual with the glasses stubbornly sticks. This perhaps even deters some people from switching from glasses to contact lenses. It is surprising that there is still a relatively low number of contact-lens wearers, even though one of the many benefits of contact lenses is that the wearer can finally give up wearing uncomfortable glasses that get in the way, and give his face an unfamiliar look.

Obviously, for many people, glasses become such an organic element of their external appearance that they gladly take on board their disadvantages. They even invest huge amounts of money in designer-label glasses – that is, proportionately larger sums of money than most people would ever spend on clothes. This is in the belief that our faces are the most important part of our appearance and should be particularly emphasized and accentuated by a pair of glasses. Rather than treat ourselves to a new pair of good shoes, we prefer initially to buy a trendy pair of glasses, because we see it every time we look in the mirror. In this respect, it is often forgotten that our fellow human beings perceive us as a whole. People who often experience the fact that others whom they have met only fleetingly primarily recall the pair of glasses worn (or are described as someone wearing a "big pair of glasses"), have probably chosen a model that is too conspicuous or less flattering than it could be. Naturally, everyone has their own personal preferences in terms of the molding of their appearance, and some just love glasses in the same way as others have a weakness for shoes or neckties. However, it is precisely when the weakness for a certain accessory has been established that it can be an interesting experiment to try and omit this accessory occasionally, or to discard it in favor of another detail. From a fashion point of view the spectacle fanatic could consider wearing contact lenses once a week, and confine his need for conspicuous colors to the choice of tie. Those who occasionally switch to wearing contact lenses instead of a pair of glasses may even be surprised at the number of comments about their fine eyes, well-shaped eyebrows, and passable nose. In other words, facial features that normally lead a shadowy existence beneath a dominant pair of glasses may be referred to. There are, of course, inveterate glass wearers who would feel naked without their glasses. For them there is an inexhaustible choice of spectacle frames. It ranges from models that are hardly visible, to very conspicuous and heavy models. Rimless spectacle frames and glasses with thin metal frames reduce the familiarity of the face the least. The other extreme is the thick horn-rimmed spectacles that admittedly are obviously no longer made from horn, but are plastic. In between there are all the different degrees of medium-light to medium-heavy frames made of metal, plastic, or natural materials. Brown and black are the classic colors for horn-rimmed spectacles, and silver and gold for metal-rimmed frames. Basically, every pair of glasses, and particularly a model in rather conspicuous colors, should match the style of dress, in the same way that it matches the color of the eyes, hair, and skin tone.

Despite all fashionable variations, there are only a few basic shapes that could be termed classic and these are circular shapes, semicircular

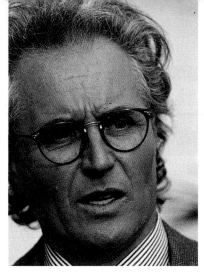

Luciano Benetton in his glasses is more reminiscent of an Italian professor of literature than a rich entrepreneur.

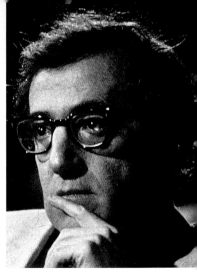

Woody Allen, the most famous wearer of horn-rimmed spectacles in the world. Instead of his favorite disguise of tweed hat, he should wear contact lenses if he wishes to remain incognito in private.

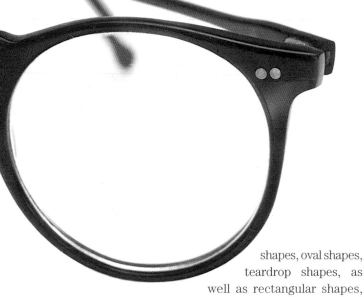

shapes, oval shapes, teardrop shapes, as well as rectangular shapes, and trapezium shapes. The choice of frame should take into account the shape of your face, so as to produce either harmony or contrast. Before you decide to buy, it is highly recommended that you take one final look in a full-size mirror for a careful judgement of the effect of the glasses in relation to your clothes, build, head shape, and hair color.

You should buy the pair of spectacle frames that stands up to all these checks, because fashions in glasses, like all fashions, are subject to rapid change. A pair of glasses can, therefore, rapidly disappear again from the range, and there is nothing more annoying than finding you have missed the ideal model. The perfect pair of glasses is almost as elusive as the off-the-rack jacket that fits perfectly.

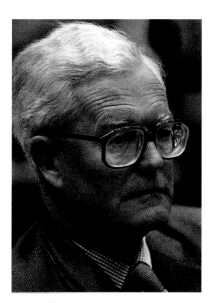

Douglas Hurd, the former British government minister and also a crime novelist, represents the anti-designer-label glasses type, something often encountered in England. In many circles there, a suit from Savile Row is considered more important than a modern spectacle frame.

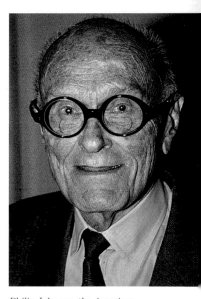

Philip Johnson, the American architect, has chosen a round horn-rimmed spectacle frame as his distinguishing feature. Its pure form is definitely a good choice for a designer.

Not only when the Sun Shines

Sunglasses fulfill many different functions. On the one hand, they protect your eyes from sunlight, and particularly from harmful UV rays. In the last few years, the latter aspect has gradually become the main focus. On the other hand, they are a fashionable, and, from time to time, expensive accessory that some wear more on their heads than on their noses. Yet, ultimately, dark glasses are an expression of the wish for anonymity, since a person who hides his eyes cannot be easily recognized. Nevertheless, however well sunglasses may avert intrusive looks, they can simultaneously draw attention to the person wearing them; anyone wearing sunglasses in a confined space becomes so conspicuous that any attempt at disguise is immediately blown. Would-be stars, however, also use this ploy to gain some attention, though with the excuse, of course, of wishing to remain incognito. No one knows how to cope so well with sunglasses as a fashionable accessory as the people in those countries in Europe where the sun shines most of the time. Sunglasses are really crucial there, and form part of the basic equipment, like a watch and mobile phone. Away from southern Europe, sunglasses were previously worn particularly when driving a car, originally only in blazing sunshine. It was not until the 1980s that people slowly started to discover and accept sunglasses as everyday objects – and, more importantly, as status symbols too. Ray Bans by Bausch & Lomb have definitely achieved cult status in Europe, not merely because of their outstanding lenses, but also because of their high price that caused Americans just to shake their heads in amazement. For a long time, therefore, Ray Bans brought back from the USA were similarly coveted, just like *501 Shrink-to-fit* Levi jeans or the tassel loafers by Alden. Yet these cult sunglasses deservedly enjoy their almost legendary reputation; after all, the first American pilots' sunglasses came from the firm of Bausch & Lomb. Although tinted glasses had been in existence since the nineteenth century, they could not withstand heights above cloud level. The US Army Air Corps, therefore, turned to Bausch & Lomb, a leading American manufacturer of optical lenses. This firm developed a totally new type of sunglasses and unveiled it to the military in 1930 – Ray Bans were born. To be absolutely precise, it must be added that these sunglasses were initially labeled "Anti-glare Goggles," and were not rechristened "Ray Bans" until a year later. Six years later, that is, in 1936, these sunglasses were also released to the general public, since when they have enjoyed enormous popularity, although most people certainly do not wear them in the cockpit of an aircraft. The famous teardrop shape, moreover, is not an arbitrary design, but corresponds to the field of vision of the human eye. Nowadays, sunglasses are rarely still designed according to such absolutely scientific criteria. They have become a fashion element, and the shapes change from season to season. Every self-respecting fashion designer has his own collection of sunglasses and, depending on your taste, you will always find a model that appeals to you. Whether this model is long lasting is dubious. Sunglasses from classic suppliers are more likely to come with a guarantee and, therefore, a make like Ray Ban is often the choice of the man who favors a timeless style. Ray Ban have their imitators, but any true observer of style can easily identify a fake, and as such they are best avoided.

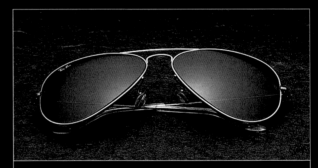

This pair of sunglasses is a direct descendant of the first pair of pilots' sunglasses by Bausch & Lomb. It is an absolutely timeless design. It suits the Harley of the 1950s just as well as the latest Ferrari. It can also be fitted with special earpieces for sport.

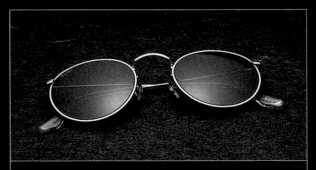

Not every pair of sunglasses by Ray Ban automatically resembles the Wayfarer. A whole series of classic but discreet models with metal-rimmed frames that are not immediately recognizable as expensive Ray Bans have been available for a long time.

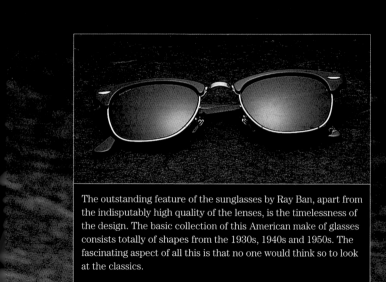

The outstanding feature of the sunglasses by Ray Ban, apart from the indisputably high quality of the lenses, is the timelessness of the design. The basic collection of this American make of glasses consists totally of shapes from the 1930s, 1940s and 1950s. The fascinating aspect of all this is that no one would think so to look at the classics.

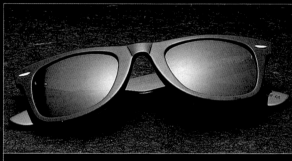

Both the black and also the brown Wayfarer perfectly suit the faces of Mediterranean types, but black is often too hard a contrast in the case of sometimes rather pale northern or central Europeans. The latter therefore prefer the brown model that goes particularly well with a smart Italian casual look and perfectly convey a sense of style.

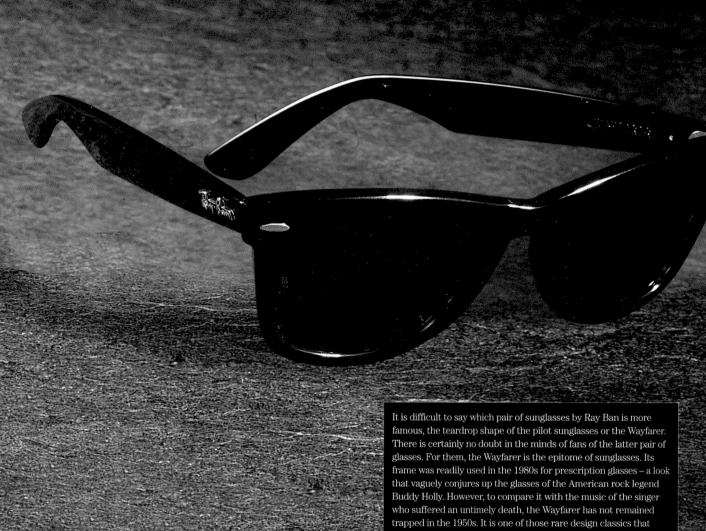

It is difficult to say which pair of sunglasses by Ray Ban is more famous, the teardrop shape of the pilot sunglasses or the Wayfarer. There is certainly no doubt in the minds of fans of the latter pair of glasses. For them, the Wayfarer is the epitome of sunglasses. Its frame was readily used in the 1980s for prescription glasses – a look that vaguely conjures up the glasses of the American rock legend Buddy Holly. However, to compare it with the music of the singer who suffered an untimely death, the Wayfarer has not remained trapped in the 1950s. It is one of those rare design classics that every generation can rediscover for itself.

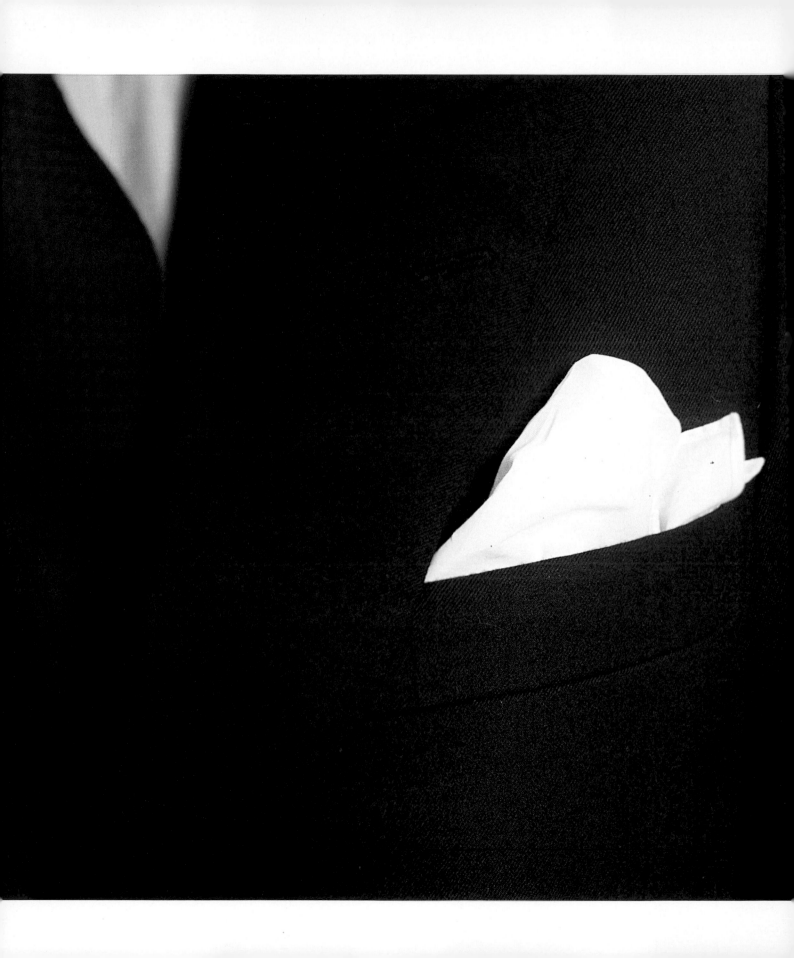

The Handkerchief

Hardly any accessory demonstrates the degree of security or insecurity in a man as happens in the case of the dress handkerchief. This relates to his self-confidence as well as to his sound judgement in matters of style. An insecure and shy man is deterred from using a dress handkerchief by the least little thing. It is either too conspicuous, difficult to coordinate with the rest of his clothes, difficult to fold into the right shape, or it could look excessive. When is it appropriate and when not, and when is it worn? The question of "when" can be answered quickest. It is always appropriate, when you are wearing a jacket – that is, both a suit jacket, and also a casual jacket or blazer, even if you are wearing jeans or chinos. Dress handkerchiefs are, therefore, not linked at all to the wearing of neckties. On the contrary, a dress handkerchief can often convey an air of relaxed elegance to a casual outfit that is worn without a tie. The remaining question concerns "how." This is also fairly easy to answer. A handkerchief that somehow picks up the colors of the rest of the clothes, thereby producing an interesting harmony, is tucked into the breast pocket, as demonstrated on the next page. You may now be thinking that you would need a gigantic selection of handkerchiefs, but in fact you should manage with relatively few. A blue and red paisley-patterned handkerchief can be coordinated with several ties, for example, if they contain the colors red or blue. The best thing to do next time you go shopping is simply to take a few handkerchiefs with you, and then try out different combinations in peace in the mirror at home. With a little bit of practice, the handkerchief will soon appear to be as elegant and relaxed as if it had been tucked into the breast pocket of a meticulously clothed tailor's dummy in the display window of a very good gentlemen's outfitters.

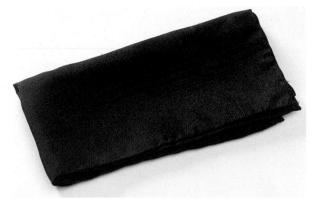

A silk dress handkerchief should be hemmed by hand. Since this means additional time-consuming work during manufacture, it is regarded as a sign of quality. If it were made of poor-quality silk, makers would not bother with this time-consuming work. Good quality, however, is particularly important in terms of dress handkerchiefs, since they are permanently creased, folded, and squashed. Poor-quality silk would not cope with this for long.

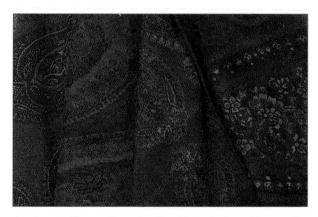

A patterned silk or cashmere handkerchief looks best with a casual jacket. Any good outfitter should have a large selection of different designs in stock.

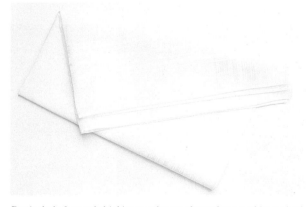

A white linen handkerchief is appropriate for all formal occasions. The rule of thumb is that a white linen handkerchief is a safe bet whenever a white shirt is appropriate. Like the silk handkerchief, it should be hemmed by hand. Some gentlemen also have their initials embroidered on it. A white cotton handkerchief "for practical use" is tucked into the pants or jacket pocket. To be absolutely sure, I would like to stress once again that you never blow your nose on a silk dress handkerchief. The white cotton handkerchief is used for this purpose. It is a peculiarity of the British to pull from the pockets of their dark suits not a white linen handkerchief but a brightly patterned one.

Particularly forward-thinking gentlemen always have a white and, of course, clean handkerchief on their person, to be able to offer it in an emergency to a lady. Many people, however, totally reject fabric handkerchiefs, preferring to use paper tissues. This is an easy-to-comprehend and equally acceptable attitude.

From Hand to Breast Pocket

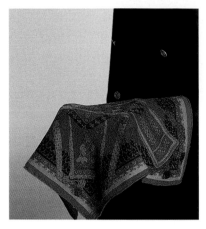

Spread the handkerchief out over the flat of your hand.

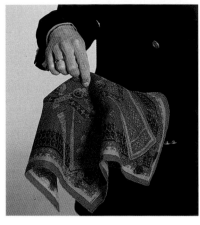

Take the handkerchief gently between the index finger and thumb of the right hand.

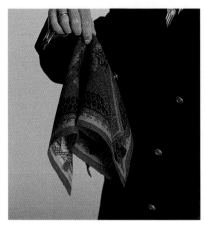

Hold the handkerchief up with the right hand and shake it gently.

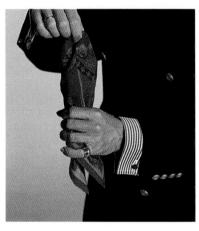

Loosely grasp the bottom of the handkerchief with the left hand.

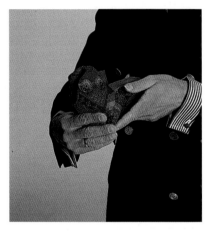

Take hold of the lower half with the right hand and fold it widthwise.

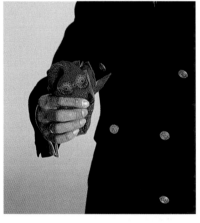

Hold the folded handkerchief in the right hand, but do not squash it together.

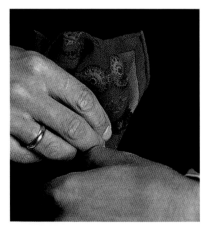

Hold breast pocket open with the left hand and tuck in the handkerchief with the right.

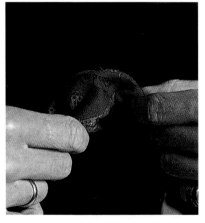

Rearrange it with the thumbs and index fingers of both hands.

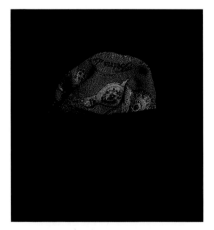

The finished dress handkerchief in the breast pocket – as if "molded."

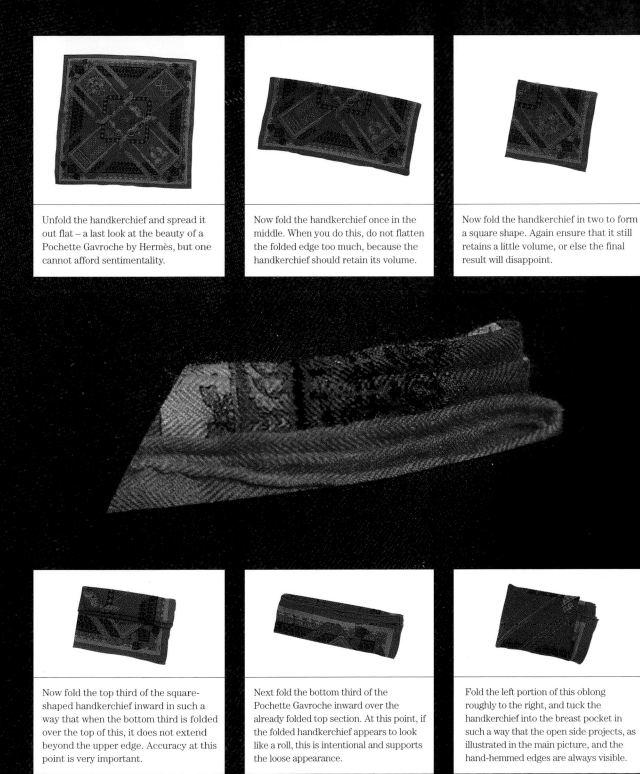

Unfold the handkerchief and spread it out flat – a last look at the beauty of a Pochette Gavroche by Hermès, but one cannot afford sentimentality.

Now fold the handkerchief once in the middle. When you do this, do not flatten the folded edge too much, because the handkerchief should retain its volume.

Now fold the handkerchief in two to form a square shape. Again ensure that it still retains a little volume, or else the final result will disappoint.

Now fold the top third of the square-shaped handkerchief inward in such a way that when the bottom third is folded over the top of this, it does not extend beyond the upper edge. Accuracy at this point is very important.

Next fold the bottom third of the Pochette Gavroche inward over the already folded top section. At this point, if the folded handkerchief appears to look like a roll, this is intentional and supports the loose appearance.

Fold the left portion of this oblong roughly to the right, and tuck the handkerchief into the breast pocket in such a way that the open side projects, as illustrated in the main picture, and the hand-hemmed edges are always visible.

The Right Combination

In terms of dress handkerchiefs, anything goes, as long as it looks good. However, avoid the "ex works" ready-folded variety of dress handkerchief, and also those that turn up in a supposedly stylistically safe pack combined with a tie. They are simply a little too boring. The whole point of the dress handkerchief is the interesting interplay between the latter and necktie, shirt, jacket, and the rest of the outfit. How this is achieved is left to each individual. Some have the dress handkerchief coordinating with the color of their socks, others select a handkerchief in a color that contrasts with all the other colors. A third section of people perhaps even daringly select a mixture of patterns. The latter, however, is usually the reason why many men recoil from wearing a dress handkerchief. Admittedly, skillful coordination of different designs and colors is difficult, not because of countless secret rules that are only known by insiders, but more precisely because of a complete lack of any valid rules for a guide to what is a good mixture of patterns and what is not. Skill in mixing patterns simply depends on your personal interpretation of style, and on the courage to stick to what appeals to you. Inevitably, it must not be the same thing that appeals to colleagues, and for every four people who agree on a certain mix of patterns, there is always a fifth person who disagrees. Some people may now like to maintain that there are indeed rules. For example, there is the rule governing the fact that similar patterns should not be combined, that is, no check tie with a check shirt, and no striped shirt with a striped suit. Yet, basically, this is a weak kind of rule. Of course you can combine similar patterns, only, as mentioned before, they must coordinate. Only you can decide whether you have achieved a coordinated look or not. Therefore, three cheers for the joy of experimenting. It is only by this means that the classic style can be further developed, and only in this way that style itself can further evolve. Moreover, you can gain inspiration for mixing patterns from anywhere, whether you are leafing through high-quality art books, strolling through a good furniture store, or at an art exhibition. There are many opportunities for acquiring an expert eye, so that during the selection of a dress handkerchief (or putting together a complete outfit), you will find the ideal

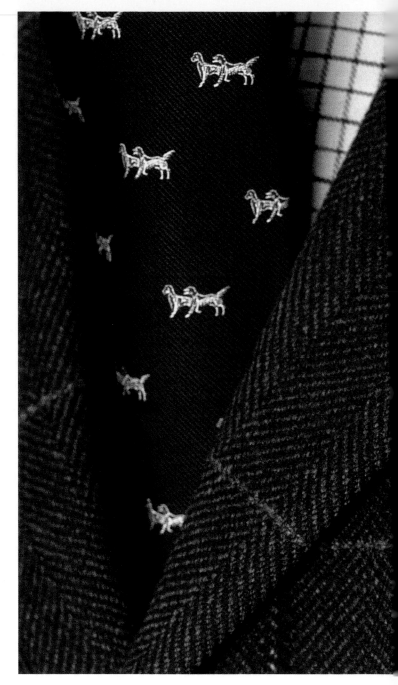

combination that is simultaneously both harmonious and interesting, both classic and innovative, and both elegant and modern. In view of the large number of potential combinations, those shown here are of course only a small sample of what is possible. Many combinations are possible. As already mentioned, anything goes, as long as you like it, and if you have good taste, you can't go wrong.

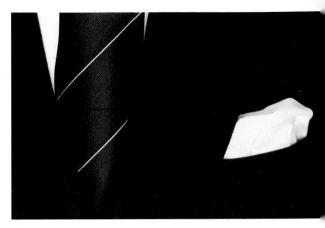

A plain but not at all bad combination is a white handkerchief with white shirt, discreet necktie, and blue blazer.

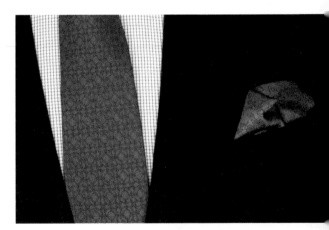

A somewhat more courageous mixture of patterns in terms of shirt, necktie, and dress handkerchief. The whole is set against the reassuring framework of a dark gray suit.

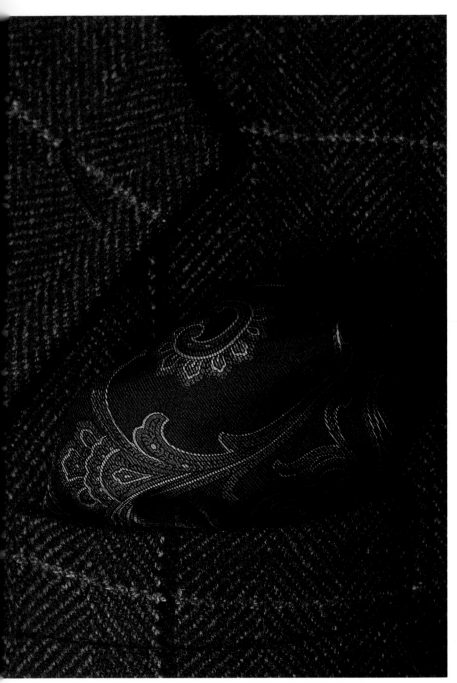

Color and shine of tie and dress handkerchief are especially emphasized by the rough surface of the tweed. Conversely, the woolen fabric has an almost pleasingly three-dimensional effect compared with the smoothness of the silk. The light horizontal stripe of the jacket is picked up in the shirt, in the motif on the tie, and in the Paisley of the silk handkerchief that visually holds the pattern together.

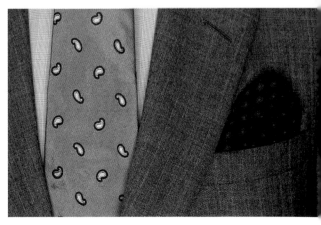

Suit, shirt, necktie, and dress handkerchief all show patterns. Thus, the overall picture is harmonious and yet interesting.

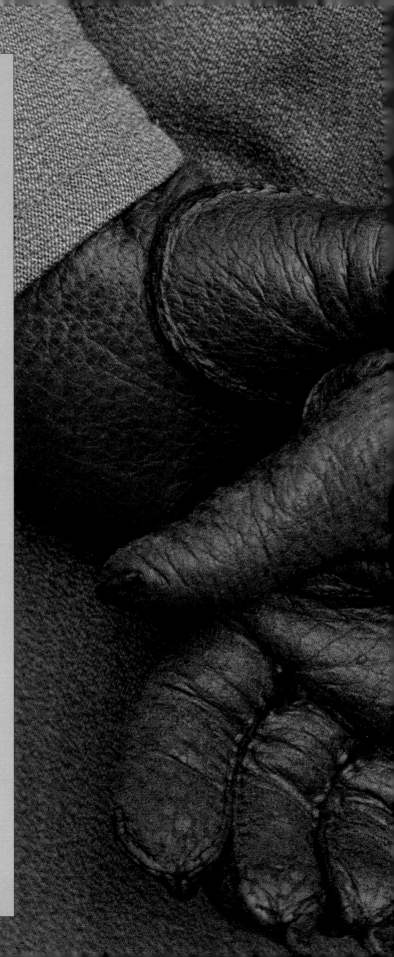

The Glove

Sport and leisure nowadays give people plenty of opportunity to be seen in light clothing or even without any clothes on at all. Eras such as these alternate in the history of man with phases of great reserve, or even prudery. In the eighteenth or nineteenth century, it would have been unthinkable for men and women to do sport or even sit in a sauna together. This would only have happened in extremely dubious establishments, and even many married people never saw their partners fully unclothed. During these times, you also wore gloves as often as possible, and especially in public. It was simply considered impolite to extend a bare hand when greeting a person, and especially a lady. Therefore, you needed to own the appropriate gloves for every occasion during the day, evening, and night, and a gentleman kept a correspondingly large stock of these. In former times, people used to glance critically at your gloves, the way we nowadays make a mental note of the cut of the suit, or the shoe leather. Gloves had to be made of the finest leather and be a perfect fit, and were never allowed to show even the slightest trace of dirt. The demands we make on gloves today appear very minor compared with former times. This can be attributed to the fact that gloves are nowadays only worn on the street. The only exceptions are white gloves with tails that are also kept on in confined spaces. During the course of the last century, gloves became further removed from their original role as protectors, and developed to become increasingly a ritualistic and strongly symbolic piece of clothing. Now they have returned to their original state. They are currently leading a modest existence preventing chilblains on fingers. Yet possibly it will soon be fashionable again to wear gloves; perhaps this will also be made absolutely necessary by external influences, as has happened with the sunhat that has simply become an intrinsic factor in many parts of the world. In terms of the protecting role of gloves, they do not merely have to be confined to assisting in heavy work or keeping you warm in winter. It can be perfectly appropriate not to seize hold of doorknobs, handles and staircase banisters, on public transport, or in buildings, with your bare hands. For sports car enthusiasts, driving gloves are essential items, and drivers of more simply functional automobiles may find them advantageous. In this case, the gloves are fulfilling a useful role, and are not simply fashion accessories.

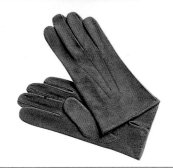

Buckskin still recalls the variety of leather types that used to be available to gentlemen for their gloves, and they are a classic style.

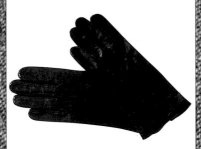

Black or at least dark gloves go with black shoes. They are available both lined and unlined. They should always be made of leather.

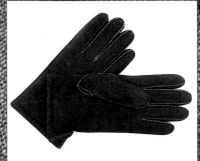

Lambskin gloves are classic for the cold season. The wooly interior keeps your hands outstandingly warm. Brown is the popular color here.

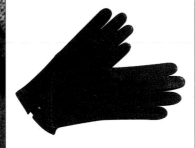

Brown grained pigskin-leather gloves coordinate well with brown shoes and casual clothes. They are the proverbial gentleman's gloves.

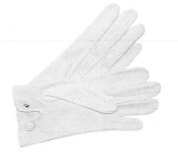

Even today, you can still wear white gloves with evening dress. In the absence of white goatskin gloves they are usually made of cotton.

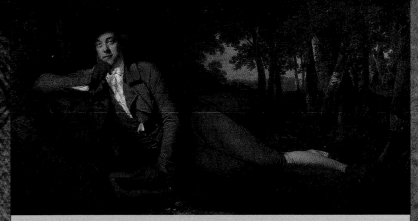

In this painting from 1781 by the English painter Joseph Wright of Derby, we see Sir Brooke Boothby occupied reading Rousseau. Although it seems mild enough for the amateur philosopher to lie full length on the forest floor, he is nevertheless wearing gloves. Obviously you did not wear gloves exclusively against the cold, but because it would have been inappropriate to show your bare hands.

Scarf Refinement

The forerunner of today's warm scarves is generally known as the "focale." It was worn by Roman legionaries as a protection against the unfamiliar cold in Gaul and Germania. In terms of any identity of form and function it may have had with the scarf of today, it is questionable whether the "focale" really was the forerunner or it represented a development of much earlier models. However, there have been no further changes to the principle of the scarf down to the present day. It generates warm air that protects us from cooling down. Heat is retained to a greater or lesser extent, depending on thickness, type, and processing of the wool. As so often in life, coarse woolen scarves are regarded as unrefined and fine woolen scarves as refined.

The more casual the occasion, the coarser, thicker, and also more colorful the scarf. Formal occasions, on the other hand, call for fine cashmere scarves that can be lined with silk in addition. There are even samples made of the finest silk that are almost merely symbolic of scarves; compared with their loose-knit, woolen cousins, they only generate a very inconsequential amount of heat. The above-mentioned cashmere scarves are the best compromise between thermal effect and formal appearance. They are accessories, similar to neckties or dress handkerchiefs, and you can stand out from the masses by ensuring your choice of scarf is made with meticulous care. When in search of something special, you should look out for scarves by Drake's. This English manufacturer produces them for the best men's outfitters in the world, but they are also sold under their own name. Connoisseurs maintain that in high-quality products they can immediately recognize the work of Michael J. Drake, who is designer and co-owner of Drake's.

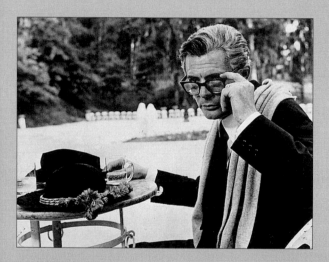

Marcello Mastroianni was typical of film stars who enjoyed being seen wearing scarves, and artistically draped them round their necks – something they have in common with many of those who are artists or who regard themselves as such.

Scarves should not only be geared to the outside temperature, but should also be coordinated with the style of the coat (which is also geared to cold temperatures). That is, a fine silk or cashmere scarf, or a combination of both, should be worn with an elegant coat. The scarf must also match the occasion – a red scarf would be inappropriate at a funeral. Apart from the common combination possibilities, there is of course always the unusual and eccentric combination too. On the one hand, a deliberate contrast can be produced between coat and scarf, for example, because you might be bored with harmony. However, a somewhat unusual combination is often deliberately done to reveal something about yourself. A coarse, even hand-knitted, scarf worn with an elegant city coat could mean: "I am a successful businessman or politician, yet I cling to the good old things, like this scarf that my wife knitted for me 20 years ago." An elegant silk-lined cashmere scarf worn with a duffel coat could be saying: "I do not attach great importance to elegance in general, but I do have one or two good items…." Like any other item of clothing, scarves often also send out a clear message, which is unlikely to be ignored. As with most other accessories, the important thing to remember about scarves is to get the right balance between style and practicality.

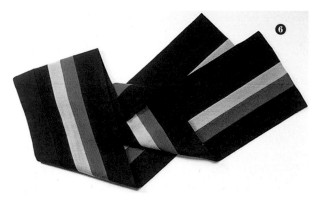

❶ Thick, warm, and wooly – the best thing to have with you in winter. Yet this woolen scarf is wholly inappropriate for formal occasions and for wearing with a city coat – even in very cold weather.

❷ This silk scarf is definitely the most elegant scarf. It is used primarily in a visual way to close the gap caused by the neckline of the coat, since the neck of the wearer otherwise projects and looks bare. It also helps to keep the collar of the coat clean.

❸ These are thin woolen scarves made from the same material used for light wool ties. They are particularly suitable for the interim periods in spring and fall.

❹ Cashmere scarves are often lined with silk. They thereby make an elegant impact on the outside, yet keep the neck and chest warm.

❺ Cashmere scarves are available in a similar variety to silk neckties. They can look casual or formal, depending on the color and design, as well as their thickness and roughness.

❻ Like a regimental necktie that displays the colors of the wearer's military unit, the college scarf is also in the colors of the respective school, and is thus a kind of "proof of identity."

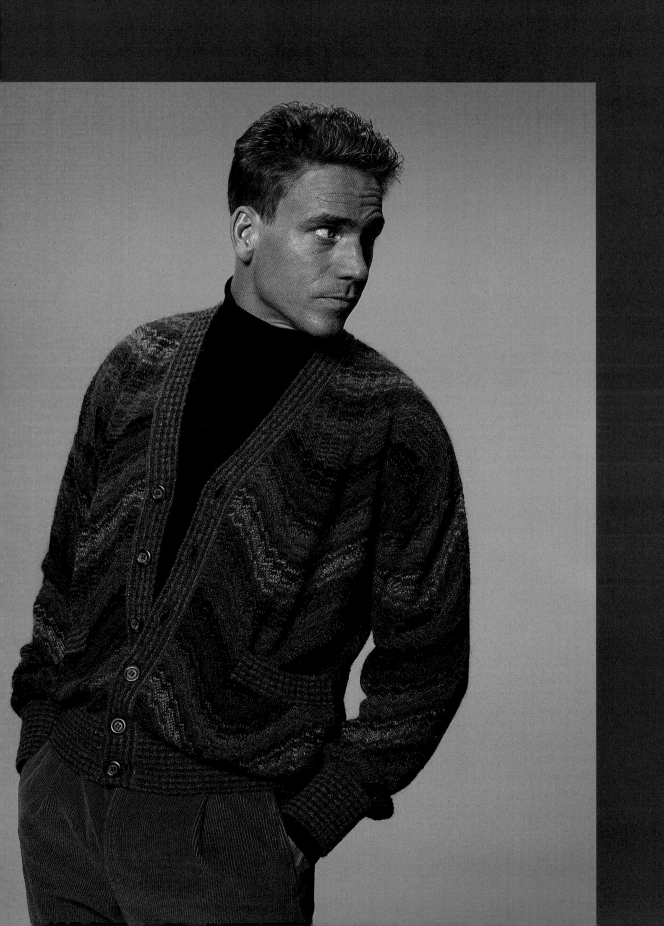

Knitwear

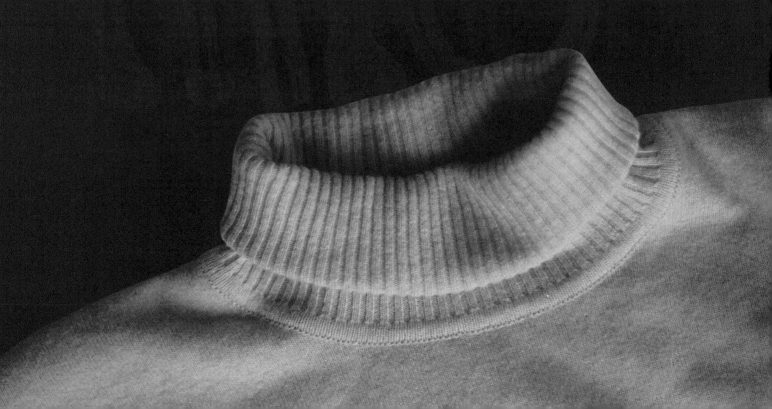

In the far north beyond Scotland lie the Shetland Islands. Here live the sheep whose wool is processed to make Shetland wool. The thinly populated islands still provide plenty of the pasture that has become rare in densely populated parts of Europe.

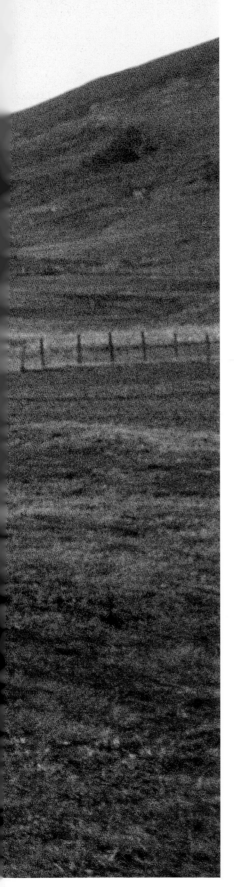

In the Beginning Was the Sweater

Until well into the middle of the nineteenth century an English gentleman had no reason to wear anything knitted. Only simple people wore something of the sort as a form of robust and particularly affordable work clothes. Not until the middle classes too began to discover sport as a form of physical exercise for themselves, did the demand for fine knitted goods emerge. They were worn, for example, for bicycle riding; for all kinds of ball games, including cricket; and for the game of polo. The article of clothing made of wool was given the name of "sweater," referring to the "sweat"-inducing effect of the wool. Initially, sweaters had simple round necklines, then came the V-neck sweaters that looked good decorated with club colors. In order to satisfy the increasing demand, sweaters soon became mass produced. For this purpose, they were cut to size from readymade webs of knitted wool and then sewn together. This is called the "cut and sew" method. The more expensive option was the "fully fashioned" method. In this case, every article of clothing was machine knitted individually and as a whole. Knitwear is still differentiated, even today, according to these two general manufacturing methods. The sweater shapes resulted from well-known examples of menswear. The V-neck pullover is an adaptation of the vest. The similarity is even more obvious in the sleeveless and buttoned version. The round neckline recalls a collarless shirt that in those times was still pulled over the head (like the pullover today). Naturally, shapes were also borrowed from traditional home knitwear, as were patterns and colors that occurred in great variety throughout the British Isles.

Since the sweater was designed for sport and leisure activities, it became integrated into the outfits that were worn at the weekend and in the country. For example, a knitted vest was designed for wearing under a tweed jacket when out riding or hunting.

All attempts to introduce the sweater (or "pullover," as the Germans prefer to call it) into the dress code in terms of formal clothing have so far remained unsuccessful. At best, a sweater is accepted as being analogous with a vest for a suit, but only in exceptional situations – as for example, on journeys, or if the heating breaks down. It can be better coordinated with a casual jacket, as is common practice in Italian style.

The real achievement of knitwear still lies in elegant casual clothing. Italians have perfected this look like no other nation. The sweater belongs here, worn or casually draped around the shoulders, both in summer and winter alike, on a shopping trip, visiting a museum, or having an aperitif in a bar. The sweater is meanwhile understood worldwide as being symbolic of freedom. As soon as politicians want to show themselves as private individuals, you can guarantee they will wear something knitted. A sweater is also an ideal companion for businessmen who want to travel light. After completing his tasks, he merely needs to remove the jacket of his suit and necktie, open the collar of his shirt, and drape a sweater around his shoulders, and the informal part of the evening is ushered in. He can feel relaxed and yet be aware that even in an informal guise he is recognized as a gentleman, very conscious of style.

From Sheep to Wool

Man has used the wool from different animals for thousands of years for making himself clothes. In this connection, wool was the most important raw material right from the start. Today there are around one billion (thousand million) sheep worldwide that supply approximately 2.2 billion US tons [2 billion kg] of wool annually. Herds of sheep need a lot of room; therefore intensive sheep breeding is only carried out in low-population regions. In this respect, Australia is in first place, with a population of 156 million sheep, of which approximately two-thirds are merinos. The extremely frizzy merino wool is the most highly prized sheep wool in the world, and most suit materials are produced from it. Apart from this, there is the lower quality and not so frizzy wool from crossbreeds. This is the raw product for coarser materials and knitted goods. Supreme quality hairs are, however, obtained from goats (cashmere and mohair), llamas and their relations (alpaca and vicuña), camels (camel hair), and rabbits (angora). These hairs

can also be blended with pure new wool. They can be further processed like sheep's wool, yet extracting them is more expensive than is the case with sheep's wool, since the hairs are not shorn, but have to be combed out. The way vicuña is obtained is even more laborious – hair caught on bushes is collected by hand. Only hair that has been obtained from the living animal can be labeled pure new wool. The shorn wool of a sheep can weigh between 2 and 11 pounds [1–5 kg] (the annual yield of vicuña per animal is only about a half pound [240 grams] by comparison). After shearing, the wool is washed, dyed, and spun to make yarn. Thinner yarns are usually woven, whereas thicker products can be used for knitting. The quality and price of the resulting knitted goods depend on the type of hair and the spinning method. The labels "one-ply," "two-ply," or even "eight-ply" indicate the number of cashmere or wool threads spun together, and whichever applies usually depends on the type of garment.

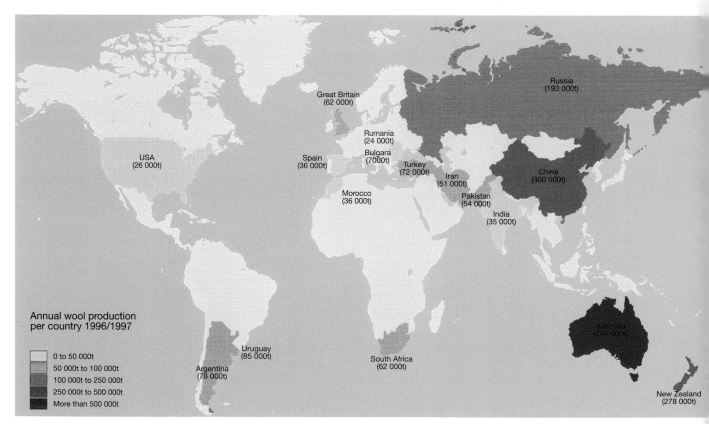

Annual wool production per country 1996/1997

- 0 to 50 000t
- 50 000t to 100 000t
- 100 000t to 250 000t
- 250 000t to 500 000t
- More than 500 000t

Great Britain (62 000t)
Russia (193 000t)
Rumania (24 000t)
Bulgaria (7000t)
Spain (36 000t)
Turkey (72 000t)
Iran (51 000t)
China (300 000t)
USA (26 000t)
Morocco (36 000t)
Pakistan (54 000t)
India (35 000t)
Uruguay (85 000t)
Argentina (78 000t)
South Africa (62 000t)
Australia (704 000t)
New Zealand (278 000t)

Sheep's wool is produced worldwide. Australia supplies the best qualities and also the biggest quantities. Here wool production is in a very favorable ratio to the number of animals, since the majority (over 60 percent) of the sheep are merinos that supply more wool than any of the other sheep varieties.

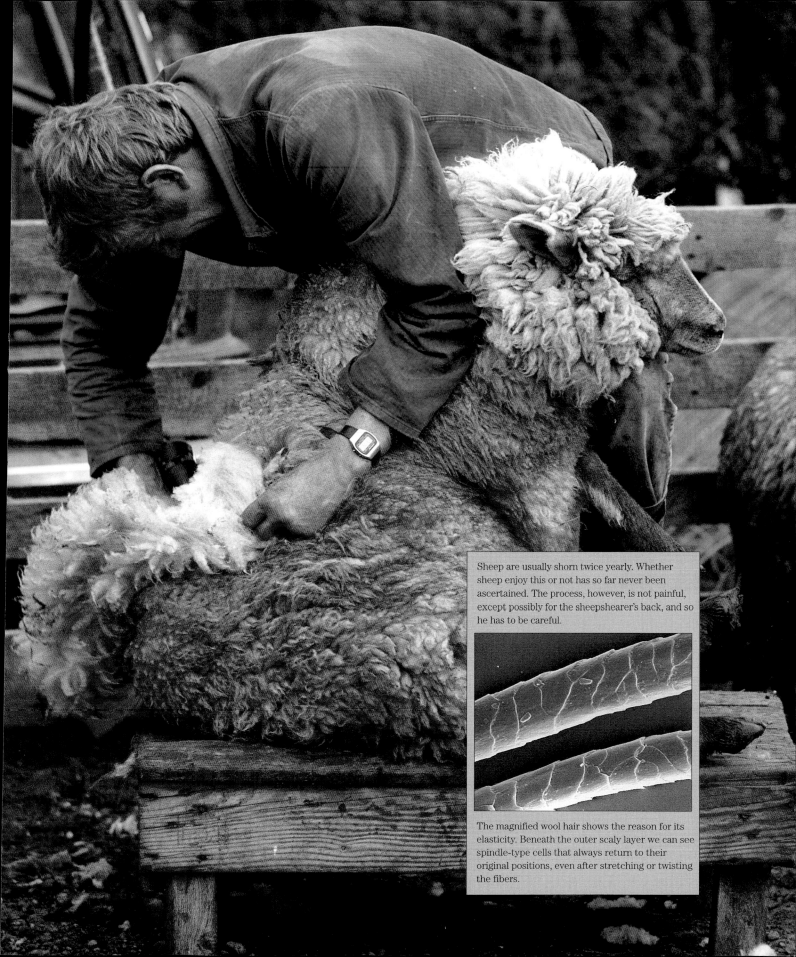

Sheep are usually shorn twice yearly. Whether sheep enjoy this or not has so far never been ascertained. The process, however, is not painful, except possibly for the sheepshearer's back, and so he has to be careful.

The magnified wool hair shows the reason for its elasticity. Beneath the outer scaly layer we can see spindle-type cells that always return to their original positions, even after stretching or twisting the fibers.

Classic Knitwear

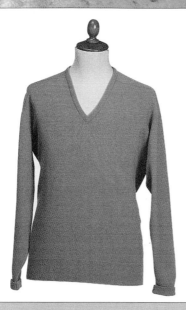

The V-neck sweater looks good worn under a sports jacket. Sweater and necktie worn without a sports jacket are problematic and can easily look boring.

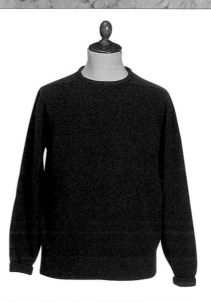

If the round-neck sweater is worn over a shirt, the shirt collar belongs under the sweater. The latter looks very good with a shirt with a button-down collar.

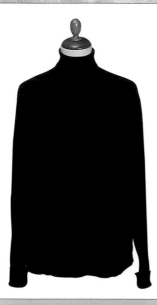

The polo-neck sweater is pleasant for winter walks, since it is a substitute for a scarf. You should wear a shirt underneath so that you can take off the sweater if necessary. Creative professional groups wear the black polo-neck sweater almost exclusively.

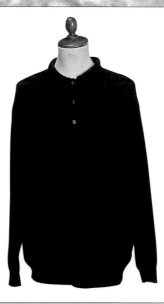

The sweater with soft collar and three-button opening has presumably developed from rugby players' jerseys. It tends to be worn as a winter version of the short-sleeved shirt with soft collar and three-button opening.

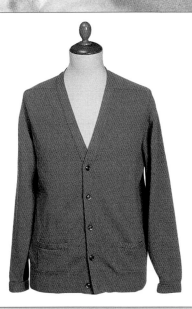

The knitted jacket has three crucial advantages over the sweater. Firstly, it can be worn open, meaning the thermal effect can be regulated. Secondly, you can take it off and put it on without disturbing your hair or knocking your glasses off your nose. Thirdly, knitted jackets often incorporate a small pocket for cigarettes, keys, or change.

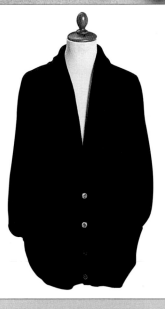

The chunky knit jacket with shawl collar is particularly suitable for those of us who are very sensitive to the cold, and also for the inhabitants of poorly heated country houses. Avoid dark-blue versions with gold buttons; these are only worn by – if you will pardon my saying so – ageing playboys.

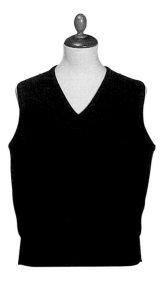

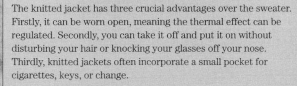

The (sleeveless) pullover is a good substitute for a vest, though it is not liked by everyone. On many men it looks too plain and conservative, yet it is ideal for keeping warm when you are sitting down. Since it has no sleeves, you also do not overheat so easily.

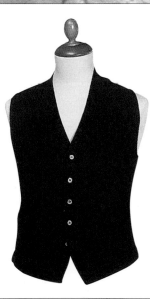

Compared to the sleeveless pullover, the knitted vest has all the advantages already described for the knitted jacket. A word of warning, however: unless the cut is right, the look can quickly misfire, just as suit vests can.

Between England and France

The knitwear industry has a long tradition on Guernsey. During the sixteenth century the island obtained permission to import wool from England and in return to supply the Crown with knitted goods. Queen Mary I and Queen Elizabeth I both owned woolen products from this Channel Island. Allegedly, the stockings that Mary Queen of Scots wore at her beheading also originated from Guernsey. The Royals at that time would hardly have worn a Guernsey (sweater), whereas nowadays, this working sweater of fishermen, mariners, and farmers is certainly sometimes worn by members of the Royal Family. The island's women initially produced the Guernseys only for their husbands. For the sweater to be able to withstand wind and surf, the woolen threads were spun to form a hard yarn and then knitted tightly, using fine-gauge needles. In actual fact the Guernsey did its job astonishingly well, even though knitted sweaters are not generally capable of being very weather resistant. Even today, only the best English worsted yarn is used for an original Guernsey. The traditional color of the Guernsey is dark navy blue, but there are also less authentic country versions available in olive green. Real Guernseys are of course "fully fashioned" and "hand-finished," that is, knitted piece by piece and sewn together by hand. Though cotton summer Guernseys have become available in recent years, they are undoubtedly not so robust as their original woolen counterparts. In the nineteenth century, Guernseys were even the subject of military approval. Lord Nelson pronounced them fit for the Royal Navy, and recommended them to the naval ministry. In 1857, the warm sweater formed part of the winter equipment for the soldiers of the garrison in Halifax, in the Canadian province of Nova Scotia.

The characteristic patterns of the Guernsey have been handed down from generation to generation, and daughters still learn from their mothers and grandmothers how to knit the weatherproof sweaters today. The decorative textured detail is supposed to represent daily objects from the lives of the fishermen. The ribbing at both sleeve ends consequently represents a ship's ladder or rigging, the hooked-up shoulder seam stands for a rope, and the garter-stitch panel around the armholes symbolizes the waves on the beach. Other details are there for practical reasons, like the square gusset under the arm that provides freedom of movement. Since the gusset folds together when the arm is in the resting position, the sweater also fits well under a jacket, provided the narrow-fitting sleeves are not too bulky. Therefore the Guernsey is an item of clothing that perfectly combines tradition and practicality. Probably that is exactly why it is so popular in many countries.

Guernsey is one of the most famous of the Channel Islands. Its reasonably small area of 24 square miles [63 sq km] offers a mixture of English snugness and French lifestyle.

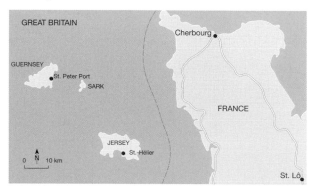

Many English people use Guernsey for short seaside breaks.

The Guernsey in Detail

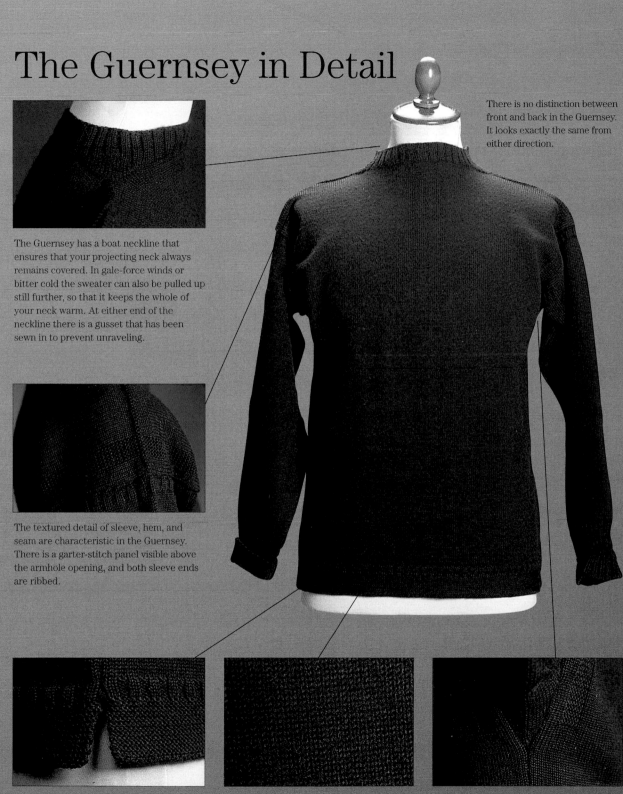

There is no distinction between front and back in the Guernsey. It looks exactly the same from either direction.

The Guernsey has a boat neckline that ensures that your projecting neck always remains covered. In gale-force winds or bitter cold the sweater can also be pulled up still further, so that it keeps the whole of your neck warm. At either end of the neckline there is a gusset that has been sewn in to prevent unraveling.

The textured detail of sleeve, hem, and seam are characteristic in the Guernsey. There is a garter-stitch panel visible above the armhole opening, and both sleeve ends are ribbed.

The bottom of the sweater is completed with a garter-stitch panel that is slit on either side to allow greater freedom of movement.

The wool of the Guernsey is heavy, hard, and tends to scratch. On the other hand, it is extremely hard wearing, very windproof, and, above all, warm. There is also a cotton version available for summer.

The armholes of the Guernsey are very narrow. This gives the advantage that it can be worn under a jacket, even if the jacket has a narrow fit. There is a square gusset knitted into the armhole underneath the arm that again allows for freedom of movement.

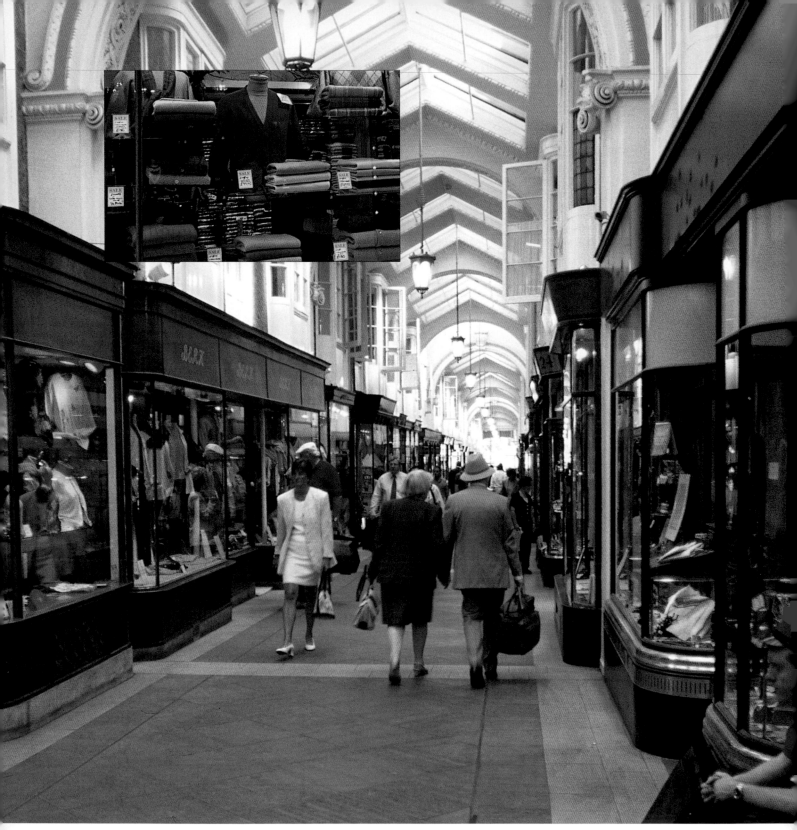

The Burlington Arcade in London's Mayfair was built in 1819, and is a good source for antique jewelry, silver, linen, shoes, and, of course, knitwear. Yet do not expect anything too flashy here; you are more likely to find classic lambswool and cashmere designs in the traditional range of colors. This shopping arcade is, moreover, a good way to get from Piccadilly to Savile Row. Upon leaving the Burlington Arcade in the direction of Burlington Gardens, the imposing façade of Gieves & Hawkes, No. 1 Savile Row, is visible on your right.

From Fine to Chunky Knit

The finest cashmere makes this sweater by John Smedley as light as a shirt made from cotton piqué. Italians tend to wear this kind of thing under a jacket instead of a shirt.

A thin lambswool sweater is extremely suitable to wear under a sports jacket, or as a substitute for a vest under a casual suit. A knitted vest does not look good with a formal business suit and so should be avoided.

A woolen sweater made of medium heavy yarn is an ideal companion for the whole year. On the other hand, very chunky knit types are only suitable for outdoor wear; they are much too warm for heated rooms.

Cotton sweaters enjoy great popularity, especially in summer, though depending on the type of knitting they are often surprisingly heavy, yet are very pleasant to wear against the bare skin.

Chunky sweaters for country pursuits, or walks in the city park, are often knitted in rib. These sweaters are heavy and warm, yet the ribbed texture means they also stretch very well, thus providing a lot of freedom of movement.

The Aran sweater is popular as leisurewear, but is nevertheless more suitable for outdoor activities than indoor ones. Although weighing surprisingly little, it is definitely too warm for confined spaces.

Correct Coordination

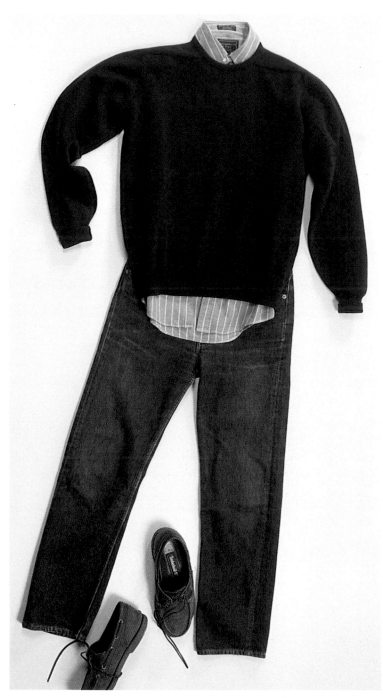

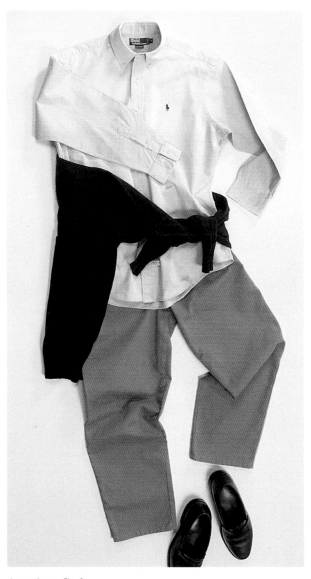

American Style

This is typical of the casual gear of an American from the East Coast. It is an absolutely timeless look, and the ingredients have been around unaltered for decades in the USA. The chinos sometimes tend to be exchanged for khaki shorts, and the "boat shoes" for loafers. A white short-sleeved shirt with soft collar and three-button opening is also popular with the sweater.

The Mediterranean Casual Look

This look is at home in Milan, Rome, Nice, and Barcelona, but you can see the combination in all other regions of Europe and in the rest of the world. Depending on the season, it will vary slightly. For instance, the button-down shirt can be exchanged for a short-sleeved shirt with soft collar and three-button opening, and the loafers for "boat shoes." However, the way the sweater is worn does not alter.

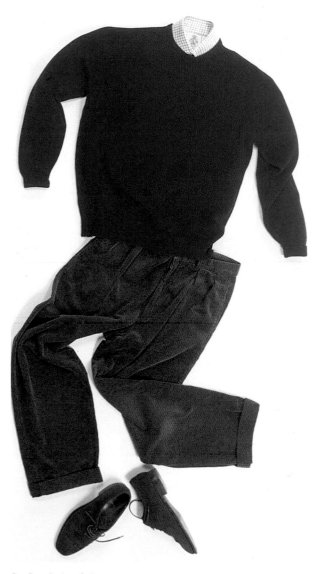

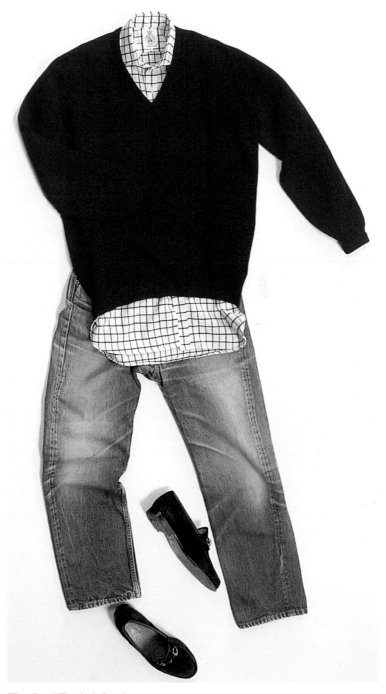

Le Look Anglais

The French interpretation of English leisurewear. A crucial feature is the fine lambswool or cashmere sweater in a classic English color like wine red, bottle green, or blue. Moreover, it is rare to find someone dressed as elegantly and well coordinated as this among the English, even though this look is named after them.

The Real English Look

Very English, but nevertheless it could be an imitation. A notable feature is the trend towards somewhat more conspicuous colors – a welcome change after the blue and gray pin stripes of the English business suit.

For Cold Winter Days

A thick woolen sweater is a crucial element in a gentleman's wardrobe, or rather chest of drawers, of clothes, whether it is brought out for settling down comfortably at home, going for an informal ride, or giving protection against the cold during some kind of outdoor activity. Since many of the old manor houses that are still inhabited in Great Britain are inadequately heated, even the thickest sweater is only just thick enough. In Italy too, really warm sweaters are enthusiastically welcomed, especially in the northern part of the country. It can get really cold in winter in these areas, so the people of Milan or Turin wrap themselves up in thick sweaters and scarves. It is interesting that hardly anyone nowadays is aware of the fact that classic knitwear from the British Isles was originally once the clothing of poor people, and gave them essential protection against the rigors of the weather.

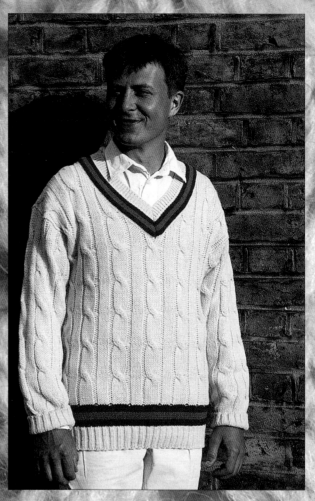

The cricket sweater is available as an original from an English sports store, or in innumerable more or less authentic varieties from different sportswear labels.

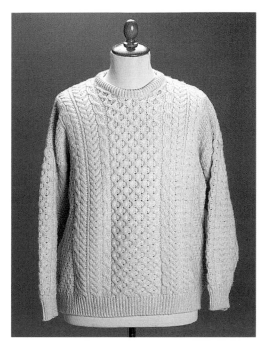

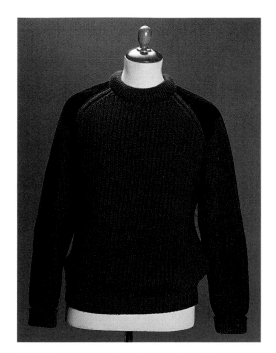

The Irish Aran sweater is one of the oldest known forms of the sweater. The textured detail is all highly significant. The zigzag pattern represents the deeply indented coastline that the fisherman hopes to return to. The tree of life, with branches growing out of the trunk, symbolizes family cohesion. The cable pattern stands for safety and good luck while out fishing. The diamond pattern signifies success and prosperity. Overall there are a dozen different patterns identifiable as traditional Aran designs.

The British army sweater influenced this civilian model. Knitted in a strong rib pattern, and with characteristic suede trimming at shoulders and elbows, this "action man" sweater is a popular classic knit for outdoor activities. It is traditionally green, but is also available in beige, brown, or dark blue. The shoulder and elbow trimming can also be made of (cotton) fabric so it washes better.

A typical winter sweater is the fleur de lys sweater. It is manufactured in different color combinations – for example, white lilies on a blue, green, or red background; or red lilies on a green or blue background. The lily pattern bestows a certain nobility on this warm sweater, despite its basically informal nature, and the colorfulness of the design is a pleasant change from the muted natural tones of the other sweaters.

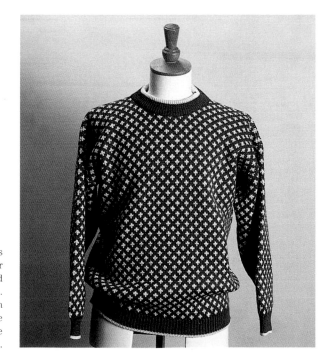

The Other Craze

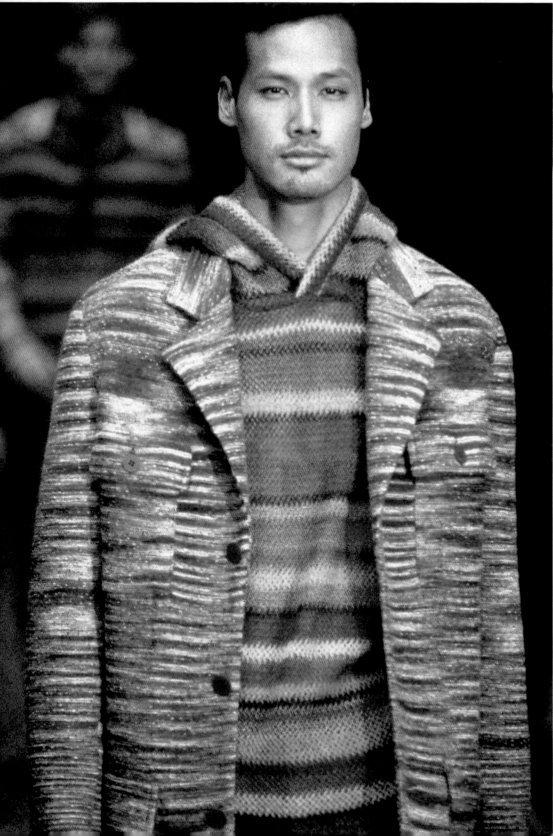

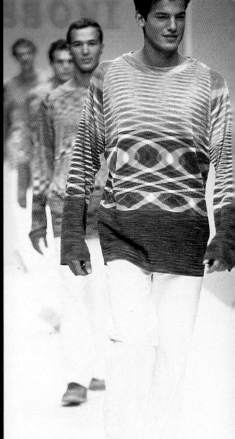

Hardly any designer label is as controversial as Missoni as far as fans of classic men's clothing are concerned. Those who think of a sweater as being something yellow with a V-neck, or as having an Aran pattern, regard the truly avant-garde creations of Ottavio and Rosita Missoni with deepest suspicion. Fans of these knitted objects bursting with color, however, consider them an ideal counterpoint to classically dark businesswear.

It is doubtful whether Ottavio and Rosita Missoni will be pleased to be mentioned in a book about classic menswear. After all, they are quoted as saying that "fashion is about wearing today what you would not have wanted to wear yesterday, and will not want to wear any more tomorrow." This definition seems a total contradiction to the idea of classic clothing, since those who advocate timeless elegance still want tomorrow what they wanted yesterday. On the other hand, the founders of the successful family business know that classic status is quite beneficial to the success of a label. Missoni has for a long time stood for more than just fashion – it is a whole philosophy. Whether you like it or not is a different matter, and opinions on the esthetics of this modern Italian classic can be quite divided. It is difficult to integrate Missoni as real English sportswear à la Cordings of Piccadilly, and the bizarre company patterns do not really seem to coordinate with the American East-Coast preppy look. Fans of these latter styles of dress will hardly ever hanker for a Missoni sweater, and will prefer to stay with the wine red, blue, bottle green, and yellow lambswool and cashmere classics. Those who positively dislike the usual leisurewear look, however, and prefer to seek out a real contrast to the dark suit in English or Italian workshops, will quickly warm to a Missoni sweater, though the Missoni look imposes high requirements in terms of a sense of style. It is relatively safe to wear a Missoni sweater coordinated with internationally accepted sportswear, preferably with an Italian note, for example, over a T-shirt in summer, with faded Levi's 501s and neutral-colored "Tods." In fall and winter a Missoni sweater looks good with a one-tone button-down shirt by Ralph Lauren or Brooks Brothers and with jeans, or with cord pants by Kiton or Barbera. To this you add winter shoes by Tods and a husky or lambskin jacket.

An American has somewhat less "awareness" than many in terms of the coordinating of clothes, and the result often mirrors this. He wears Missoni in all possible and impossible combinations, for example with his adored turtle necks, with jogging pants, or with cowboy boots. This and innumerable cheap imitations have done major damage to the reputation of this designer label. This is certainly a pity because Missoni launch an absolute explosion of new colors and patterns every year. If you can develop a feeling for the best way to coordinate these colors and show them off to their best advantage, you will find that a Missoni sweater is a really valuable acquisition, even as part of a classically international wardrobe of clothes. It is worth trying to integrate Missoni's ideas with the rest of your wardrobe for an alternative look that still exudes style.

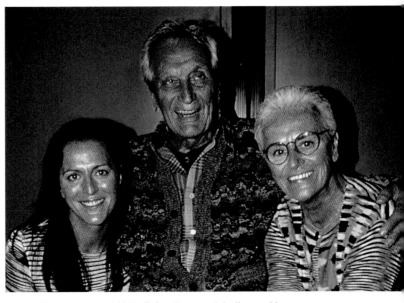

Ottavio Missoni, born in 1921 in Dalmatia, was originally an athlete, or more precisely, a 400-meter sprinter. In this capacity he participated in the 1948 Olympic Games in London, representing Italy, and promptly reached the final. One of the spectators watching Ottavio at that time was a young lady from Lombardy who was studying languages in Hampstead. Rosita Jelmini and Ottavio Missoni (seen in the picture with their daughter Angela) fell in love and were married in 1953. That same year the two of them founded a small knitting workshop at home in Italy. They did not have to wait long for success. Their knitted clothes had made the name of Missoni famous worldwide by the end of the 1960s. In 1968 a Missoni model appeared for the first time on the front cover of French *Elle*. A year later Missoni made their debut on *Women's Wear Daily*. Three years later the same publication classified Missoni among the top 20 fashion powers in the world. Numerous different awards followed, while the creative duo gradually extended their activities to include other sectors such as wall hangings, furniture, and furnishing fabrics, stockings, beachwear, neckties, and even perfume.

Missoni have produced neckties since 1984. The Missoni tie was the ideal back door by which means the company gained access to classical menswear as a maker of antinecktie fashion, that is, as a maker of sweaters.

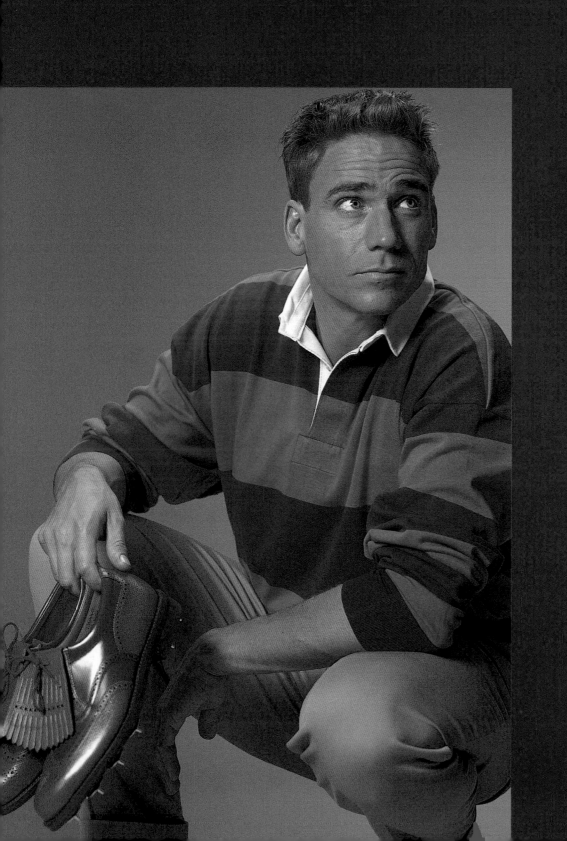

Sporting Life

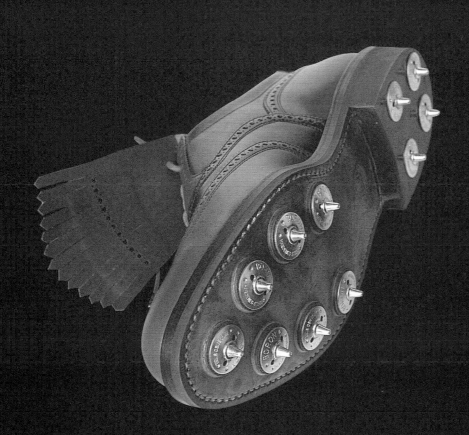

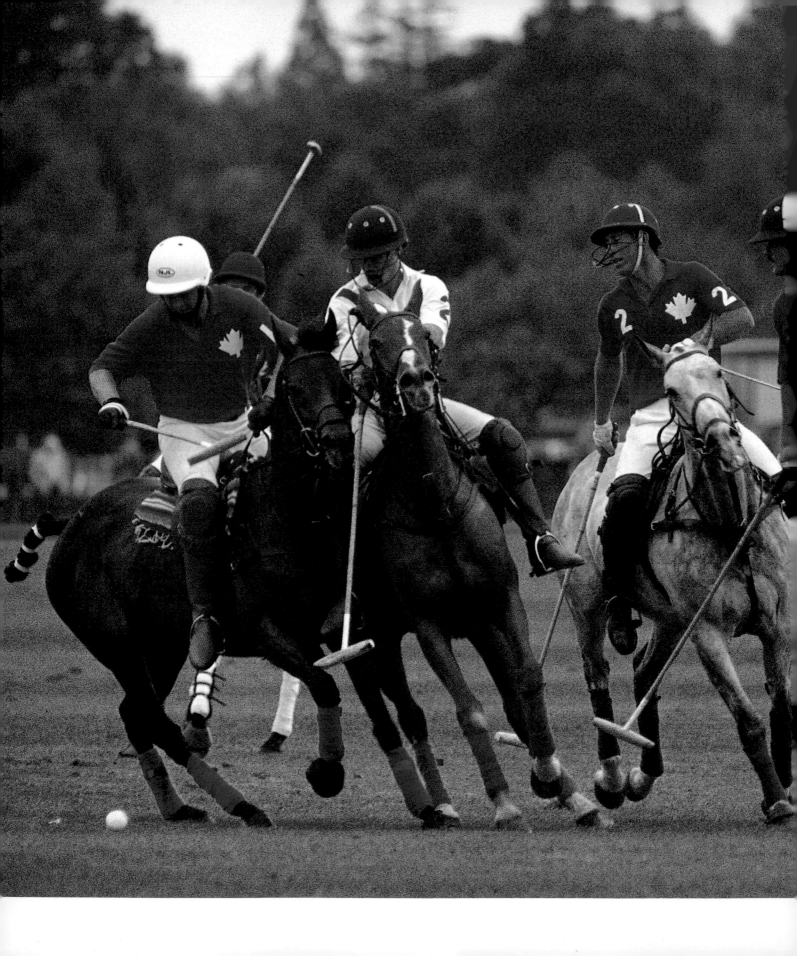

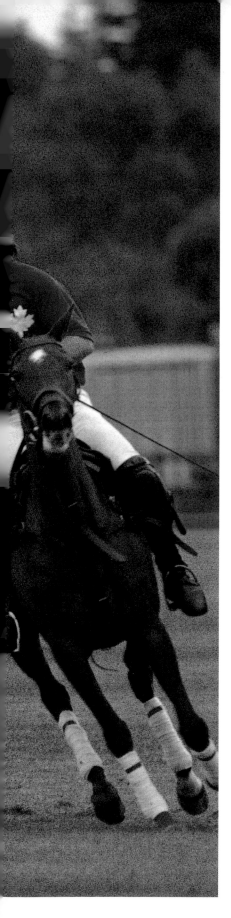

Why Sport?

It would be impossible to write a book about the components of international style in clothing without discussing sport. By this, we do not mean football, light athletics, or high diving, but the sports pursued by the English country gentleman: hunting, shooting, riding, and fishing. We have to thank these once feudal and even today only partly democratized pleasures of rural life for a style of dress that continues to demonstrate its timelessness. Other sports are also well worth looking at, particularly if their specialist clothes have been sources of inspiration for the classic wardrobe. This chapter may even inspire the reader to try out one or other of these pastimes. It certainly does us no harm to keep ourselves healthy. What use are classic clothes if they do not fit on account of an ever-expanding waistline? Of course, it could be argued that one's clothes should fit the body, and not the other way round. This is, of course, incontestable. Someone who decides not to partake in physical exercise can certainly still enjoy the pleasures of the classic sports – as a spectator. Not everyone is lucky enough to own a horse, but anyone can watch horse racing from the stands, and polo is magnificent watched from the edge of the playing area. Apart from this, several of the activities described here are not at all strenuous. For example, angling is a highly relaxing pastime, while golf, it could be argued, consists predominantly of extended walks, though of course these do demand considerable stamina.

Someone who is appalled by the stale, sweaty atmosphere of the local gym should try out one of the sports practiced in the open air. It does not even have to be shooting, though hunters always say that there is nothing finer than sitting in a hide waiting for a stag in the first light of morning. But this is a matter of opinion: regardless of whether they are in favor of blood sports or not, most city dwellers simply have no opportunity to take part in shooting. However, one does not need to be an enthusiastic hunter to take pleasure in certain pieces of clothing that were originally conceived specially for shooting. In fact, many popular elements in our leisure wardrobe – the Barbour jacket, the husky jacket, the tweed suit, moleskin pants, and the loden coat – are shooting wear. Nowadays this does not stop anyone, not even dedicated animal-rights activists or vegetarians, from wearing a Barbour or a tweed jacket. These pieces of clothing have long since spread beyond their original sphere and become general property. Here we want to show them, along with other pieces of sporting clothing and equipment, in their original environment just once before they again become quotations in our everyday wardrobe. So the photographs on the following few pages are of gentlemen wearing sports clothing for sporting activities, traditions that stretch back for generations and epitomize the English countryside. The clothes are worn for their practical value, but nevertheless are clearly stylish.

For many people polo is the noblest of all sports, but it demands more than just the financial resources required for the purchase of expensive ponies. First of all, one must be an excellent rider before it is even worth thinking about the cost of this ancient leisure activity. This probably explains the great success of the brand that has used the polo player as its symbol. When we buy a shirt by Ralph Lauren we feel we are playing a little part in that big world of which polo is an essential feature.

Hunting, Riding, Fishing...

Hunting, riding, fishing – these were the sports pursued by the landed gentry throughout Europe for many years. In England the term "hunting" means hunting with hounds, while "shooting" is what is known elsewhere as hunting. For the most part, an aristocratic family would leave the upkeep and economic management of their estate to specialists so that the gentlemen of the house could dedicate themselves undisturbed to their favorite leisure activities. The aspiring bourgeoisie saw it as completely natural to imitate this apparently ideal mode of existence. Rich merchants, bankers, industrialists, and high government officials followed the example set by the aristocracy and bought fine country residences. There they cultivated the lifestyle of the aristocracy down to the last detail, purchasing horses, going hunting, and traveling to Scotland to do a spot of salmon fishing. Despite all the fashionable opposition to hunting, for many people it is still in many ways a status symbol. The upper middle classes still take great pleasure in hunting, and in this respect they follow the example given by high society.

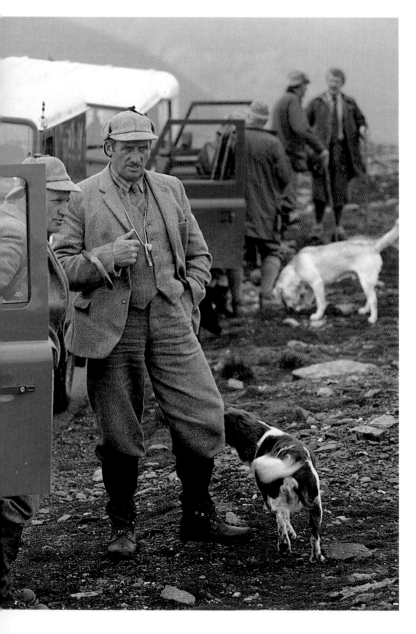

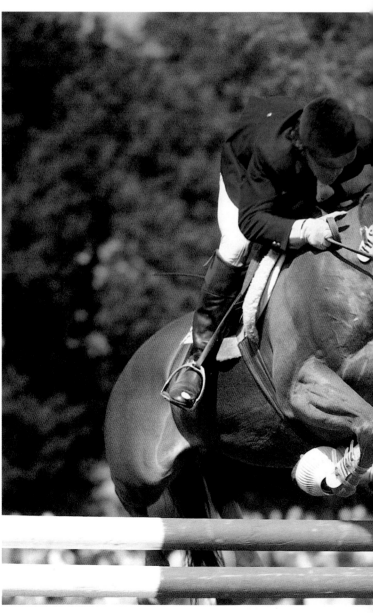

Apart from a certain prestige value, there are also other arguments in favor of hunting, riding, and fishing: contact with nature, exercise in the fresh air, the chance to relax surrounded by greenery – in short, a taste of the romance of "country life." With the right clothes and an off-road vehicle, a doctor from Nuremberg can feel like an English lord, just as a professor of history from Granada feels like a hunter from the Austrian Royal Household when he goes out hunting for quail in a loden coat and a traditional Austrian tunic. The style of modern hunting clothes is derived from two sources: English country life and the Alpine look based on loden. An English hunter will sport a tweed jacket and a deerstalker; his continental colleague wears a Janker (a loose jacket worn in the Alps) and a Tyrolean hat. Some people even combine these two very different styles. Again, this tendency to mix and match hunting wear is associated with the nobility who did so much hunting throughout Europe. In the 19th century the royal houses of Europe established much of what is now accepted in matters of style, and as they were almost all related to each other, they often made use of the regional styles favored by their cousins, uncles, grandfathers, and brothers-in-law from other countries. In consequence, the style from the British Isles and the chic of the Alpine region are both equally popular today. Which you prefer to wear yourself is just a question of personal taste.

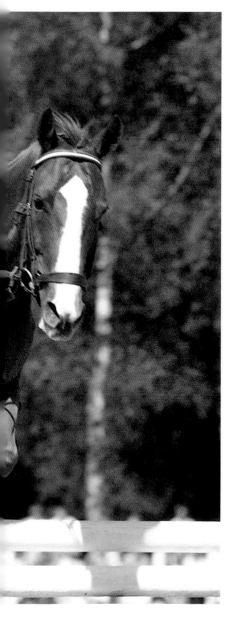

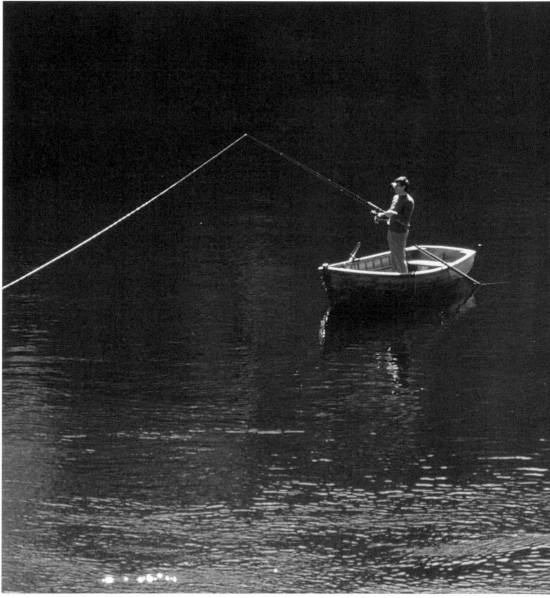

Shooting – the Outfit

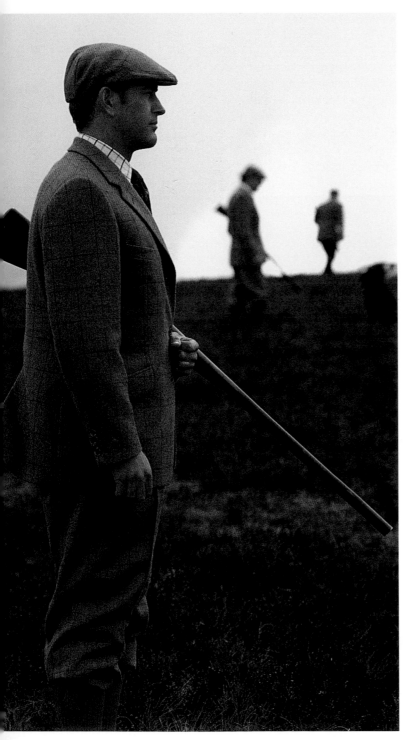

When he goes shooting an English gentleman wears a tweed suit from a outfitter like Cordings or from his own tailor. The patterned Scottish cloth is used as camouflage and, at the same time, provides protection against the cold.

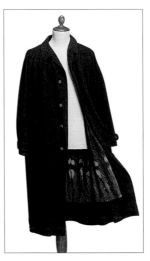

Today the loden coat is popular for both city and country wear, but, as its color suggests, it really belongs to the world of shooting. Despite the superb protection it provides against high winds, good loden is astonishingly light and even slightly water repellent. The coat's wide cut and the vertical pleat in the back give the wearer great freedom of movement.

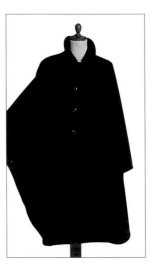

The loden cape is the poncho of the Alpine region. This green, sleeveless garment provides more freedom of movement than a coat and can also be worn over a game bag. The classic cape made by the German manufacturer of hunting clothes Kettner is only for dyed-in-the-wool loden fans, who praise it to the skies.

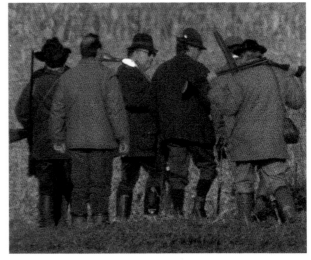

Hunters on the European mainland have a liking for Alpine loden. This look is not to everyone's taste, but even the style-conscious Edward VIII enjoyed going stalking in a Tyrolean hat. In the Mediterranean countries the style of shooting clothes is much less distinctive, which is probably a result of the high temperatures in these regions. It is too warm for loden, cavalry twill, or Bedford cord in the south of Spain, even in winter.

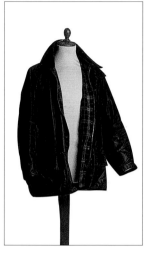

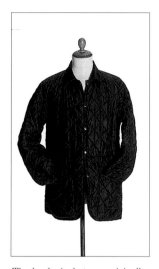

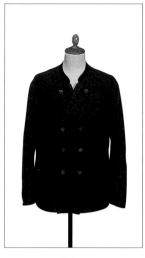

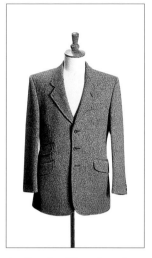

The Barbour jacket is the best protection against wet, dirt, cold, and thorns, whether you are hunting for small game or taking part in any other country activity. It needs to be rewaxed regularly because otherwise it loses its waterproofing (more about this English classic is to be found on pp. 200 ff.).

The husky jacket was originally developed as a warm, but light, shooting jacket. It has been a classic now for many years, and is worn in the city just as much as in the country. Apart from the original husky, named after the breed of dog, there are also numerous imitations – this jacket, which is equipped with a practical inside pocket, is made by Lavenham.

Shooting clothes in the Alpine style are most popular in Germany and Austria and, in truth, can only be worn in those countries. An Austrian who is invited to go hunting in Scotland would do well to exchange his Janker for a tweed suit.

A suit made of the extremely warm material Bedford cord replaces at least one coat, if not two. The material is too thick for more moderate climates, where you would run the risk of suffering heat stroke if you went shooting in Bedford cord. However, it is ideal for shooting in really cold winter conditions or waiting in a hide.

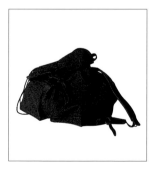

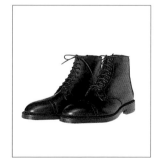

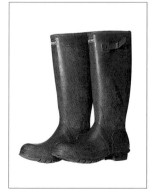

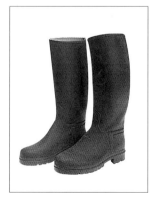

The classic game bag has remained unchanged to the present day. It has no supporting frame to hold it in shape, but molds itself to the hunter's back. Most game bags have a removable, washable compartment for animals that have been dispatched. The bottom and also the edges are reinforced with leather.

Tricker's ankle boots go absolutely perfectly with a tweed jacket and knickerbockers. They can be purchased in London at No. 67 Jermyn Street, and also outside the UK – for example, at the Cologne clothes shop John Crocket, where the shoe can be ordered in any kind of leather you specify.

Wellington boots are highly durable and the only completely waterproof footwear. They are perfectly suited to work in the yard or for a stroll in the rain. Apart from the models made by Barbour, "Hunter wellies," as the boots produced by Hunter are affectionately known, are very popular. The classic colors are green and blue.

Shooting boots made of natural rubber with a leather insert for better fit and more comfort are a French specialty.
Le Chameau have been making them since 1927 in Chateauvillain southwest of Nancy. They are particularly prized by hunters in continental Europe.

The Real Thing

Piccadilly Circus is still a favorite starting point for many visitors to London. Most start their shopping trip through Regent Street there. It is a much better idea, though, to begin by turning into the street to the left of Regent Street known simply as Piccadilly. Here there are a number of famous hotels, such as the Bristol and the Ritz. Of greater interest to someone looking for real English leisurewear is No. 19 Piccadilly, which is on the corner of Air Street. There you will find the business premises of J. C. Cording & Company Ltd., which was founded in 1839. The shop stocks everything you need to kit yourself out for English country life – or at least in order to look as though you were going to the country. Tattersall check shirts made of cotton, or mixes of cotton and wool; magnificent coarse tweed suits, perfectly styled with a single vent and three buttons; moleskin and cord pants with adjustable waistbands in typical English colors – such as rust, olive, forest, yellow, navy, or corn; neckties with country motifs, covert coats, riding macs, and much, much more. The tweed jackets are not made primarily for a Saturday stroll through Paris or Milan, but will stand up to hard wear in various outdoor activities, which is what they were originally intended to do. The clothes offer good value for money, while the tailoring is very respectable, and some of it is lavish. The jackets fit acceptably if you like a close cut that emphasizes your body shape. The pants match the jackets in being cut close to the leg. Even real plus-fours, or knickerbockers, are available. There is evidently still a demand for these seemingly anachronistic pants in England. Special orders and made-to-order adaptations of the ready-to-wear range are also among the services on offer at this traditional, but lively, outfitters. However, as mentioned above,

At No. 19 Piccadilly you will find everything you could ever need for English-style country life, whether you are going to be in Yorkshire, the Bois de Boulogne, or Tokyo. Although Cordings have been supplying style lovers from the continent and overseas for many years, you will never receive the impression that you are in a shop that could not exist without tourists. Cordings really have very little to do with the idea of the *look anglais* as it is understood around the world – they sell the undiluted original.

The Cordings label is something of a secret sign among the aficionados of English sportswear. The Royal Family wear the traditional label, and even the wife of the Duke of Windsor possessed a pair of hunting boots from Cordings, as was revealed by the auction of her belongings at Sotheby's in New York.

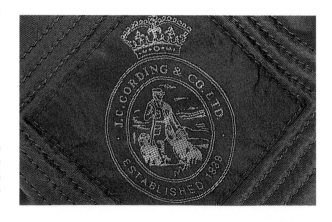

Cordings offer the unrefined and sometimes not entirely elegant original. People who like a more delicate version of the *look anglais* more oriented towards the taste of clients from continental Europe may well be disappointed. The selection held by this traditional shop has very little in common with the clothes stocked by Burberrys and similar outlets for tourists, but someone who prefers authenticity will love Cordings. It is also well worth casting an eye over the city suits there. Alongside numerous casual suits, they also stock blue and gray single-breasted and double-breasted suits cut in the Cordings house style that are very well made indeed for ready-to-wear garments. If you are looking for really warm pants made of cavalry twill, a garment that will last practically a lifetime, you will definitely find what you are looking for at Cordings, particularly if you call in at No. 19 Piccadilly in fall or winter. If you go to London less frequently, there is still no need to go without the eccentric classics. Like many other seemingly old-fashioned English manufacturers and shops, Cordings have a very efficient mail-order service that dispatches tweeds, cords, and Tattersall checks reliably and swiftly to all corners of the earth to satisfy their regular customers.

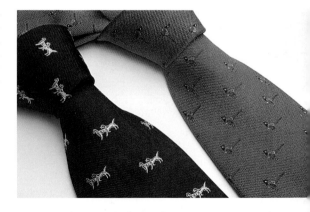

At Cordings a gentleman can fit himself out from head to foot for a weekend in the country, even with neckties.

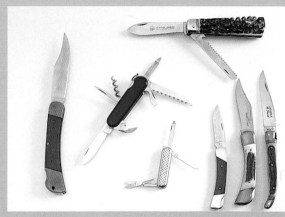

The pocketknife

A gentlemen with a pocketknife? The two go better together than many might think. After all, the Scouts' motto is "be prepared" – for anything. And men of the world also adhere to this precept.

The variety of the models on the market is large, but the choice is reduced considerably if you are looking for a knife that really is small and light enough to go in your pants pocket. Often these are models with a flexible blade that does not click into position or have to be released. The Swiss Army knife has a blade of this type, which can easily snap shut if it is used incorrectly at the wrong moment. A solid knife should be chosen if just one blade is required. A locking mechanism would make a knife with several blades or additional functions weigh too much. Someone who only wants a knife to open letters, cut pieces of string, and peel apples will be well served by the lightest model. When you buy a knife, you must make sure that all the parts fit together precisely, and the blade opens smoothly and does not wobble when it is open. The metal parts should be well polished – this costs time and money, expenditure which is

usually only made with good materials. However, as even a specialist will not be able to judge the quality of the steel in a knife by sight, the safest way to avoid disappointments is to buy a good make. it is also advisable to visit a specialist supplier for your knife. There you will be able to choose the right one for you, from the simplest to the most sophisticated, and feel confident that you have made the right decision.

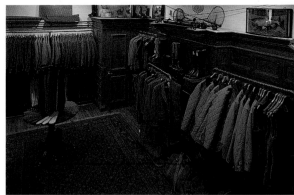

Whether the pocketknife is large or small, with one or several blades, depends on what it is to be used for.

Riding – the Outfit

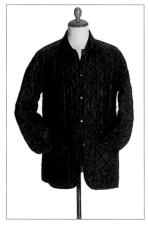

The light, but nevertheless warming husky jacket is extremely popular among riders. It can also be machine washed, which is a great advantage in view of the constant risk of getting dirty in the stable and saddle room.

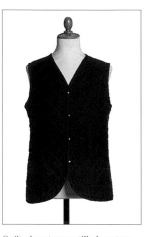

Quilted vests are still almost as popular among riders as the long-sleeved jacket. They are light as a feather, and air can circulate freely under them. A vest like this is also ideal if you want to look smart for a weekend in the country.

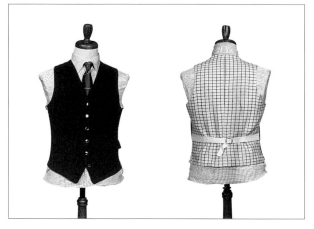

A "hunt vest," as these traditional vests are known, is essential if you want to make a stylish appearance on a ride or at a hunt meet. They are made of thick woolen felt, and the back is decorated with Tattersall check. The famous English saddlemakers and riding-tackle retailers W. & H. Gidden also sell reversible hunt vests. Apart from red, the most popular colors are green and canary yellow.

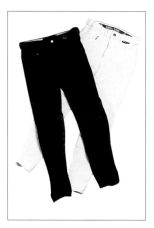

Only in England is the art of making perfect riding breeches understood – and even there only by the specialist suppliers of riding and hunting wear Bernard Weatherill. Traditional craftsmen use their mastery of the art of tailoring to achieve what is now so often done with stretchy, elastic fabrics. Prestigious customers, such as huntsmen, test the fit of their breeches on a wooden horse.

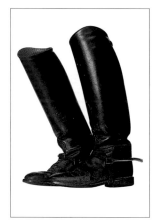

If you only go riding occasionally you are hardly likely to invest in leather riding boots, but someone who sits on a horse almost every day definitely needs a pair. Every rider dreams of a pair of custom-made boots. People who can afford it order them from Hermès in Paris.

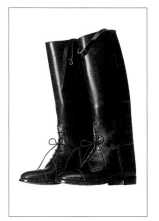

Riding boots do not necessarily have to be black. Polo players often wear brown boots. Unlike the shoes worn by other riders, these are fastened with laces. Boots in contrasting colors are the height of style.

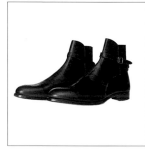

Jodhpur boots are not just popular with riders. They come with elasticated gussets or, more traditionally, leather straps. When riding they are worn with the ankle-length jodhpur riding breeches that gave these ankle boots their name.

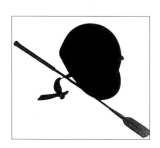

The riding cap is just as controversial in riding circles as the safety belt among automobile drivers. It is clear that it makes sense to wear one, but it is often rather uncomfortable.

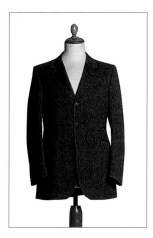

What could be better for riding in than a hacking jacket? Its close cut, high waist, long back vent, and slanted flapped pockets suggest that it was the original version of the English sports jacket. The slanted pockets are easier to reach into when sitting on a horse, and the vent allows the tails to fall elegantly over the upper thighs.

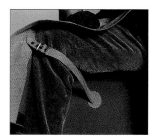

A rubberized riding mac is rather like a rubber boot covering the whole body. The rubber layer on the inside prevents any moisture getting in, and the long coat tails can be fastened to the legs with straps, which means that they remain in a protective position even when it is windy.

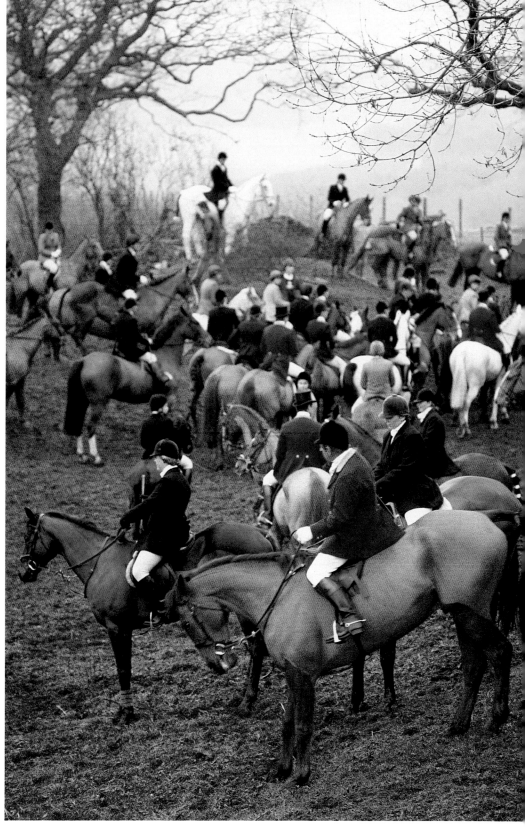

The English fox-hunting season begins on the first Monday in November and continues through to the following April. This makes it, in a sense, a winter sport, and explains the thick material used for the clothes worn by hunters. Hunting outfits are often worn for several generations, in which case the lining just has to be mended every 30 years or so by a tailor.

Spectating in Style

Someone who occasionally goes to horse races or to equestrian tournaments will probably have wondered why so many of the men present wear a hat that is far too small for them. If these hats are dark brown, you can be pretty sure they are members of the "trilby" species. The brown trilby has traditionally been worn by people who work with horses. The tradition comes from England, where the trilby is obligatory wear for all events in the equestrian calendar. This assures hatmakers like Lock & Co. a certain proportion of their turnover each year. However, it is not clear why the English like wearing their trilbies a size too small. They are definitely available in larger sizes. Maybe it is because most trilbies were handed down from father to son and have shrunk over the generations.

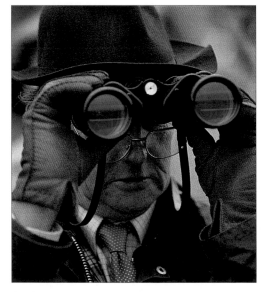 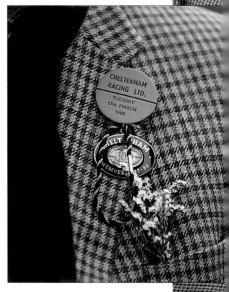

The Grand National at Aintree is a famous English "steeplechase." Its roots go back to a race between two Irish compatriots, Blake and O'Callaghan, held in 1752. The starting point and finish of the race were two church steeples, which is why this sporting competition was christened, simply enough, a steeplechase. Blake and O'Callaghan raced over 4 miles and 855 yards, and even today this is the distance that the riders have to cover. The public come in huge numbers, eager to bet on the races, and all the men, from the modest better to the rich stable owner, wear a trilby.

The classic outfit worn at race meetings consists of a brown trilby, a tweed suit or tweed jacket, binoculars, and a Barbour jacket if it is raining.

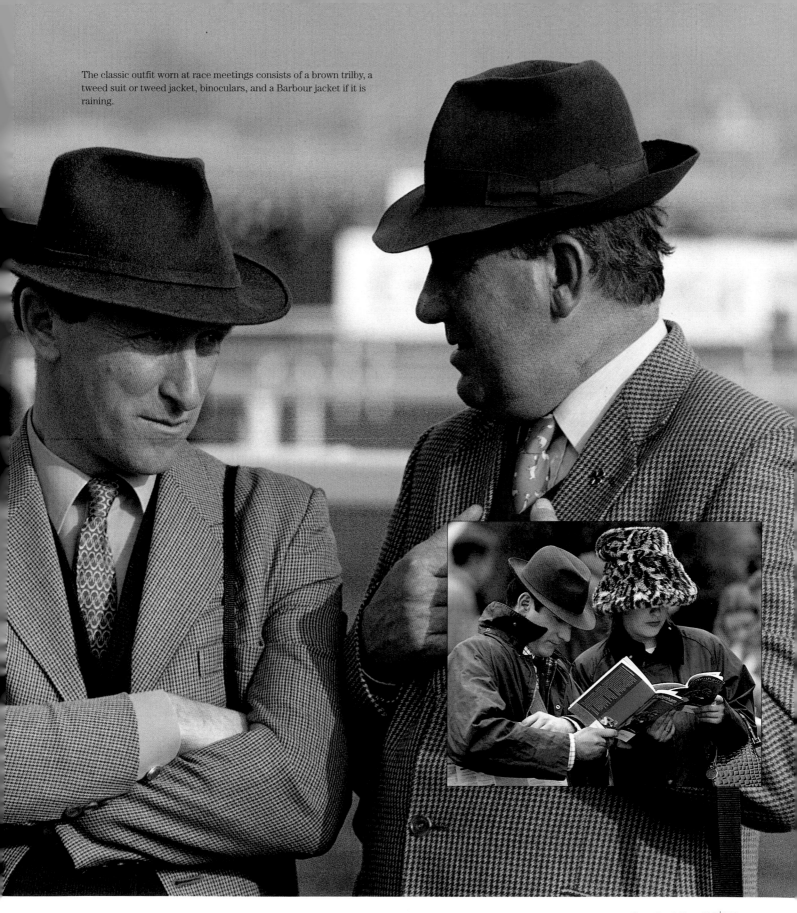

Fishing – the Outfit

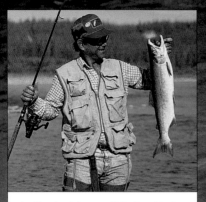

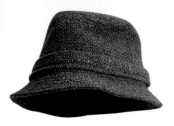

A tweed hat is not just useful as protection against cold and rain. Fly fishers also stick their bait into their hats for ease of access.

Angling is a leisure activity loved just as much by kings as by commoners. The monarch will relax by fishing the streams that flow through his estate; his subject simply sits by the nearest canal. Not much is required in order to make a start with this hobby. For the first attempts it is enough to have a simple rod with a fishing line, a hook, and a float. At this point there is no need to think much about one's outfit either. Even someone who does a lot of angling will not have to spend much money on a special wardrobe. In contrast to hunters and riding enthusiasts, anglers have no precise dress code that has to be followed. What they wear is determined mainly by practical considerations and the requirements of the chosen method of fishing. Someone who is angling for salmon will certainly need breast-high chest waders for standing in the river. Others will need just a pair of rubber boots to prevent their feet getting wet on the river bank. Angling is a much too unspectacular and solitary business for the men who love it to worry about making an impression with the elegance of their clothing. This is not to say that specialist suppliers do not stock a variety of vests, waders, rubber boots, hats, caps, and umbrellas. However, angling clothes, unlike hunting or riding wear, are difficult to integrate with normal casual clothes. This is probably why there is such a wide range of neckties with fish motifs. This, at least, is one way for a keen angler to indicate his interests by his choice of clothes. Men wearing such ties can often be heard discussing the best rivers to fish, boasting about the size of fish caught, and "the one that got away."

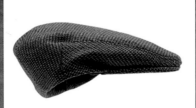

The flat tweed cap is as popular as the tweed hat, and its coarse woolen material does just as good service as a storage place for flies.

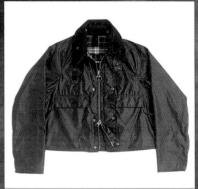

Someone who spends much time standing up to his knees in a river needs a short jacket. The jackets made by Barbour offer the best protection against rain, and, as the water level can sometimes rise more than expected, they have wide waterproof belts that stop the warm lining of the jacket becoming saturated with water from below.

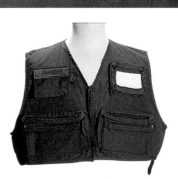

Anglers see a vest as a place to store pieces of equipment. For this reason they wear vests with low intrinsic weight and as many pockets as possible. In this way they resemble photographers.

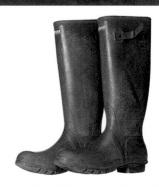

Fish live in water. Someone who wants to join them there should wear long rubber boots. They are available in various lengths.

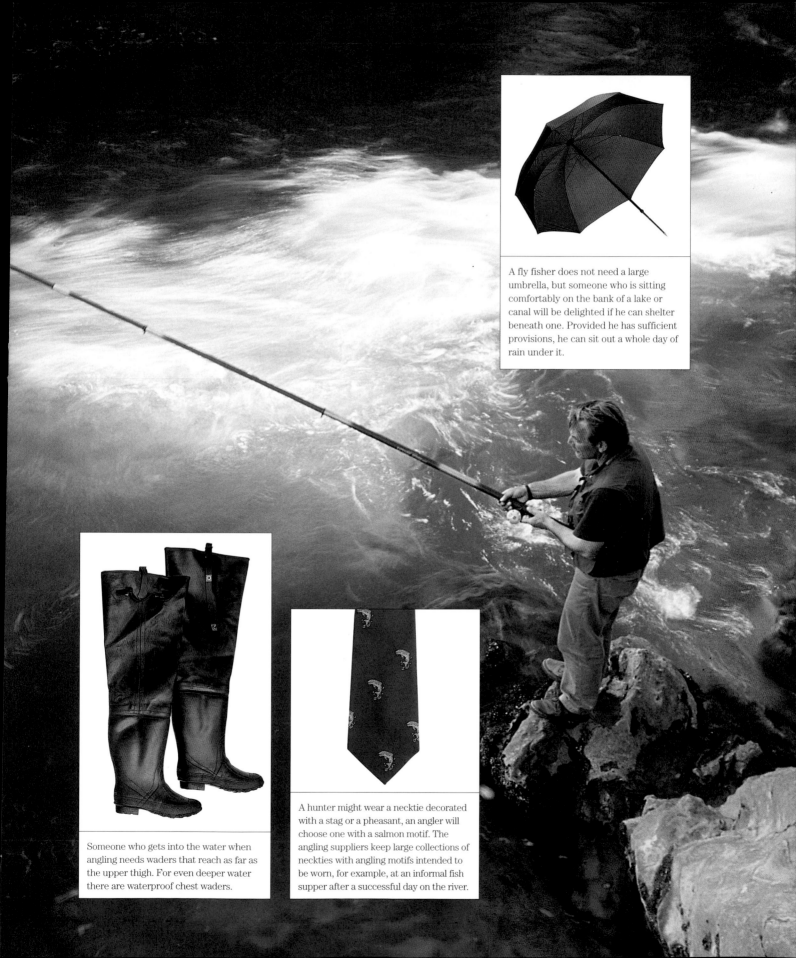

A fly fisher does not need a large umbrella, but someone who is sitting comfortably on the bank of a lake or canal will be delighted if he can shelter beneath one. Provided he has sufficient provisions, he can sit out a whole day of rain under it.

Someone who gets into the water when angling needs waders that reach as far as the upper thigh. For even deeper water there are waterproof chest waders.

A hunter might wear a necktie decorated with a stag or a pheasant, an angler will choose one with a salmon motif. The angling suppliers keep large collections of neckties with angling motifs intended to be worn, for example, at an informal fish supper after a successful day on the river.

Hole in One

There are indications that golf originated in Holland, but this thesis should never be uttered in the presence of a Scot. It is better to agree with the opinion that it was invented in his homeland. And there is some evidence for this. After all, golf was mentioned in the deliberations of the Scottish Parliament as early as 1457. The oldest golf club in the world is also to be found in Scotland: the Royal Blackheath, which was founded in 1608. All questions relating to the rules of the game are decided not by the oldest club, but by the Royal and Ancient Golf Club of St. Andrews, which was founded in 1754. With such a long tradition in Scotland, it would not be unexpected if the clothes worn by golf players included a kilt, but this is not the case. Golf is played in pants, long pants to be precise, though they are often decorated with tartan. The ancient traditions of golf nevertheless inspire such respect that the clothes worn on a golf course may be somewhat casual, but are always elegant. A careful observer can read what was regarded as casual and elegant at a particular point in the past by looking at the clothes worn by the golf players of the period. The Prince of Wales wore a necktie when he played at the Royal and Ancient Golf Club of St. Andrews in a brightly patterned Fair Isle sweater in 1922. Neckties are no longer worn today, but you will not be too formally dressed in a pullover, shirt, and ironed pants. And, as golf does not exactly bring the sweat out on your brow, there is no reason why people should not play it in suit pants. It is therefore possible to exchange your suit jacket for a cardigan during your lunch break, slip on your golf shoes, and drive quickly over to the golf club to practice a bit on the putting green. The generally relaxed outfit worn by the players should not disguise the fact that golf is an extremely difficult sport that requires intensive training, as well as talent, but the charm of the game probably lies in the fact that no one lets this show. It is not possible to make sweeping generalizations about golf as a game of the rich. In the countries with great golfing traditions it is played by people from every section of society. Happily, a low handicap is not something that can be bought, even with the most expensive equipment.

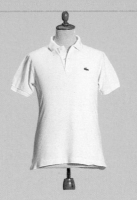

Today the polo shirt is part of a golf player's standard equipment, but an overshirt is also just as good. A T-shirt or a sleeveless jersey would not be suitable – golf is not a game played on the street.

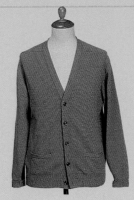

Golf is the only sport that can be played in a cashmere cardigan. Of course, lambswool or cotton are just as good.

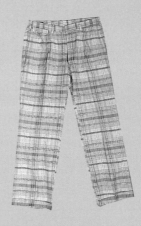

If you are going to wear check pants, you are best off with a traditional tartan. But care must be taken in Scotland. Your fellow player might belong to the very clan whose tartan decorates your pants. You will be on the safe side with Madras check, which comes originally from India.

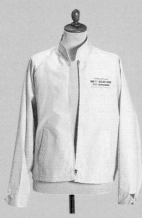

Golf is not just played in good weather. A light windcheater will keep you dry in a brief shower. If necessary a Barbour jacket will do good service, but is too heavy to play golf in for long.

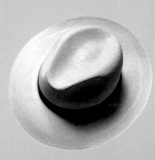

Someone who does not like baseball caps can wear a Panama hat when the sun is shining. Flat peaked caps made of light or checked material are also to be recommended because the wind cannot blow them from your head so easily.

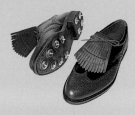

Golf shoes differ from other shoes only in that they have spikes in the sole and that their leather is particularly waterproof. Otherwise, the same heavy demands can be made on golf shoes as other shoes. Almost all manufacturers of good welted shoes have golf shoes in their range. They can also be custom made, of course.

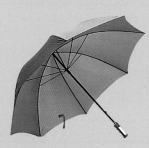

The golfing umbrella traditionally has a straight handle instead of a bent one, and there is a reason for this. It means that the umbrella can be folded up and stored in a round golf bag without getting tangled up with the clubs.

Golf provides one of the few opportunities for a gentleman to wear white shoes.

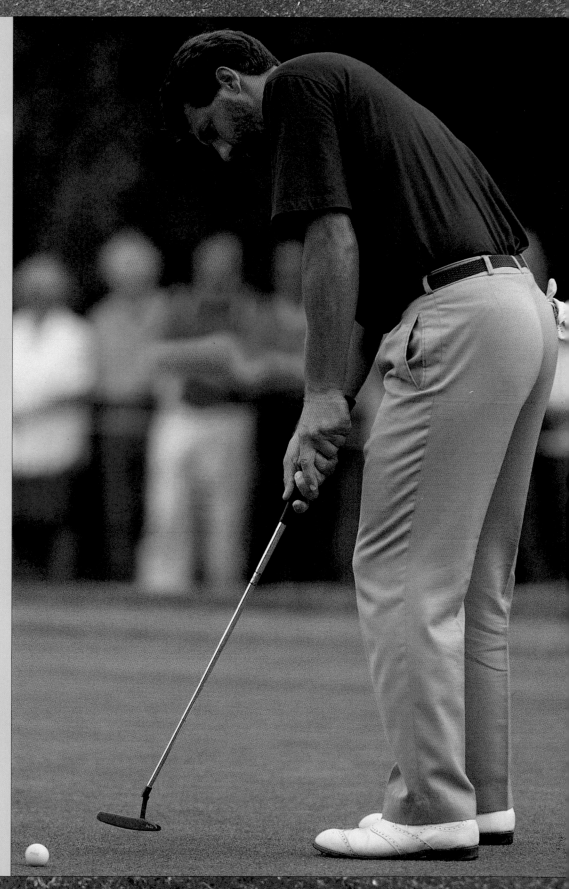

The Crocodile

The shirt that René Lacoste designed for himself in 1933 was intended to be worn when playing tennis and golf: "Pour moi, pour jouer au tennis comme au golf, j'eus un jour l'idée de créer une chemise." His design became a massive success. By 1939 up to 300,000 shirts were being produced annually. It quickly took the place of the long-sleeved overshirt as the clothing favored by tennis players. The design was based on the shirt worn by real polo players. The idea for a shirt like this was in the air at the time; Lacoste simply had the luck, or genius, to be the first person to put his stamp on the idea. The crocodile logo that he had sewn onto his shirts was intended as protection against imitations. In the 1930s everyone in France still knew why he had chosen this animal as his symbol. "Le crocodile" was Lacoste's nickname as a tennis player, and it was as "le crocodile" that he has made his reputation. The name undoubtedly did much to make the success of his shirt possible. René Lacoste would certainly not be forgotten today on account of his sporting triumphs, but his memory will endure around the world not least thanks to the popular shirts that bear his name.

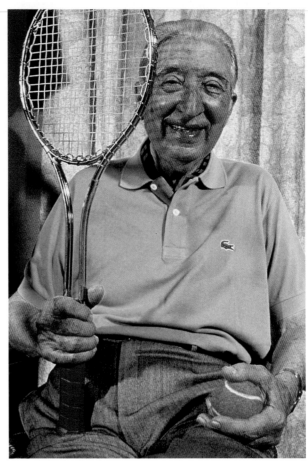

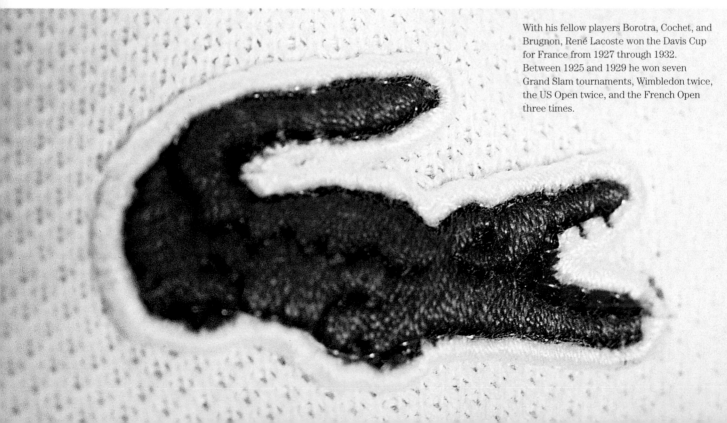

With his fellow players Borotra, Cochet, and Brugnon, René Lacoste won the Davis Cup for France from 1927 through 1932. Between 1925 and 1929 he won seven Grand Slam tournaments, Wimbledon twice, the US Open twice, and the French Open three times.

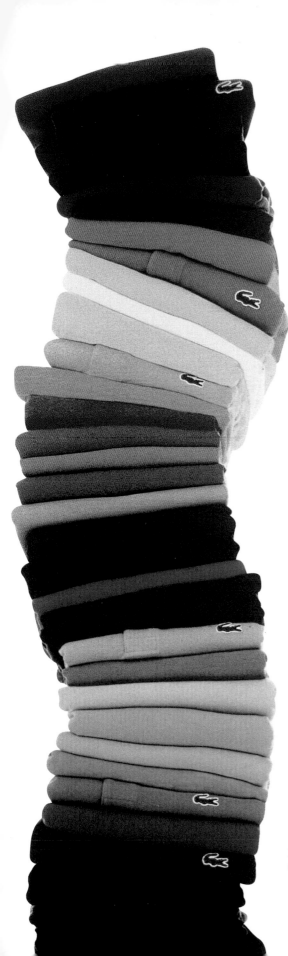

The Other Polo Shirt

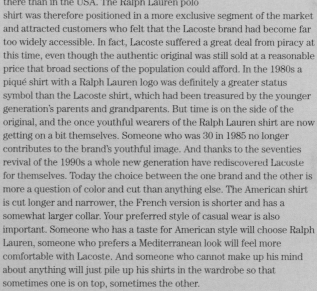

There are a few American classics that are essential for a wardrobe in the international style. Levi's 501s, Bass Weejuns, and Sperry Topsiders are originals that we really cannot do without. The polo shirt is not a member of this group. Nevertheless, the piqué shirt by the American designer Ralph Lauren is a great success around the world. Many people who buy this polo shirt probably do not even know that *la chemise Lacoste* was there first. The shirt with the crocodile had already been on the market for 33 years by the time Ralph Lauren founded his company. But this may have added to the latecomer's appeal. In the 1980s the piqué shirt with the polo-player logo became the preferred wear of the young, aspiring generation. In Europe it owed much of its success to the fact that Ralph Lauren clothes are sold at considerably higher prices there than in the USA. The Ralph Lauren polo shirt was therefore positioned in a more exclusive segment of the market and attracted customers who felt that the Lacoste brand had become far too widely accessible. In fact, Lacoste suffered a great deal from piracy at this time, even though the authentic original was still sold at a reasonable price that broad sections of the population could afford. In the 1980s a piqué shirt with a Ralph Lauren logo was definitely a greater status symbol than the Lacoste shirt, which had been treasured by the younger generation's parents and grandparents. But time is on the side of the original, and the once youthful wearers of the Ralph Lauren shirt are now getting on a bit themselves. Someone who was 30 in 1985 no longer contributes to the brand's youthful image. And thanks to the seventies revival of the 1990s a whole new generation have rediscovered Lacoste for themselves. Today the choice between the one brand and the other is more a question of color and cut than anything else. The American shirt is cut longer and narrower, the French version is shorter and has a somewhat larger collar. Your preferred style of casual wear is also important. Someone who has a taste for American style will choose Ralph Lauren, someone who prefers a Mediterranean look will feel more comfortable with Lacoste. And someone who cannot make up his mind about anything will just pile up his shirts in the wardrobe so that sometimes one is on top, sometimes the other.

Of course, the first Lacoste shirt was white because it was designed for tennis players. Even today there are a number of traditionalists who simply ignore the enormous selection of colors and insist on the original white shirt. But even if there are disagreements over the color, there is only one choice as far as material is concerned. A Lacoste shirt must be made of cotton piqué. Only then will it have the qualities that make it so ideal for sport and leisurewear. It is breathable, it stretches, and it can absorb plenty of moisture. Piqué shirts do not necessarily need to be ironed. If they are hung up smooth after washing they can be worn straight away once they have dried.

Water Sports – the Outfit

The heavy demands of competitive sailing have created a style of clothing that has to provide protection against wind, cold, and sea water. Pieces of this wardrobe have been found suitable for extreme weather conditions on land. This is why some items of sailing wear are popular in fields for which they were never intended, but in which they nevertheless do excellent service. For example, the Henri Lloyd jacket was originally developed solely for the demands of yachting, but is now extremely popular among motor cyclists. Like the Barbour jacket, it went through a process of assimilation as it was accepted by new groups.

By contrast, the less athletic style of summer sailing in the comparatively peaceful waters of the Mediterranean gave rise to a completely different way of dressing based on the simple clothes worn by fishermen. This is a casual style with a maritime accent and is not particularly suited to extreme weather conditions. This look was pioneered in holiday resorts on the Côte d'Azur, and is still perfectly acceptable today with its classic combinations of blue and white. No one should worry that this style of dress is too casual, as many well-known personalities have been seen wearing it.

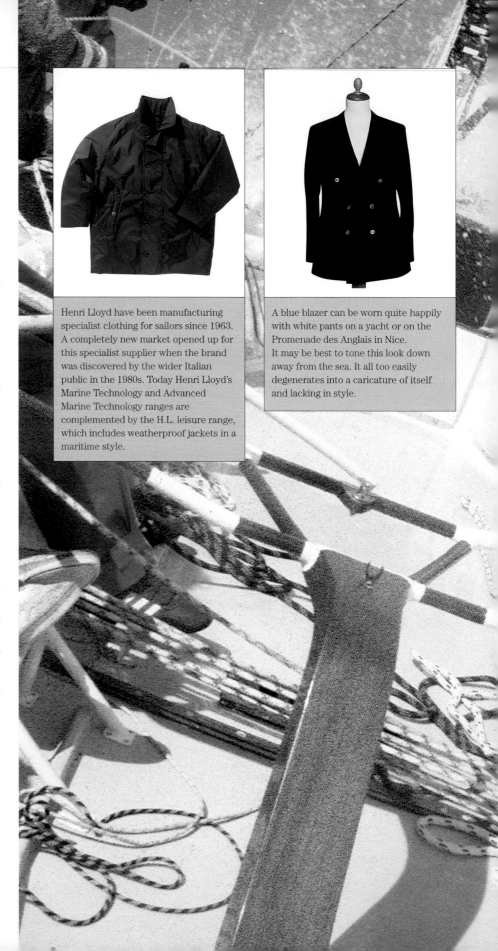

Henri Lloyd have been manufacturing specialist clothing for sailors since 1963. A completely new market opened up for this specialist supplier when the brand was discovered by the wider Italian public in the 1980s. Today Henri Lloyd's Marine Technology and Advanced Marine Technology ranges are complemented by the H.L. leisure range, which includes weatherproof jackets in a maritime style.

A blue blazer can be worn quite happily with white pants on a yacht or on the Promenade des Anglais in Nice. It may be best to tone this look down away from the sea. It all too easily degenerates into a caricature of itself and lacking in style.

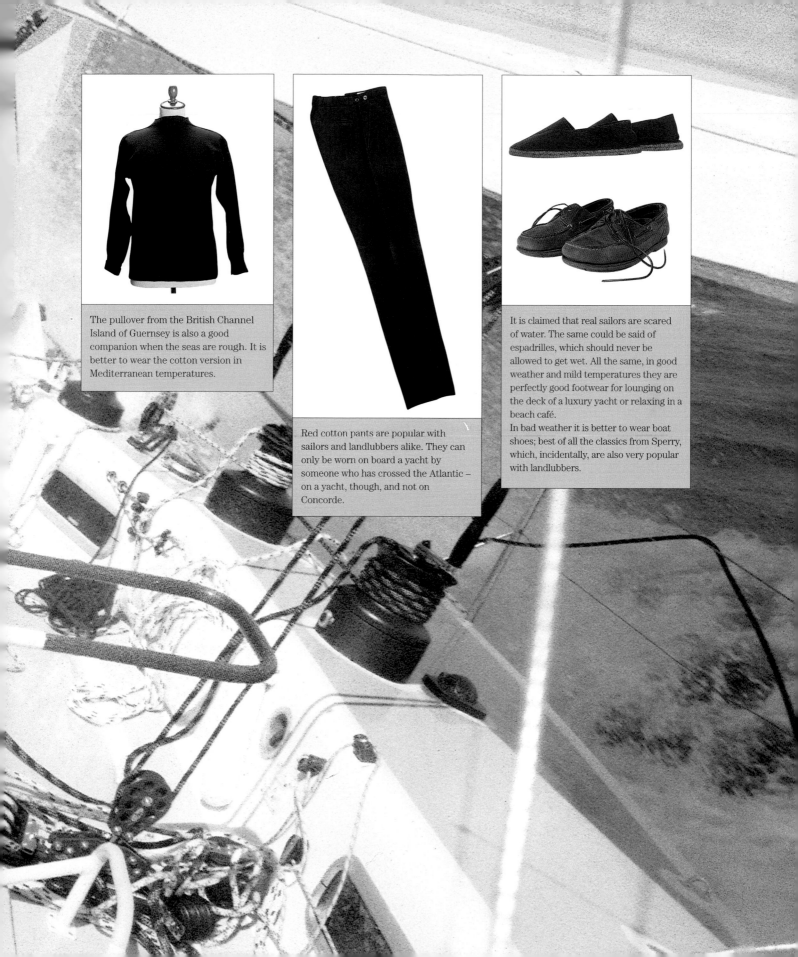

The pullover from the British Channel Island of Guernsey is also a good companion when the seas are rough. It is better to wear the cotton version in Mediterranean temperatures.

Red cotton pants are popular with sailors and landlubbers alike. They can only be worn on board a yacht by someone who has crossed the Atlantic – on a yacht, though, and not on Concorde.

It is claimed that real sailors are scared of water. The same could be said of espadrilles, which should never be allowed to get wet. All the same, in good weather and mild temperatures they are perfectly good footwear for lounging on the deck of a luxury yacht or relaxing in a beach café.
In bad weather it is better to wear boat shoes; best of all the classics from Sperry, which, incidentally, are also very popular with landlubbers.

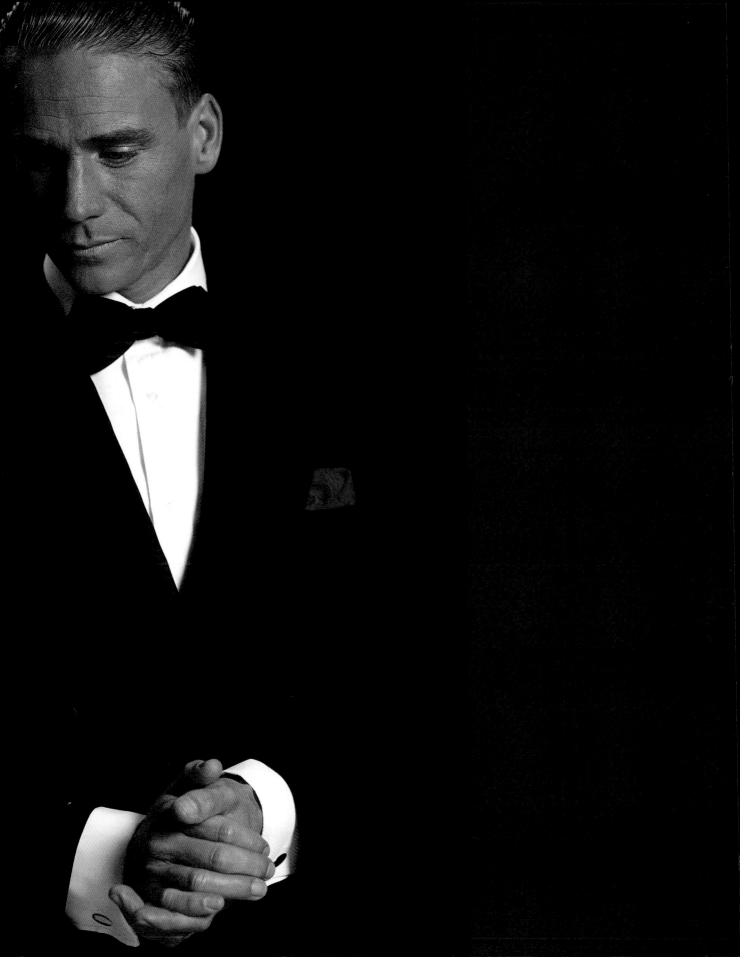

Formal Dress

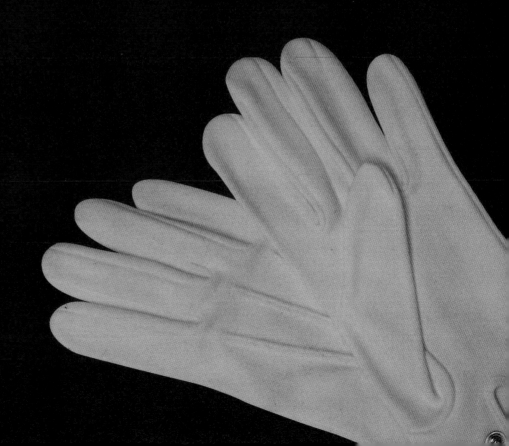

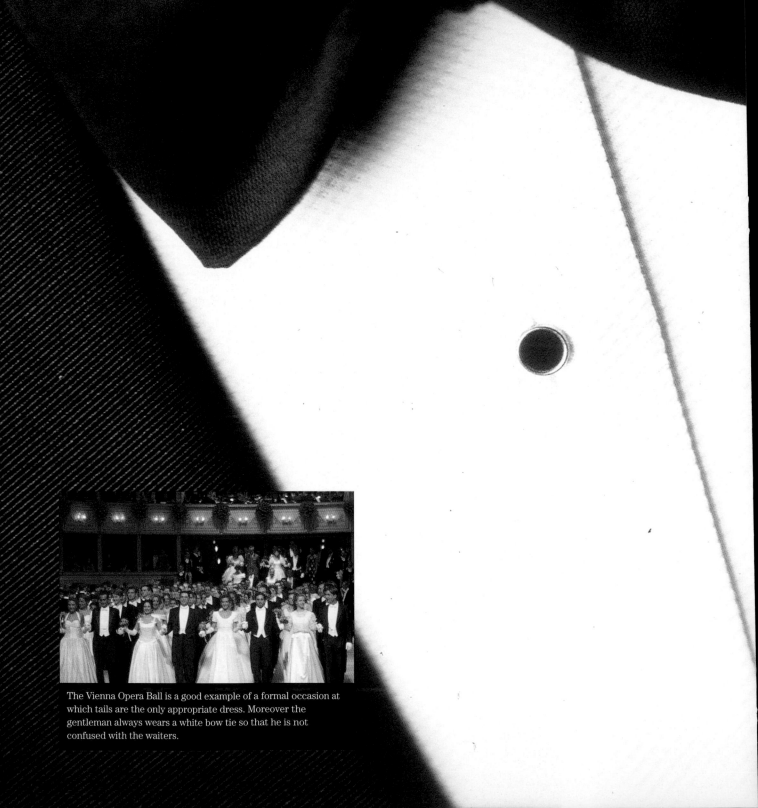

The Vienna Opera Ball is a good example of a formal occasion at which tails are the only appropriate dress. Moreover the gentleman always wears a white bow tie so that he is not confused with the waiters.

White or black?

"White tie" or "black tie," tails or tuxedo – the invitation to a formal occasion always indicates what the guest is expected to wear. If it says "white tie," "cravate blanche," or "full evening dress," then tails must be worn. But more usually you see "black tie," "cravate noire," or "evening dress," which means a tuxedo.

"Tuxedo" is in fact an exclusively North-American term, the name coming from Tuxedo Park, New York, where the jacket is said to have been first introduced in 1886 (for more on this contentious point see page 325). It is called a "smoking" in German-speaking countries and a "dinner jacket" in England. Though strictly speaking all three terms denote only the jacket, they naturally also cover the pants. To add to the confusion, what the Germans call a "dinnerjacket" is actually a *white* tuxedo (in England a white dinner jacket).

But let's return to the invitation. The type of evening dress required is made quite clear by the color of the bow tie specified. As a black bow tie is traditionally worn with a tuxedo, the indication "black tie" means that this is the correct form of evening dress to wear. A white bow tie, conversely, is worn with tails, so "white tie" indicates that tails are what you must wear. It must be said, however, that occasions to which either tuxedo or tails must be worn are becoming increasingly rare, so that many men no longer have any evening clothes at all.

In most countries in the world you would indeed be overdressed if you wore evening dress to go to a restaurant, the cinema, or a bar – particularly as formal clothes no longer necessarily conform to present-day ideas about how our leisure time should be spent. But opportunities to wear a tuxedo do still occur, though their frequency will depend on the circles you move in. If you stay at the Waldorf when you visit New York you can certainly dine in a tuxedo, and in Europe's best hotels – if in doubt – it is still the safest choice. In any case nobody who often wears suits should be afraid of the tuxedo. That's all it is, after all, just a suit – though it's only worn in the evening. Full evening dress is slightly different. It really is an awe-inspiring outfit – and at the same time there is no more elegant way for a man to dress. This will be confirmed by anybody who has admired himself in well-fitting tails with a white bow tie, a wing collar, and patent shoes. Everyone should have this pleasure at least once, even if it is just for a few minutes in front of a dress-rental company's mirror. Investing in tails only really makes sense for men whose profession frequently requires them to attend official functions. Most wearers of tails these days are politicians, ambassadors, and conductors of orchestras. Even some of these will have rented their outfits if the occasions for which they are required are rare.

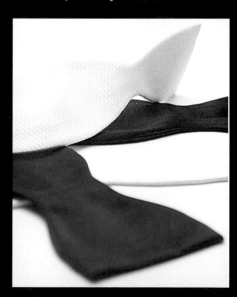

A gentleman's wardrobe should contain both white and black bow ties. The "black tie" is naturally worn more often.

The Tuxedo

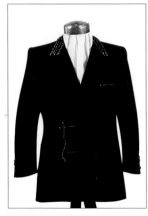

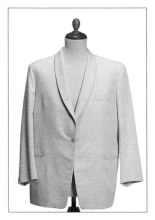

A tuxedo jacket can be either single or double breasted and usually has silk faced peaked lapels. A shawl collar is an acceptable alternative. The color is black or midnight blue. The fabric is generally lighter than that of a suit for day wear, as it can often be very warm at evening occasions.

The white tuxedo is worn at open-air evening parties and on cruises. It is either genuinely white or écru, a shade between natural white and light beige. The cut and fabric of a white tuxedo are subject to the same rules as its black equivalent. It's very stylish to wear an heirloom.

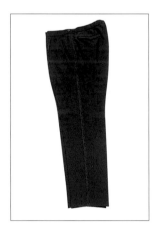

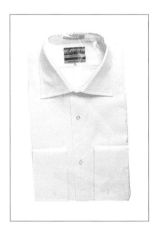

The pants are black or midnight blue, like the jacket. The outside seams are embellished with a plain silk stripe, which is called a braid. They have no cuffs, because cuffs are felt to be informal. The pants worn with a white tuxedo are also black or midnight blue, never white like the jacket.

A tuxedo requires a dress shirt, which is white and has French cuffs. Sometimes dress shirts have a fly front. The front often has vertical or horizontal pleats, or it is reinforced with cotton piqué. So that the front does not bulge upward when the wearer sits down, this trimming should not extend as far down as the waistband.

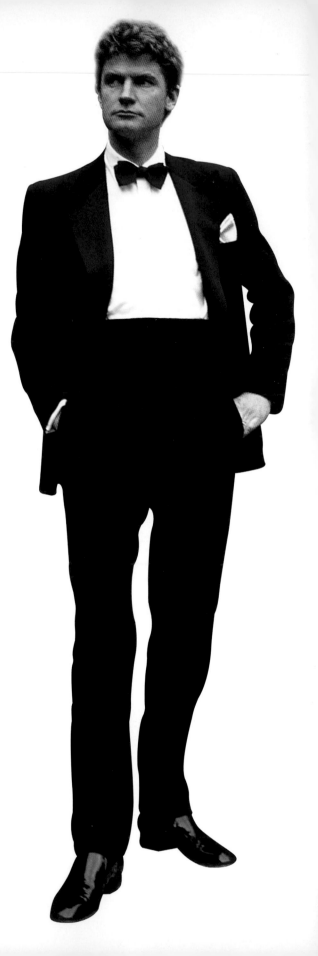

– and What Goes With It

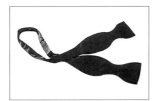

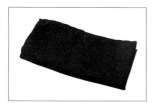

If the invitation says "black tie," then the bow tie really should be black. White is out of the question; the white bow tie is reserved for tails. It must be the sort you tie yourself – see how on page 86.

A dash of color is enormously effective with a black tuxedo. A red silk handkerchief, for example, looks splendid against the black of the jacket. A simple white linen handkerchief is also correct, and very appealing

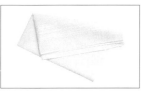

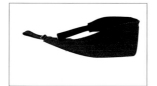

The handkerchief in your pocket should be cotton, white, and clean. You can use it to dab away the perspiration if dancing or eating becomes too strenuous – and to come to the aid of a lady who has nowhere to put one in her evening gown.

The cummerbund covers the area where the shirt tucks into the pants. It's an adaptation of the sash worn round the waist in India, which in Hindi is called a "kamarband." It used to have a little pocket sewn into it, which is why it is put on with the folds pointing upward.

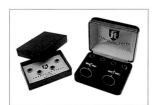

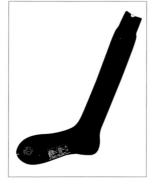

As a dress shirt has French cuffs, cuff links are essential. Gold is very appropriate, as are combinations of gold and black semiprecious stones. Many dress shirts fasten with studs, and these are sometimes available to match the cuff links.

Black knee-length socks should be worn with a tuxedo. They should be in wool or silk, depending on the weight of the tuxedo fabric.

Black & White

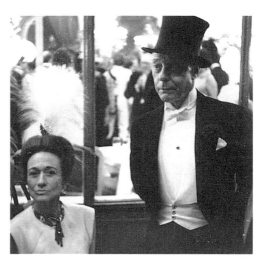

The Duke of Windsor – seen above in formal garb, full evening dress with the obligatory white tie, and below in tuxedo and black tie – popularized the tuxedo with shawl collar in the 1920s. The Americans are often credited with the invention of the tuxedo, and they themselves seem convinced that this thesis is correct: the 100th anniversary of the tuxedo was celebrated on 10 October 1986. The American Formalwear Association even marked the occasion with an advertising campaign extolling tobacco heir Griswold "Grizzy" Lorillard, who is supposed to have been the inventor. When he entered the Tuxedo Club in Tuxedo Park, New York, on 10 October 1886 his evening-dress jacket lacked its characteristic tails. This date went down in history as the birthday of the "tuxedo," and in America the name has been retained in honor of its place of birth. In the year of the purported jubilee Angus Cundey, managing director of Henry Poole at No. 15 Savile Row, merely remarked discreetly: "We made a short smoking jacket for the Prince of Wales as early as 1865."

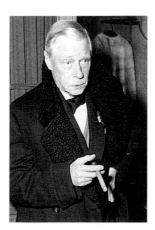

What you wear over the tuxedo depends on the weather. On winter days in New York the Duke of Windsor used to favor a fur-lined overcoat that had been in his wardrobe since the year 1934.

White Tie

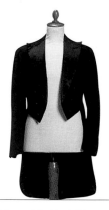

Tails must be black. The jacket is always single breasted – indeed it cannot be buttoned up. The facing lapels are silk covered, as in the tuxedo.

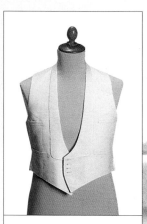

The evening waistcoat is in white cotton piqué. It has lapels, and depending on the cut it can be single or double breasted.

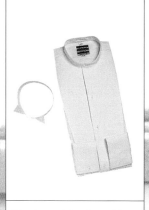

The front of the dress shirt is either pleated or trimmed with cotton piqué. It has a wing collar and single cuffs fastening with cuff links. This classic style seems destined to last forever.

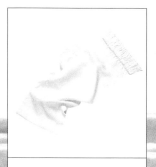

The white silk scarf is worn only with an overcoat, so the two are taken off at the same time. Under no circumstances should it be tied theatrically round the neck.

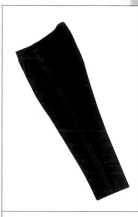

Full evening-dress pants have double braids – two parallel silk stripes – on the outside seams. This distinguishes them from tuxedo pants, which have only one. Like tuxedo pants, these never have cuffs. Since a belt cannot be worn under the full evening-dress waistcoat, the pants are held up by suspenders, which tend to be more comfortable anyway.

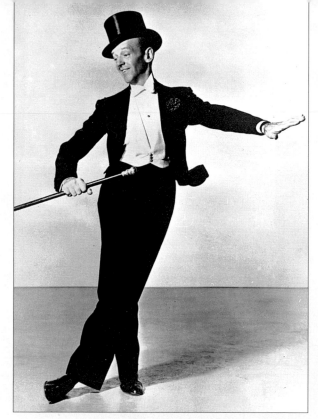

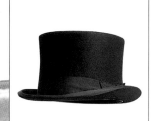

A black top hat should really be worn with tails, but the practice has virtually died out. You have to take off your hat when you arrive at a party in any case, so nobody would see it but the hat-check girl and your companions.

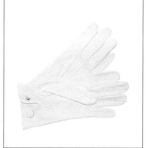

White gloves are not obligatory on every white-tie occasion; they need not be worn at a ball, for example. They may be appropriate at a state banquet, and care should be taken on such occasions to ensure that etiquette is not breached.

Fred Astaire was among the most famous wearers of tails; in his movies he wore them in countless dancing scenes. On him tails certainly looked particularly elegant, but he wasn't entirely responsible for that – it was largely due to their cut. The waistband is cut very high, and the vest – also high – is covered by the sides of the jacket. This cut has the effect of elongating the figure, because the white of the vest does not divide it into two unflattering halves. Fred Astaire got this idea from the Prince of Wales, whose vest had caught his eye. "The waistcoat did not show below the dress-coat front. I liked that." Fred found out that Hawes & Curtis had made this attractive item, but they declined to make one for him. He later found more compassion in Savile Row: Kilgour, French & Stanbury made him the evening dress that he wore in the 1935 movie *Top Hat*.

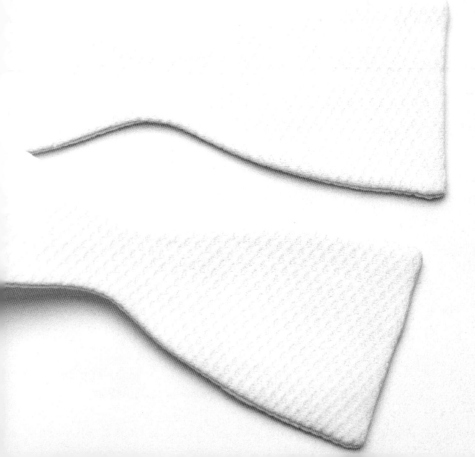

The bow tie worn with tails is always in white cotton piqué. It must be the sort you tie yourself – see how on page 86.

A Jacket for Smoking

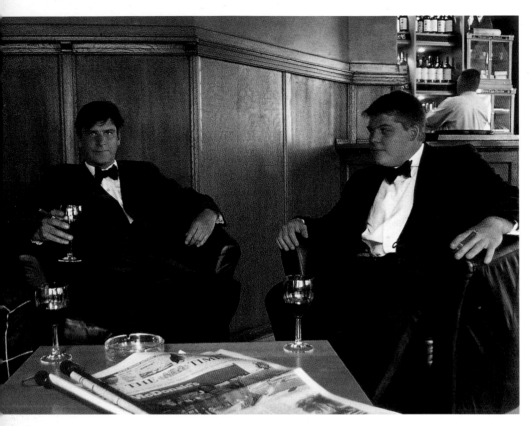

A close relative of the tuxedo (which the Germans call a "smoking," remember) is the true smoking jacket, which is worn in England to parties in homes and to country balls. The name denotes its original function: gentlemen would don their smoking jackets before withdrawing to the smoking room for a cigar, and afterwards they would put their "dinner jackets" on again. This had the advantage that the ladies present were not forced to endure tobacco fumes, either directly or from the smoke-impregnated jackets of the gentlemen. It used to be considered unseemly to expose the female nose to such offense.

In contrast to the black "dinner jacket," the "smoking jacket" is made of colored velvet, generally with a shawl collar. The collar is sometimes in a contrasting color, for example black silk. A smoking jacket is worn with velvet slippers, embroidered with rural motifs or the wearer's initials, sometimes matching the jacket's color – typically dark green, dark violet, burgundy, or blue. The "dinner-jacket" pants, a dress shirt, and of course a black bow tie complete the ensemble. There is no doubt about the pleasing elegance of the outfit, and the slightly more relaxed feeling that a smoking jacket gives the wearer.

Available to Rent...

It is understandable these days that only very few men own a smoking jacket; they hardly ever have the opportunity to wear one. And if you really need one, you can rent it. Anybody who has a problematical figure or is of an unusual size should seek out the local dress-rental firm in good time so that the availability of the required size can be checked in peace and quiet, otherwise he may find himself on the night before the big occasion with nothing to wear. But what is on offer at the dress-rental firm may not be up to the requisite standard, and in this case it is worth considering buying your own smoking jacket. When you have one, you will find more and more frequent opportunities to wear it: dinner in a good restaurant, a theatrical première, simply going to a bar. It is often exactly right for private functions, as long as they are held in the evening – though the tuxedo is completely wrong for a wedding. In any case, you should buy a pair of patent shoes in good time, because although a jacket can be rented if necessary, shoes can't. You should wear them for a few evenings at home before going out in them, otherwise the big event may end with painful blisters, making walking difficult and dancing impossible. As can be seen on the following page, there are different designs of shoe possible for wearing with tuxedo or smoking jacket. It is important for a gentleman to choose the right style for him.

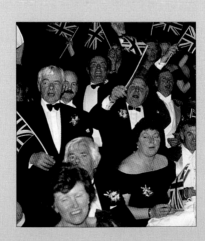

The Right Shoes

Opinions differ on the subject of patent shoes. Traditionalists advocate pumps with silk bows, not only with a tuxedo but with full evening dress as well. The design of pumps goes back to the sixteenth century, which makes them one of the oldest items in the gentleman's wardrobe to have survived virtually unchanged. But this is not a sufficient argument to induce many men to put them on; a man really does need a little courage to wear gleaming shoes with silk bows on. It is no *faux pas* to wear patent shoes in the Oxford design instead. This is certainly correct with a tuxedo, as Oxford shoes are its contemporary, and there is not really anything to be said against wearing them with full evening dress either. As long ago as the 1930s pumps were widely felt to be an anachronism. In his famous book, *All Creatures Great and Small*, the English writer James Herriot describes an amusing incident when he was lent a pair of patent pumps by his future father-in-law. "I ... shrank back when I saw the shoes. They were a pair of dancing slippers from the early days of the century, and their cracked patent leather was topped by wide, black silk bows." James Herriot's attitude is by no means unusual so choose Oxfords if in any doubt.

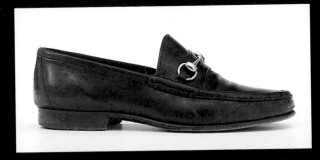

Black Gucci loafers are a popular alternative to patent shoes. This variant first appeared in England, but it has now achieved international acceptance. In highly traditional surroundings, however, such extravagance should be eschewed and patent shoes chosen instead.

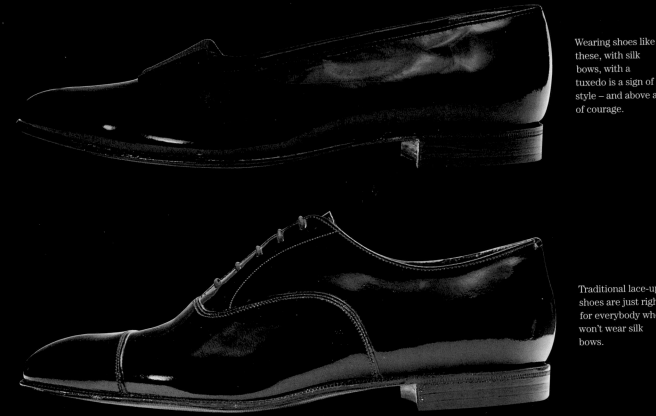

Wearing shoes like these, with silk bows, with a tuxedo is a sign of style – and above all of courage.

Traditional lace-up shoes are just right for everybody who won't wear silk bows.

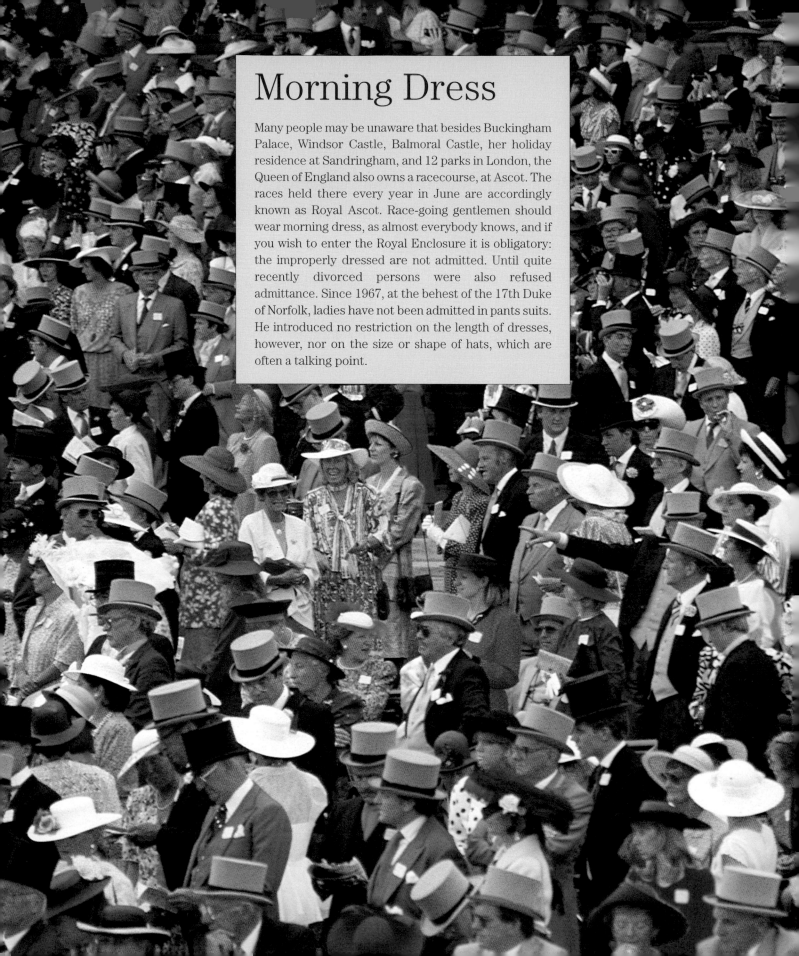

Morning Dress

Many people may be unaware that besides Buckingham Palace, Windsor Castle, Balmoral Castle, her holiday residence at Sandringham, and 12 parks in London, the Queen of England also owns a racecourse, at Ascot. The races held there every year in June are accordingly known as Royal Ascot. Race-going gentlemen should wear morning dress, as almost everybody knows, and if you wish to enter the Royal Enclosure it is obligatory: the improperly dressed are not admitted. Until quite recently divorced persons were also refused admittance. Since 1967, at the behest of the 17th Duke of Norfolk, ladies have not been admitted in pants suits. He introduced no restriction on the length of dresses, however, nor on the size or shape of hats, which are often a talking point.

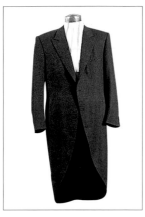

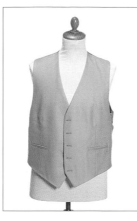

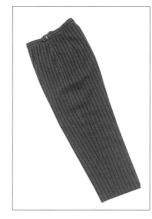

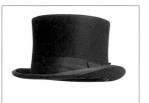

The morning coat is black or gray. At traditional weddings only the groom and the bride's father may wear gray. If in doubt, black is never wrong. Basically the morning coat is a frock coat with the corners cut away – hence the alternative English name of "cut-away coat," which the Germans adopted and shortened to "cut." The morning coat is worn only during the day.

The morning coat must be accompanied by a vest, which may be single or double breasted. Its color is either light gray or buff (the more traditional color), which can be described as a yellowish beige. Less traditional, but very popular with young men, are vests in colored silk.

The morning coat is worn with striped pants, but there is always somebody determined to be different. There have been sightings of pants in Prince of Wales check, houndstooth, and even Scottish tartans (which really ought to be reserved for the Scots). At weddings the groom and the bride's father may wear light-gray pants to match their morning coats.

Morning dress is often accompanied these days by a gray top hat. At most occasions – weddings, for example – this is correct, but at funerals it should be black. Good top hats are made of silk, and are no longer easy to come by. Anybody who lacks an exquisite and appropriate heirloom must content himself with a modern felt creation.

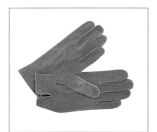

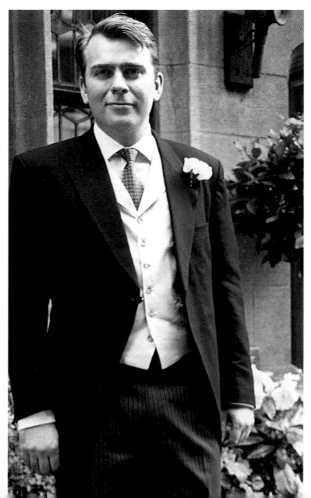

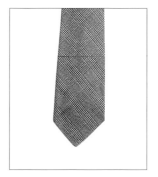

A pair of gray buckskin gloves should be worn with morning dress.

Those inclined to nostalgia enjoy accompanying a morning coat with a necktie like this, recalling the "cravate" of the nineteenth century. A silver-gray necktie is less romantic, but absolutely correct. Colored ties may also be worn if the occasion allows. A bow tie, however, is never worn with a morning coat.

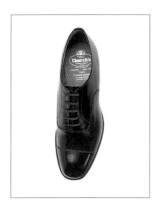

Black Oxfords are the classic shoes with a morning coat, but monkstraps and loafers will do.

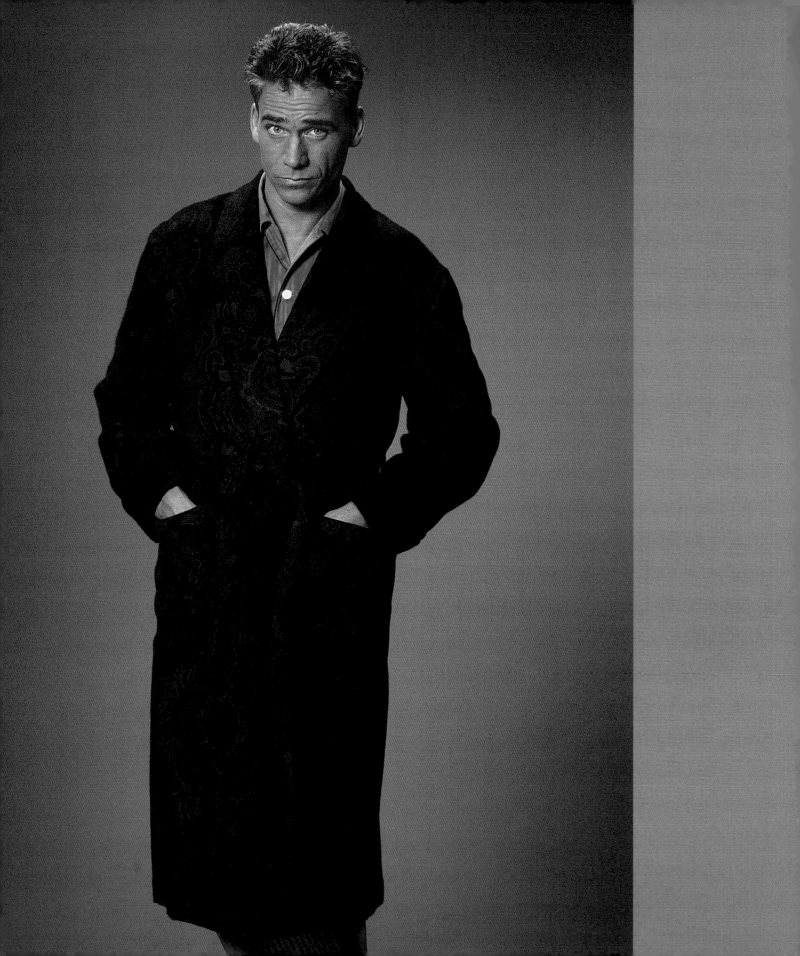

Home Comfort

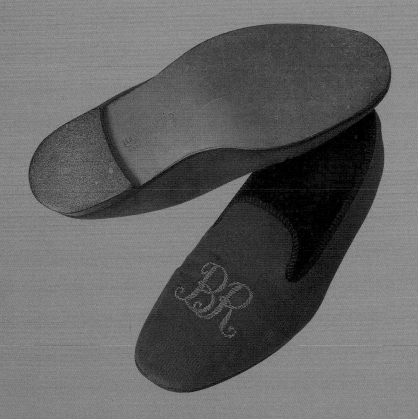

A Hint of Decadence

America has always held a fascination for Europe. Even now that everyone has long been aware of the dark side of the American dream, Europeans still look to America for inspiration. Television acts as their principal source of information. International news programs give them an insight into a society that they previously knew mainly from TV series and movies. But anybody wishing to form a picture of America between 1930 and 1960 can do so with the assistance of art books. Illustrator Norman Perceval Rockwell's collected works are a real treasure trove for the study of menswear styles. Take the cover of the *Saturday Evening Post* on 16 May 1959, for example. Here we see how the modern middle-class American male began his Sunday mornings: reading the paper in his Eames chair, drinking tea from a Wedgwood porcelain cup, and smoking a cigarette. But above all, look at his clothes: they are the most timeless of all the objects depicted. What this man is wearing can still be purchased today in New York, London, Paris, and Barcelona. It is another example of the fact that to this day countless clothing styles from the 1930s remain unchanged, and are still attractive. Indeed, they still have style, which is the most important thing for a gentleman, whether in public or in private, when only his family may see him.

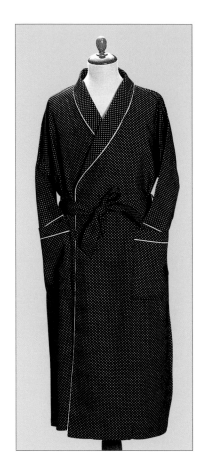

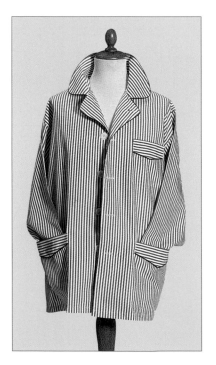

Cotton pajamas, generously cut, are far more becoming than tight jersey. The only better way to sleep is wearing nothing at all.

A dressing gown or robe and fine pajamas are so elegant that in principle you could wear them to fetch the bread for breakfast. It would certainly give the baker a shock.

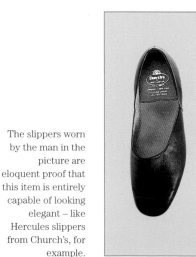

The slippers worn by the man in the picture are eloquent proof that this item is entirely capable of looking elegant – like Hercules slippers from Church's, for example.

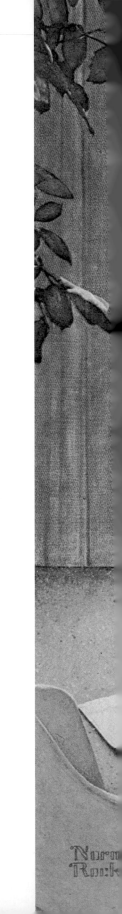

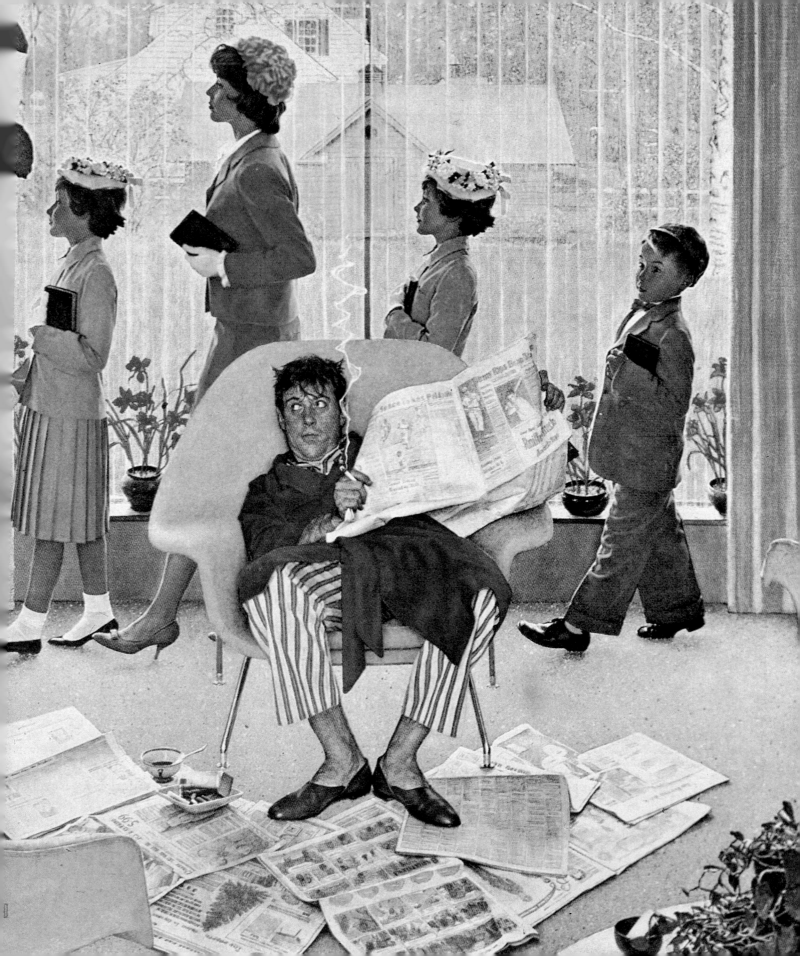

Breakfast with Style

Style is revealed in little things. Like how you dress when there's nobody to see you. A gentleman's clothing is not a costume. He wears what he wears because he likes it. And not in order to impress anybody. The only external constraint to which he will defer is the occasion. And the first occasion every morning is breakfast. Regrettably, fewer and fewer people these days take the time for this first – and, as many think, the best – meal of the day. They prefer to stay in bed as long as possible, then rush off at the last minute – and breakfast, what with showering and dressing, falls by the wayside. Of course it takes willpower and discipline to set the alarm half an hour earlier. But that half-hour is a good investment if it is used for a breakfast that is stylish in every respect. For a meal in the morning fortifies us for the demands of the hours that lie ahead. Freshly brewed tea and a Wedgwood or Spode tea service, your favorite jam from Fortnum & Mason on a slice of toast precisely the right shade of brown. A gentleman may also wish to take his time reading the morning newspaper while drinking his second or third cup of tea. A man who believes he owes it to himself to go to all this trouble will not profane his frugal but perfect breakfast by consuming it in a baggy T-shirt, boxer shorts, and rubber bathroom slippers. A man with style will always keep himself dressed as is appropriate to greet the woman he loves: in a dressing gown that is right for the occasion.

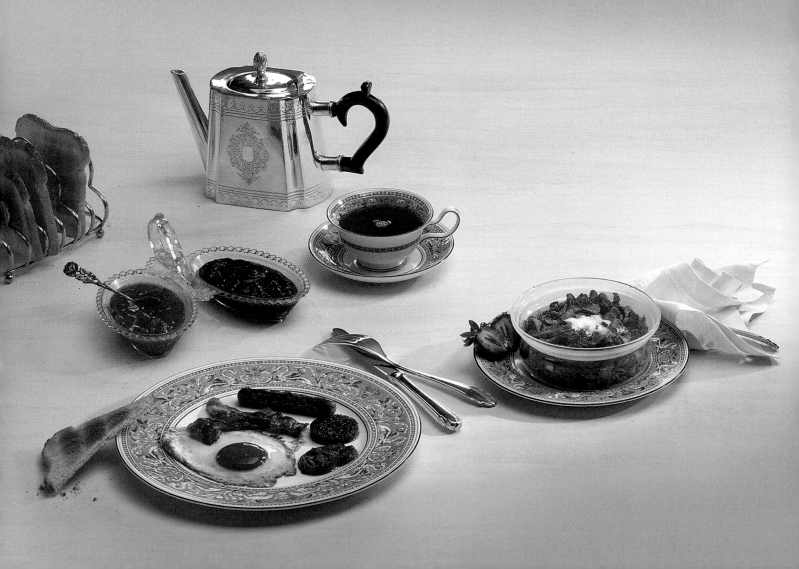

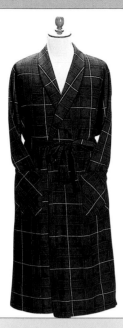

You need not abandon all thoughts of elegance at the breakfast table just because you think a silk dressing gown is overdoing it. There is as wide a choice of dressing gowns in cotton flannel or wool as there is of pajamas.

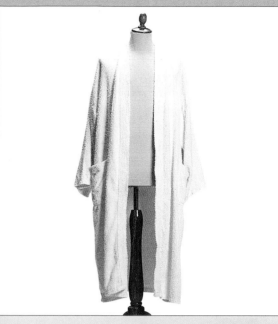

For many years white terry-toweling bathrobes were a favorite "souvenir" of top-class hotels, and consequently they are now often available only on request. The Plaza in New York even sells them in its own souvenir store. White terry-toweling bathrobes are in fact freely available in the stores, but of course without the prestigious hotel name.

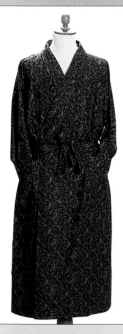

There is always an aroma of decadence about a silk dressing gown. It is hard to imagine Hugh Hefner, the legendary publisher of *Playboy*, wearing anything else. It used to be customary to receive persons of equal or inferior status thus attired, and in some quarters this tradition is still observed.

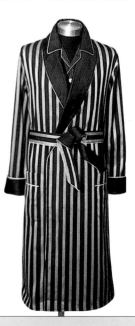

The silk dressing gown in regimental colors is a real evergreen in the range of the famous English Derek Rose brand. It is available in all the color combinations found in regimental ties. The selection of striped robes is just as extensive, and many gentlemen have a Derek Rose in their wardrobe.

A Souvenir from the Colonies

What distinguishes pajamas from a nightshirt is the presence or absence of pants. And, strictly speaking, that's exactly what pajamas are: pants. The word is a corruption of the Persian term "pae jamah," which means a garment covering the feet or legs. Pajamas are thus modeled on the pants that used to be worn in India and the Middle East – by day, that is. British colonialists adapted them as nightwear and took the new bedroom fashion back to England with them under the name of pajamas. This was competition for the nightshirt, but it was not until after 1930 that pajamas took the lead. Today the stiffest competition probably comes from the combination of boxer shorts and T-shirt, and many men sleep in the raw. Actually there is really no compelling reason to wear pajamas, though some do. Perhaps because they provide the opportunity to wear all those colors that have no place in a classic wardrobe. Certainly they come in a range of colors and patterns that can have no place in everyday wear.

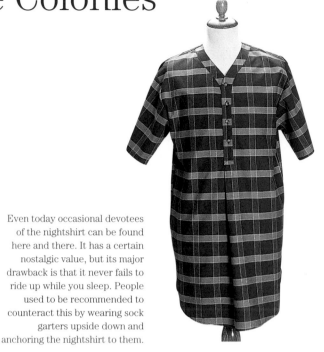

Even today occasional devotees of the nightshirt can be found here and there. It has a certain nostalgic value, but its major drawback is that it never fails to ride up while you sleep. People used to be recommended to counteract this by wearing sock garters upside down and anchoring the nightshirt to them.

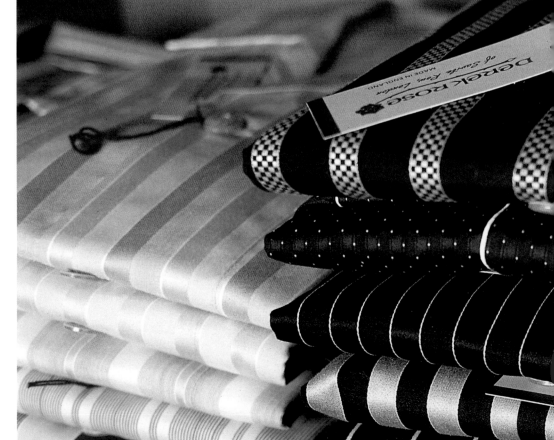

Striped pajamas are a specialty of the Derek Rose brand. Originally founded in 1925 as H. H. Winder Ltd., the company made pajamas which were then sold under the names of numerous Jermyn Street shirt-makers and department stores like Harrods and Simpsons. Since 1975 these pajamas have been sold under the "Derek Rose, Savile Row" brand name, together with dressing gowns and nightshirts.

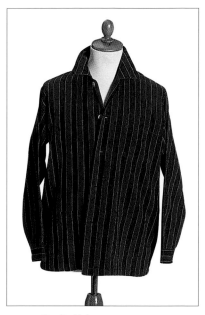

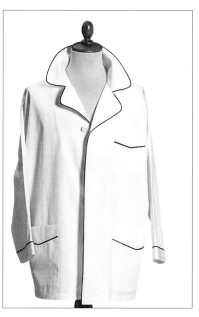

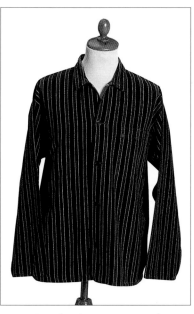

Most pajamas are made of cotton. They come in the same diversity of color and pattern as shirts. They can be custom made, with matching dressing gown and boxer shorts if required. All custom shirt-makers offer this service, for example Charvet in Paris and Hilditch & Key in London.

Silk pajamas are extremely comfortable to wear; they are warm in winter and cool in summer. And nothing is smoother and softer on the skin than silk, as long as it is of outstanding quality. Silk pajamas should thus only be bought from suppliers of the best cotton pajamas.

Anybody who tends to feel cold in bed will be more interested in woolen pajamas. And anybody who cannot stand the thought of new wool next to the skin, but still needs something warm, is recommended to consider Viyella – that blend of cotton and merino wool familiar to us all from shirts.

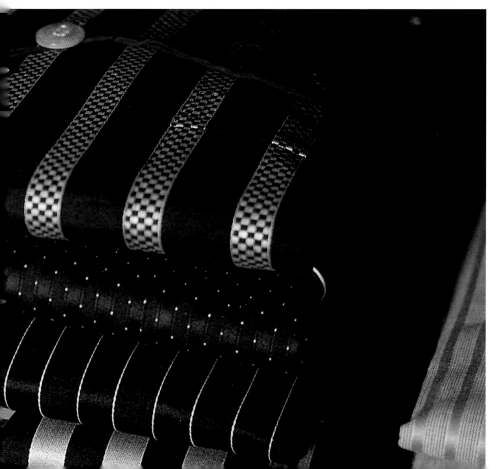

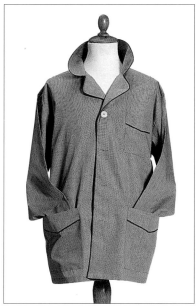

Cotton flannel is a popular fabric for warmer pajamas with people who dislike wool and Viyella. These slightly thicker pajamas often come in cheerful wintry patterns like tartan, and in colors like cozy burgundy and bottle-green.

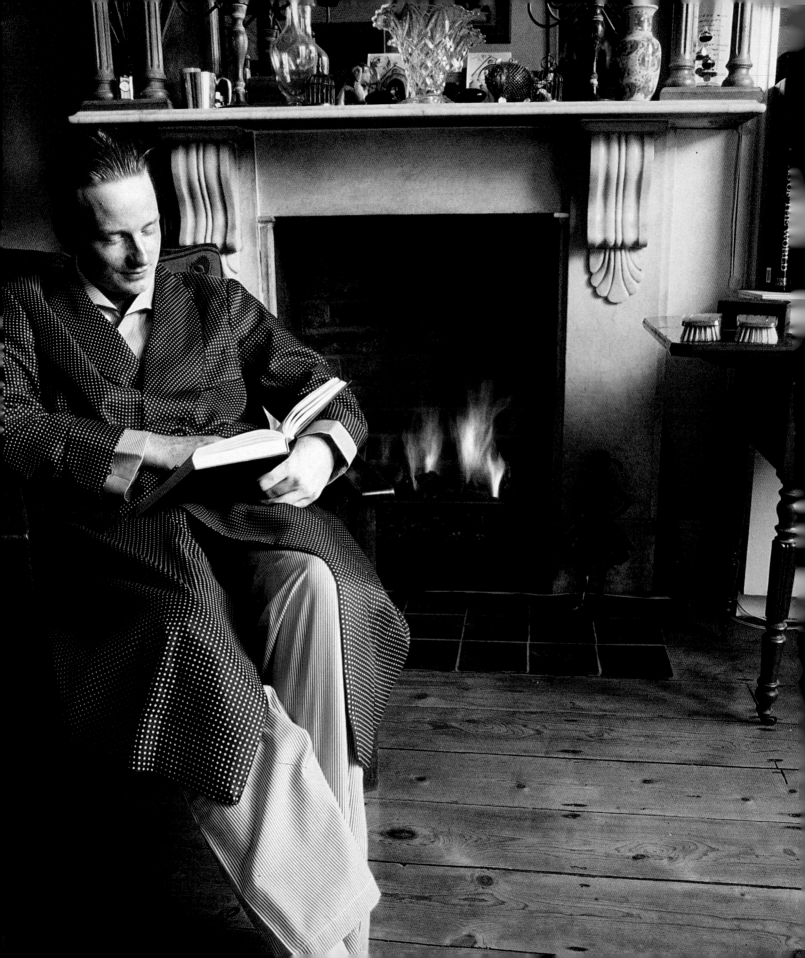

Home Comfort

In the late nineteenth century the silk dressing gown, shimmering in all the colors of the rainbow, offered a remarkable contrast with the dark and serious everyday clothing of the English gentleman. This colorful indoor garb doesn't seem to fit in with the overwhelmingly black wardrobe of the Victorian period. But if you consider the interiors of the time, you will be struck by the general preference for an opulence that is almost oriental. In our mind's eye we can see Oscar Wilde, casually reclining on the divan, receiving visitors in a silk dressing gown.

Not only England was fascinated by the exotic allure of the East, with all its stereotyped ideas about hookahs, ladies of the harem, and the Thousand and One Nights. The continent of Europe was also acquainted with the phenomenon of exoticism, in fashion as well as in architecture and the plastic arts. Again and again nineteenth-century literature, too, fled the rational modern world to return to themes from the realm of the crescent moon. In the acclaimed novel Oblomov by Russian writer Ivan A. Goncharov, the protagonist's silk dressing gown plays a central role as a symbol of his indecision and withdrawal from the world. And though the description of the hero in his dressing gown may not be all that flattering to him, this passage may well be the best-known literary tribute to the garment: "He wore a robe of Persian silk, a true oriental robe making not the slightest concession to Europe, with no tassels, no velvet, no waist – and very wide and comfortable, so that Oblomov could wrap it round himself twice. The sleeves, as unequivocally prescribed by Asiatic fashion, grew wider and wider from the fingers to the shoulders. Although this robe had long since lost its original freshness, and in places replaced its initial natural gleam by a different sheen, honestly acquired, its fabric was still sound and its oriental colors were resplendent. In Oblomov's eyes this robe had a plethora of inestimable advantages: it was soft and supple, he could hardly feel it on his body, it complied like an obedient slave with the tiniest movements he made."

Surely there can be no other passage in world literature that more effectively urges the reader to acquire a silk dressing gown than these lines in the first part of Oblomov. And indeed, how splendid to sit by the fireside, wrapped in such a masterpiece of the silk weaver's art, reading – perhaps a novel, perhaps the book that you now hold in your hands, from which at this point we respectfully take our leave.

Appendix

Looking after your Wardrobe

The Suit

If you want to look after your suit, you have to begin by handling it with care. This does not mean treating it with kid gloves. On the contrary, you will only look good in a suit if you move quite unaffectedly when you wear it. Careful handling is just a matter of treating a suit with love and attention. As the product of great craftsmanship and many hours of work, it has earned a certain degree of respect. Anyone who has seen how much work goes into a good suit and how long it takes for a two-dimensional strip of fabric to be shaped into a piece of clothing that fits the wearer perfectly will regard the garment with new eyes. In practice, this means that the suit should be hung up on a broad, well-shaped clothes hanger after it has been worn. Ideally, the hanger should be shaped like a pair of shoulders. The hanger does not need to be made of wood as long as it is the right size and fills out the jacket.

The hangers on which suits are hung in shops are narrow so that more clothes can be fitted onto the rails and into the display units. In order to prevent the sensitive shoulder seam from stretching out of shape while the jacket is hung up on these narrow hangers, it is fixed with white cotton thread, which is removed after the suit has been purchased. Good hangers can be bought in a department store.

Pants should hang on a pants hanger, which clamps onto the bottom hem so that they are pulled into shape by their own weight. If you place great store on an immaculately ironed crease, you can put your pants in a pants press, or iron your pants by hand. When you do this, always lay a piece of damp, white cotton cloth between the iron and the material. Otherwise, the suit will be shiny after it has been ironed.

Do make sure you have emptied the pockets before you hang up a jacket. After a day in action a suit needs a day of rest. If it has been worn for several days in succession, the rest period should be lengthened to match. Before the suit is hung away it should be given a quick brush. This should be done with a clothes brush made of natural bristle. Clothes brushes are available in various grades for different types of material. For example, particularly soft goat's hair brushes are used for sensitive cashmere. It is best to buy English brushes, such as the ones produced by G. B. Kent & Son. You would be well advised to avoid the sticky rolls that are supposed to pick up fluff. They leave behind traces of adhesive on the material, which can cause considerable damage. It is much better to simply remove hairs and fluff with your fingertips.

Go gently when you brush your suit. Do not pull off the buttons! The pockets also require careful treatment. Dirt really builds up in the cuffs of a pair of pants. They should be emptied and brushed as often as possible. You should turn your trousers inside out now and then in order to brush them from the inside. A suit should not disappear into the wardrobe straight away after it has been brushed. It is better to let it air for a while in an open window, on a balcony protected from the rain, or in a bathroom. Wool fibers need moisture to maintain their elasticity. A steam bath is just as beneficial to a suit as a Turkish bath to its owner. Clothes can be steamed easily in any bathroom. Close all the windows and air vents, run hot water until steam forms, and then hang up the suit for a while in the misty atmosphere you have created. This gets rid of creases and unpleasant odors.

The experts are not in agreement about dry cleaning. The traditionalists of Savile Row say that it is unnecessary: brushing, airing, and steaming are quite sufficient, while stains should be treated individually. Others see no danger in dry cleaning: the real problems are associated with how a garment is ironed afterwards. Anyone who has seen how a suit is treated at the dry cleaners round the corner will definitely stick to brushing and airing. Ironing a suit is a highly skilled task, and getting a suit ready to be worn with an iron takes a very long time. Bad ironing can practically destroy a suit. It is best to ask the leading gentlemen's outfitters in your area which dry-cleaning company offers the best service.

Custom-made clothes can be taken to a tailor to be cleaned. He will also send your suit away to be cleaned, but will get it back unironed, and then iron it to a professional standard. In any case, if the suit fits well and the material is of the right weight for the time of year, it will not even need to be cleaned. After all, a suit hardly ever comes into direct contact with bare skin.

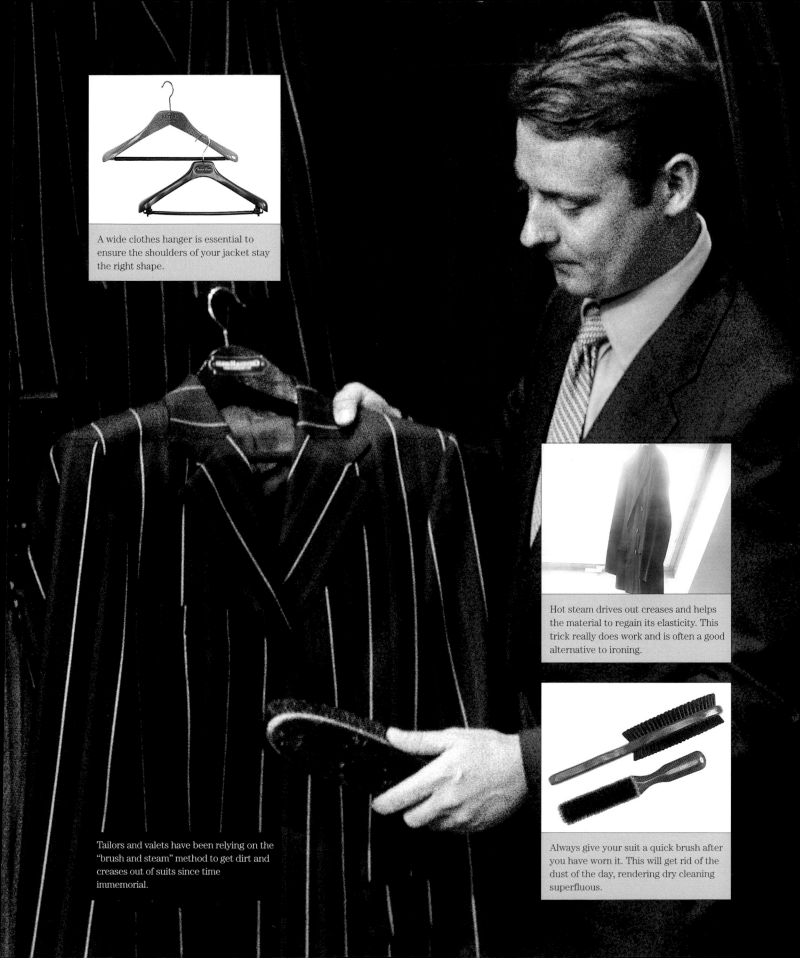

A wide clothes hanger is essential to ensure the shoulders of your jacket stay the right shape.

Hot steam drives out creases and helps the material to regain its elasticity. This trick really does work and is often a good alternative to ironing.

Tailors and valets have been relying on the "brush and steam" method to get dirt and creases out of suits since time immemorial.

Always give your suit a quick brush after you have worn it. This will get rid of the dust of the day, rendering dry cleaning superfluous.

The Necktie

Neckties are put under quite enough stress as it is when they are knotted. This is why they should be spared any further rough treatment if at all possible.

A necktie is not a piece of string round a parcel that you have to pull with all your might. It should be knotted and unknotted gently. It is also better not to wrench your necktie energetically to one side in order to remove it from your collar once it is open. Instead, open the knot, turn up the collar, and then take the necktie off over your head. If your necktie is creased, the specialists recommend holding it by the thin end, rolling it round your fist, and then leaving it to rest overnight. The next day all the creases will have disappeared.

Neckties should never be washed. Stains can be removed as and when necessary. It is worth trying out stain remover before you

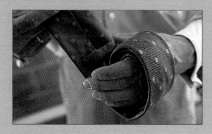

use it on a piece of the material that will not be seen.

Neckties are as sensitive to dry cleaning as suits. Poor ironing can destroy the appearance of valuable, handmade neckties, which have rounded edges that must never be ironed flat. In any case, as we do not usually wear the same necktie every day, cleaning is very rarely necessary. The best option is to own many neckties, so that cleaning is not often required.

Shoes

Everyone knows how to clean shoes. What is not generally known is that they should never be worn on two successive days. A pair of shoes needs at least a day of rest, and if your lower extremities tend to generate a lot of moisture, you should really leave them to air for a couple of days. Shoes are only comfortable when they have dried out completely. Slipping your foot into a damp, clammy shoe is unpleasant and also extremely uncomfortable. What is more, if you follow this general principle you will automatically double or triple your shoes' life expectancy.

As has been noted above, everyone knows how to clean shoes. This is why we will confine ourselves to commenting on shoe creme and wax polish.

Shoe creme is used on fine leather. Wax polish is equally suitable for fine and thick leathers. Shoe cremes are essential for ladies' shoes. Most men's shoes can bear wax polish. Just as it is difficult to spread ice cold butter onto bread, cold wax polish is difficult to rub into leather. For this reason shoes and wax polish should be placed in the sun for a while before cleaning in summer, and in winter shoes should be polished in a warm room. The polish penetrates the leather more quickly and is easier to brush up to a shine. Do not forget the bottom of the sole and the inner edge of the heel when you apply wax polish or shoe creme. Otherwise the leather may begin to crack in these places.

The longer you leave wax polish on leather, the quicker the shoes can be polished to a shine with a brush. This is partly because brushing forces the polish into the pores of the leather, and partly because it also removes superfluous polish from the surface. The more wax polish has penetrated into the leather before it is brushed, the better. When you have finished brushing you can go over the shoe quickly with a cloth to remove the last remains of the polish, which would otherwise end up smeared onto the bottom hem of your pants. Shoe creme should not be left on leather for so long. Many people have learnt by experience how quickly it can dry and harden. When this happens, it is very difficult to polish it off.

Shoe trees should be inserted into your shoes when you have taken them off. Loafers have to be stretched more than laced shoes because loafers are bent more as the foot rolls forward when you are walking. Shoe trees do not necessarily have to be made of cedarwood. Plain wooden shoe trees are just as good.

If your shoes get very wet, they should be stuffed with newspaper to dry out. Wet shoes should never be placed directly against a source of heat. Shoe trees can be inserted when the shoes are reasonably dry. There are specialists who recommend applying wax polish to shoes while they are still wet. Against this one might argue that leather saturated with water is hardly in a condition to absorb water-repellent polish. Opinions are just as divided when it comes to how shoe trees should be inserted into shoes. Some say that they should be put into the shoes while they are still warm; others advise that the shoes should be allowed to air first. As a general rule, we can only recommend that shoes should not be stretched excessively by the shoe tree and that the upper should not be stretched too much at the heel.

Shoe Repair

Shoe repair could also be discussed under the heading "after-sales service." If you live in England or the USA you can take your shoes to a shop, which will then send them back to the factory for repair. There they will be repaired by experienced craftsmen using original materials. All the major manufacturers of welted shoes offer this service, but, unfortunately, not usually for customers outside their own country, who are left to deal with the holes in their shoes as best they can. This means that they take a pair of shoes that cost the equivalent of a cheap flight from Frankfurt to New York to the local cobbler on the corner, where they are ruined by amateurish repair work. There is nothing wrong with most cobblers, but they should not be allowed anywhere near welt-stitched shoes. Unfortunately, the shoe retailers do not show the least concern about this problem. Church & Co. are the only company to offer a worldwide repair service. Their shoes can be taken to the nearest outlet selling Church's shoes. They will send them off to England. The shoes come back two to four months later and are just as good as new. This service obviously has its price, but the repair work is carried out to perfection. However, shoes are only accepted if no alterations have been made to the sole by a cobbler. The repair of the heel should be entrusted to a good master shoemaker, a specialist who can build shoes himself. Only a craftsman will repair shoes expertly. For example, moccasins with glued or through-stitched soles cannot be mended at a factory for reasons connected with their design. A master shoemaker will grind down the sole and stick a new leather sole over it. In this way even lightweight mocassins can be mended several times.

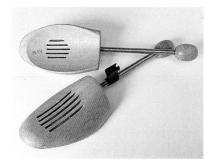

The sole should also be treated occasionally with shoe creme. Otherwise it may dry out and become brittle.

Shoe trees are indispensable. Inexpensive shoe trees are quite sufficient. They should always be made of wood, which is able to absorb moisture from the leather.

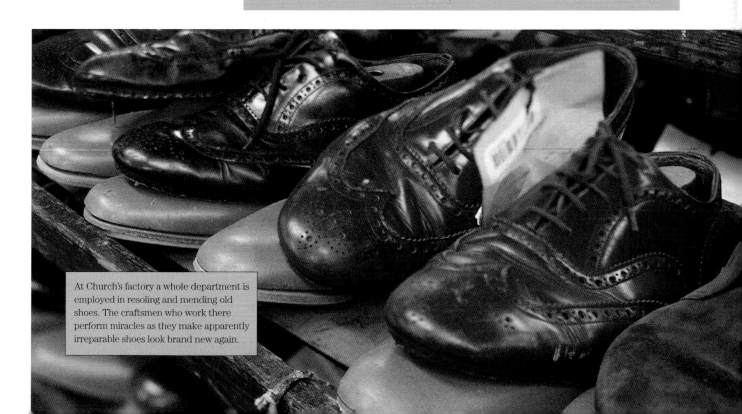

At Church's factory a whole department is employed in resoling and mending old shoes. The craftsmen who work there perform miracles as they make apparently irreparable shoes look brand new again.

Glossary

A

Adjustable Waistband
A pants waistband with an adjustable device inside it that can be used to vary the waist measurement. Pants with an adjustable waistband do not need to be worn with a belt. Adjustable waistbands are usually found on pants that are held up by suspenders.

B

Balmoral
In America the Balmoral, sometimes shortened to "Bal," is a shoe with closed lacing. The most formal of all Balmoral shoes, the Oxford, is called the "Balmoral Oxford" in the USA.

Bedford Cord
A thick woolen material that makes extremely warm, durable jackets, suits, and pants. It is often used in shooting wear.

Beefroll
An American loafer.

Belt
A strip of material, usually leather, that is fed through loops on the waistband and is used to hold pants in position. It should match the wearer's shoes. Belts replaced suspenders as the favored means of holding up suit pants after the Second World War.

Bemberg Rayon
The manufacturer's name for a silky material made of cotton and used as a lining.

Bengal Stripes
Narrow stripes on a white shirt, usually dark blue, deep red, or dark gray. A classic pattern for business shirts.

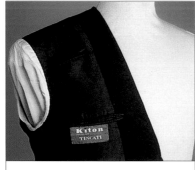

Bemberg Rayon

Bespoke Tailoring
An English term for what is known in American English as "custom-tailoring." One definition is: "a garment cut by an individual, for an individual, by an individual."

Blazer
1. A dark-blue double-breasted jacket with two side vents and gilded brass buttons (the navy-blue blazer).
2. A single-breasted club jacket, usually with sewn pockets and brass buttons. Traditionally, club jackets were striped and came in the colors of a club. Today they are usually single-breasted versions of the navy-blue blazer.

Blucher
An American-English term for a shoe with open lacing. The quarters of a Blucher are stitched onto the vamp. The vamp, the part of the shoe that covers the instep and the toes, is made of the same piece of leather as the tongue.

Boater
A hard straw hat with a flat crown and round brim.

Boat Shoe
A moccasin with leather laces and a non-skid plastic sole. The Sperry Topsider is the original boat shoe.

Bowler Hat
A stiff hat developed in the workshops of the legendary hat makers Lock's, better known in the US as the "derby." It was commissioned by William Coke, and intended as a form of headwear for gamekeepers. It was originally called the "coke hat," and only became known as the bowler when the company Bowler & Son began producing the new hat around 1850. See also Derby.

Braid
A silk stripe along the outer seam of the pants leg. A single braid is worn with a dinner jacket, a double braid with tails.

Breeches
An English term for riding pants.

British Warm
A short, sand-colored, double-breasted woolen coat with leather buttons and epaulettes. Originally a British military coat.

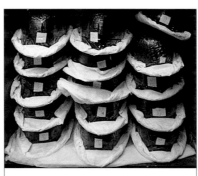

Bowler hats

Budapests
Wingtip shoes. A version of the British brogue developed in Budapest.

Buffalo Horn
A material used for the buttons of suits and sports jackets.

Button-down Shirt
A shirt with collar tips buttoned to the breast. The original version is the button-down shirt with a soft-roll collar made by Brooks Brothers of New York.

C

Canvas
Canvas is used in traditional tailoring to give shape to a suit jacket. A custom tailor will sew it in by hand, but in industrial manufacturing it is stuck in with adhesives. Canvas that has been fused in stops the material of a garment falling loosely, reduces the breathability of the suit, and is less durable than hand padded canvas.

Cashmere
Yarn or weave made from the fine hair found under the coarse winter coat of the Cashmere goat.

Casual Suit
A suit that is not worn to work in the city, but for leisure activities and days in the country. Casual suits are usually made of rustic woolen cloths in natural shades, often checked. A casual suit could be described as a sports jacket with matching pants.

Cavalry Twill
A warm, extremely long-lasting woolen material with a characteristic diagonal structure. It is mostly used in the beige and brown pants traditionally worn with sports jackets and blazers.

Chalk Stripe
A classic pattern used in suit-making, with white strips on a gray or blue background. It is often used for double-breasted suits.

Chesterfield
A city coat with a fly front. Traditionally, a Chesterfield is single breasted, comes in a gray herringbone pattern, and has a black velvet collar. The Chesterfield is also available in blue, black, or beige.

Cheviot
A robust, but very coarse, worsted fabric made from the wool of the Cheviot sheep. A typical material for English sporting suits.

Club Tie
Originally a necktie in the colors of an English club that was only available to club members. Today it is used as a general term for the striped necktie.

Coat
The word used in Savile Row for a sports jacket or the jacket of a suit.

Coat-maker
A tailor who specializes in making jackets.

Coke Hat
See bowler hat.

Cordovan
A term for horse leather, a rare and expensive raw material used in shoemaking. Only the leather from the hind parts of the horse can be used. One hide supplies two round pieces of leather, just enough for two or three pairs of shoes. The best Cordovan shoes are considered to be those made by the North American manufacturer Alden.

Cotton
The most important textile commodity. Cotton is even more widely used than natural wool. Underclothes, overshirts, jeans, chinos, and Gabardine raincoats are typical garments made of cotton.

Covert Coat
A single-breasted coat made of covert cloth, a medium twill, and reaching as far as the knee. Its typical features are a fly front and four simple parallel decorative seams above the cuffs and along the bottom hem.

Crombie Coat
A dark-blue single-breasted city coat with an open button facing.

Cuff Links
Two identical objects shaped so that they pass through the button holes of the cuff to fasten it. They are secured in place with a bar, a chain, or an elasticized ribbon.

Cuffs
A relatively recent invention, pants cuffs have only been worn since the first half of the nineteenth century. Originally, pants really were rolled up to prevent the hem getting wet or dirty. Today most pants have cuffs. The pants worn with very formal clothes, such as the morning coat, tuxedo, or tails, are not made with cuffs. In British English cuffs on trousers are called turnups.

Cutaway Collar

Also generally known as the "spread collar." The tips of the collar are "spread" far apart on shirts that have cutaway collars. It is a classic among shirt collars, and is second only to the broad turndown collar.

Cutter

In English custom tailoring the tailor who advises the customer, takes his measurements, drafts the pattern on manila paper, cuts the cloth, and fits the suit.

D

Deerstalker

A shooting cap with ear flaps. It is famous as the hat worn by Sherlock Holmes.

Denim

A blue cotton material used for jeans.

Derby

A term that has never been defined conclusively. It is commonly understood to mean shoes with open lacing, but is also the name of a brogue, or wingtip, shoe. In the US it is also the name for a bowler hat.

Dinner Jacket

An English term for what is known in the USA as a tuxedo, and in Germany as a *Smoking*. In German-speaking countries *Dinnerjacket* is used to refer to a white or ivory dinner jacket only.

Donegal Tweed

A coarsely flecked Irish tweed.

Double-breasted Jacket

A jacket with two rows of buttons, usually three pairs. The two upper buttons are purely decorative. A double-breasted jacket should always be fastened up when you are standing. Otherwise, the jacket opens out very wide, which does not look flattering

Dress Shirt

A shirt to be worn with a tuxedo or tails. For a tuxedo it can have either a wing collar or a turndown collar. For tails it has to be a wing collar.

Dress Waistcoat

A white backless vest made of piqué and worn with tails.

Dry Cleaning

A cleaning technique using chemicals that dissolve fats and stains. Traditionalists reject it outright because it destroys the natural moisture of the material. They prefer brushing, airing, and steam ironing. If clothes are to be dry cleaned, only the best specialists available should do the work.

Duffel Coat

A short, single-breasted hooded coat with horn toggles.

Dusty Madder

A traditional technique for dying silk. It is also used to describe necktie patterns with a dusty, powdery look that softens what are, in fact, glowing colors. Dusty Madder and Heavy Dusty Madder neckties usually have Paisley or foulard patterns. The most important manufacturers of Dusty Madder and Heavy Dusty Madder are David Evans, a company based in England that supply all the major necktie manufacturers of the world.

E

Elasticized Waistband

The elasticized waistband is typical of pants that are worn with suspenders. When the wearer is standing, the pants are held in place and do not get any tighter where the suspenders are fastened. When he sits down, the pants fit snugly round his stomach. Elasticized waistbands are also found on pants that can be adjusted at the side to suit different waist measurements.

F

Fishtail

The rear part of a pair of pants cut specially for wearing suspenders. The rear is divided and pulled upwards so that the vest does not ride up onto the waistband of the pants when the wearer bends over.

Fitting

In modern custom-made tailoring three fitting sessions are usual and sufficient to make sure the necessary adjustments are made before a garment can be finished. Trying on ready-to-wear garments is not fitting because the clothes are already finished.

Flannel

The word comes from the Welsh *gwalen*, and means an object made of wool. The soft, smooth feel of flannel is created by a special manufacturing process, in which the wool is fulled until it turns felty. A pair of pants made of gray flannel can be worn with a sports jacket, or a shirt and pullover.

Four-in-hand

A simple necktie knot named after an English club that existed in the early nineteenth century.

French Cuff

Known in England as the "double cuff." French cuffs are worn on traditional men's shirts and fastened with cuff links. A French cuff is the perfect way to finish off a sleeve, and looks particularly good worn with a suit or sports jacket.

G

Gabardine

A waterproof, wind-resistant cotton weave with a characteristic diagonal structure. A British patent was taken out in 1879 by Thomas Burberry, who retained the exclusive manufacturing rights for the material until 1917. Gabardine is the material used in the raincoats made by Burberry and other manufacturers.

Galoshes

Rubber overshoes that protect the shoe and foot against wet and cold, and prevent the wearer's feet skidding.

Gingham Check

A fine checked material used in shirts. The word derives from the Malayan word *ging-gang*, which means "striped."

Glencheck

See "Prince of Wales Check."

Guernsey

Island in the English Channel, home of the pullover of the same name that was originally worn there by fishermen. A popular and extremely hard-wearing pullover for leisure activities.

H

Hacking Jacket

A riding jacket. The name derives from the verb "to hack," meaning to ride. Its typical features are its close-cut, high waist, long rear vent, and slanted flapped pockets. The hacking jacket is one of the precursors of the modern sports jacket.

Harris Tweed

One of the most famous varieties of tweed. Only tweed woven on the Outer Hebrides is allowed to bear this much sought-after label. It comes in various vivid colors and is particularly suited to robust sports jackets.

Herringbone

A type of diagonal weave, in which the yarn is woven into a diagonal structure. In order to create the characteristic herringbone effect, the direction of the weaving is changed at set intervals to create a zigzag pattern. Herringbone is used to make light and heavy fabrics. Fine gray herringbone fabrics are made into business suits, while heavy herringbone tweeds are used for sports jackets.

Homburg

A hat with a stiff, curved brim. It was discovered by King Edward VII in the German spa town of Homburg. The Homburg is now the most formal hat after the top hat and comes in black, gray-blue, and dark or light gray.

Horsehair

Canvas with horsehair is used to reinforce and shape a suit, usually at the breast and lapels.

Houndstooth

A casual pattern in two colors for woolen fabrics. A popular choice for sports jackets and coats.

House Check

A checked pattern that is only used by one brand and serves to identify their products. It is often used as a lining material. The most famous house check is the Burberry check.

House Style

Stylistic features that identify very different garments as the work of particular custom tailors. There is, for example, no mistaking the soft, rather shapeless jackets made by the Savile Row tailors Anderson & Sheppard.

J

Jermyn Street

A street near Piccadilly Circus that links Regent Street with St. James's Street, the home of the most famous shirt-makers in the world. "Jermyn Street" sums up the style and origins of the English tradition of shirt-making. Well-known names on Jermyn Street include Turnbull & Asser, Harvie & Hudson, Hilditch & Key, New & Lingwood, T. M. Lewin & Sons, and Thomas Pink.

K

Kipper Necktie

The famous wide necktie of the late 1960s and 1970s, supposedly named after Michael Fish. Kipper is the name of a smoked fish, usually a herring. Fish is claimed to have

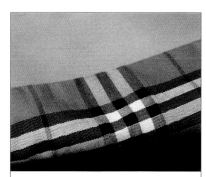

House check

introduced this necktie style into England when he worked at the shirt makers Turnbull & Asser.

L

Last

A simplified model of the human foot made according to average dimensions and used in the manufacture of ready-to-wear shoes. The shoe is built up around the last. The wooden handmade lasts used for custom-made shoes reproduce the unique dimensions of the customer's feet.

Lining

A layer of material usually made of cotton or silk on the inside of a garment. The lining covers the padding of a jacket, prevents sweat staining the outer material, and ensures that the garment glides elegantly over the wearer's other clothes. Most half-lined summer jackets are lined at the shoulders to give as good a fit as possible. Pants are usually lined as far down as the knees. Sometimes the lining even reaches the calves if the pants are made of very coarse woolen material. The lining of a durable custom-made suit can be renewed after several years if it is torn.

Loden

A fulled, napped woolen weave that is relatively waterproof and windproof, and not easily damaged by bushes, branches, and thorns. Loden is a typical material from the Alpine region. The green loden coat is regarded as an international classic – even though it has strong European associations.

M

Macintosh

Also shortened to "mac." A raincoat named after the inventor of India-rubber cloth, Charles Macintosh. In 1822 he invented a special, waterproof material made of two layers of cotton with a layer of rubber in between. Originally "Macintosh" was a brand name, but later it became the generic term for waterproof raincoats.

Made-to-measure

A compromise between ready-to-wear clothing and custom tailoring. This is really a contradiction in terms, since ready-to-wear clothes are made following average dimensions and not "custom-made" for individual requirements. In order to make a garment that looks as though it has been custom made, the customer selects one pattern that fits him particularly well from a number of ready-to-wear designs. The manufacturer then uses this pattern to make a single garment using the customer's measurements for the sleeve, leg, and waist. Many people confuse made-to-measure clothes with the products of real custom tailoring because it is possible to select the material used in both types of product.

Madras Check

A check pattern that originates in India and is used for light cotton fabrics. A popular pattern for casual shirts, sports jackets, and golfing pants.

Master Tailor

Anyone can call himself a master tailor. The term originally meant a tailor who had finished his training. Today it refers to the best, most experienced tailor working for a gentlemen's outfitters, but is often used purely in order to impress customers. The owner or manager of a tailors' firm is known as the "guv'nor," and

addressed by his first name, preceded with "Mister." Someone who asks for Robert Gieve at Gieves & Hawkes will hear the call go out for "Mister Robert."

Merino Wool

The tightly curled hair of the Merino sheep is the finest wool in the world. It is used in many suit fabrics. The main country producing Merino wool is Australia.

Moccasin

Originally the footwear worn by the North American Indians. Today it is the term for a shoe made by pulling

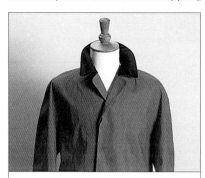

Macintosh

the leather upper onto a last from below. Gucci loafers and boat shoes are types of moccasin.

Mohair

A shiny, extremely crease-resistant fabric made from the wool of the Angora goat. Ideal for tuxedos and summer suits.

Moleskin

Soft, warm cotton cloth in a satin weave, a favorite material for casual pants in England.

Monkstrap

A shoe that is not laced, but fastened with a buckle.

Morning Coat

A coat worn on special occasions. It is also popularly known as the "cutaway coat."

Mufti

A word borrowed from Arabic and the term for the clothes worn by off-duty soldiers, officers in particular. Mufti is often equated with the traditional English style of clothing that is kept alive in Savile Row.

N

Necktie

Alongside the suit, shirt, and shoes, the most important element of the formal outfit. More than any other piece of clothing, a necktie is a sign of respect for western social norms. It has been widely worn in its current form since about 1925.

Norfolk Jacket

A tweed jacket with three or four buttons, a belt or half-belt, pleats for ease of movement, and roomy bellows pockets for bullets and provisions. It is regarded as a precursor of the sports jacket. It was first worn in the nineteenth century on the estates owned by the Duke of Norfolk.

O

Ostrich Leather

The skin of the ostrich. It has a unique texture and is popular for small leather goods, such as wallets and straps for wristwatches. It is also used to make shoes.

Oxford

1. A fabric that makes soft, but hard-wearing, shirts. It is made by weaving together dyed and undyed cotton yarns. Oxford weaves always look rather less refined and formal than batiste or poplin. The material is often used in the Brooks Brothers shirt.
2. The most formal men's shoe, with closed lacing and undecorated toe caps. Black Oxfords are the traditional shoe worn with a pinstripe suit, or a morning coat at state functions, weddings, and funerals. Brown Oxfords are worn with sports suits.

P

Pajamas

A suit of night clothes with a generously cut pair of pants. The word is derived from the Persian expression *pae jamah*, meaning "foot wear" or "trousers." In the colonial era the British imported these comfortable pants from India and the Middle East. They did not seem suitable for wear during the day, but proved ideal for restful nights asleep.

Penny Loafers

In the 1950s students at the Ivy League universities would place a penny under the strap of their loafers to bring themselves good luck. The Bass Weejun is regarded as the original of this style of shoe. It has remained practically unchanged since its introduction onto the market in the 1930s.

Pigskin

A naturally grainy leather made from the skin of wild pigs and used traditionally for making gloves.

Pinstripe

A woolen fabric with thin white stripes on a dark, usually gray or dark-blue, background. The traditional suit worn in the City of London is made of blue pinstripe.

Plus Fours

A particularly voluminous variety of knickerbockers, so called because 4 inches are added to the knee length to create the overhang. (The famous Duke of Windsor claimed to wear "plus twenty-fours.") These pants are still often worn with a casual tweed suit, when shooting, for example, but only in Great Britain.

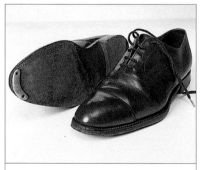

Oxford

Polo Shirt

A short-sleeved sport shirt made of cotton piqué. It was designed by the French tennis player René Lacoste in 1933 for his own use, as he explained: "Pour moi, pour jouer au tennis, comme au golf, j'eus un jour l'idée de créer une chemise." His design was a massive success. By 1930 as many as 300,000 shirts were being made each year. Today the Lacoste shirt is an international leisure classic.

Poplin

A cotton weave made with fine warp yarn and a thicker filling. The filling is responsible for the character of the material. It is often used in shirts.

Prince of Wales Check

Known in German-speaking countries as *Glencheck*. A colored overcheck, usually of blue or red stripes, on a background of Glen Urquhart plaid. Patterns of this type were designed for rich English landlords who settled in Scotland and had no clan tartan of their own. Their employees wore these fantasy tartans, which were called "district checks." The Glen Urquhart plaid belonged to the estates of the Countess of Seafield. This robust patterned material is ideal for school, work, and travel. In England it is used for casual suits.

Pump

Flat men's shoe, often with a black bow. Traditionally, they are worn with tails, and sometimes with a tuxedo.

R

Raglan Sleeve

On a coat with Raglan sleeves the sleeve and the shoulder are made from one piece of cloth. The Raglan sleeve was named after Lord Raglan, a commander during the Crimean War (1853–1856), and is typical of raincoats. There are one-piece and two-piece Raglan sleeves. The one-piece Raglan sleeve lies flatter on the shoulder, and is used, for example, in the Moorland jacket by Barbour.

Ready-to-wear

Clothes that are not cut following individual measurements, but for a notional average figure. The advantage of ready-to-wear clothing is that it can be used straightway. Its disadvantages are the limited choice of cuts and materials available in any one season, the fact that it is pure chance whether the garment fits, and, most of all, the poor standards of tailoring.

Regimental Tie

A necktie in the colors of an English regiment that is worn with civilian clothes. Today it is a general term for the striped necktie.

S

Saddle Shoe

A traditional American shoe with closed lacing. The quarters are made of a single piece of leather laid over the instep like a saddle. The saddle is usually different in color from the rest of the upper leather. The saddle shoe has not so far become popular outside North America.

Savile Row

A street in London's Mayfair, the home of the most famous men's tailors in the world, and a synonym for the English suit. The most respected addresses are Henry Poole at No. 15; H. Huntsman at No. 11; Anderson & Sheppard at No. 30; Kilgour, French & Stanbury at No. 8; and Gieves & Hawkes at No. 1. There is a multitude of other excellent companies in Savile Row and the surrounding streets.

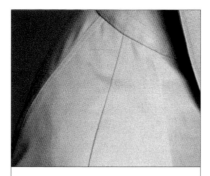

Raglan sleeve

School Tie

A necktie in the colors of a school or an institution of higher education. In English-speaking countries it is worn by pupils and old boys as a sign of loyalty to their place of education. A famous example is the Old Etonian necktie.

Sea Island Cotton

The most expensive of the cotton materials used in shirt-making. This material has a particularly silky feel because it is woven from a higher number of yarns than poplin. While poplin has about 100 yarns per inch (40 per cm), Sea Island cotton has 140 (56).

Silk

A fine material traditionally made into neckties, shirts, suits, and pajamas. It is also used as a lining material or yarn in men's tailoring. It is obtained from the cocoons of various types of silkworm, such as *Bombyx mori*, which feeds off mulberry leaves.

Shetland Wool

Wool from the Shetland Islands off Scotland. A popular material for rustic pullovers, often in a cable knit. Also a flecked carded fabric used in casual suits, sports jackets, and coats.

Shoe Tree

A piece of wood shaped like a foot that is inserted into the shoe to fill it out when it is not being worn. It serves to keep the leather in shape and absorb moisture.

Single-breasted Jacket

A jacket with a single button facing and two or three buttons. If the jacket has two buttons, only the upper button is fastened. If the jacket has three buttons, the middle button, the upper pair, or all three can be fastened.

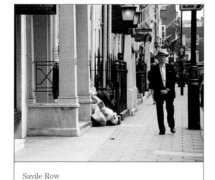

Savile Row

Slip-on

A raincoat with Raglan sleeves, a fly front, and small lapels, usually made of gabardine.

Sports Jacket

A single-breasted jacket, usually checked, that is not part of a suit. It is a descendant of the English hacking jacket and the Norfolk jacket, and is often made of tweed, though versions for town wear may be of cashmere or other woolen materials. It is not to be confused with the blazer (see above).

Suit

A suit consists of a jacket, a pair of trousers, and a vest of the same material. Its precursor was a combination of a frock coat or morning coat, vest, and trousers all made of different-colored materials. After the First World War the suit became accepted as the normal clothing for a man at the office and on important occasions.

Super 100

Light, crease-resistant natural wool that keeps its shape and is used to make summer clothes.

Suspenders

Known as "braces" in England. Shoulder straps that are used to hold up pants. They make the figure look taller and keep the pants in the right position.

T

Tailcoat

A black tailcoat worn with a white bow tie is the classic evening wear for celebrations and special occasions. It is worn if the invitation specifies "white tie," "cravate blanche," or "großer Gesellschaftsanzug."

Tartan

A massive variety of check patterns that were used by the Scottish clans for identification purposes. Today a general term for all kinds of checked patterns in traditional Scottish colors.

Tassel Loafer

A loafer on which the shoe laces are fed once round the shoe through a series of eyes or a "tunnel," and then tied in a bow on the instep. The ends of the laces are decorated with leather tassels. The original tassel loafer is the one made by Alden.

Tattersall Check Shirt

A casual shirt with mesh check of dark brown, green, burgundy, blue, or black stripes on a cream or light beige background. This pattern is named after the horse market run by a man called Richard Tattersall, where the horse blankets were decorated with this very check. The Tattersall check shirt is often worn with a sports jacket.

Ticket Pocket

A small extra pocket over the right pocket of a jacket. Most often found on sports jackets.

Top Hat

The most formal of all the hats. It is now only worn with a morning coat at functions during the day, or with a tailcoat in the evening, but is no longer obligatory. One variation is the collapsible top hat, the *chapeau claque*, as it is known, which can be folded flat for transport and storage.

Trench Coat

A belted, double-breasted gabardine coat first worn by British troops during the Boer War (1895–1902). Pieces of equipment were attached to the epaulettes and the D-shape metal ring on the belt, which still serve as reminders of the garment's military past.

Trilby

A narrow-brimmed felt hat with a hat band. The brown trilby is the typical hat worn by English people (and anglophiles) interested in horses.

Trimmer

In English custom tailoring the trimmer selects all the additional features of a suit, such as the buttons, padding, thread, and lining materials. If a customer expresses no particular wishes, the trimmer decides on these important details. Young tailors train their feel for style by working as trimmers.

Trouser-maker

A tailor who specializes in sewing trousers.

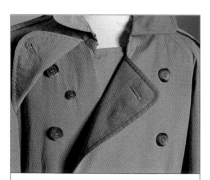

Tassel loafer

Turnups

See Cuffs.

Tuxedo

Often shortened to "Tux." This is the American term for the dinner jacket. It supposedly commemorates a historical event that took place on 10 October 1886, when Griswold "Grizzy" Lorillard, an American tobacco heir, appeared at the Tuxedo Club in Tuxedo Park, New York, wearing a tailcoat without tails.

Tweed

A woolen fabric from the British Isles, generally from Scotland. It is woven from woolen yarns of several different colors. The name is probably a corruption of the Scots word *tweel*, which means "twill."

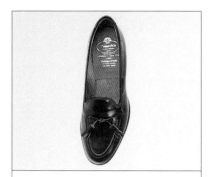

Trench coat

V

Vest

A common men's garment since the seventeenth century, the vest was originally a component of the suit as it developed at the end of the nineteenth century. Since the Second World War it has not been a compulsory part of the suit.

Vest-maker

A tailor who specializes in making vests.

Vicuña

The very expensive inner hair of a humpless South American camel related to the llama. Hairs that have been left hanging in bushes are gathered by hand. This is exceedingly expensive and yields are very low. Many people see a suit or coat made of vicuña as the epitome of luxury.

Viyella

A warm shirt material invented in 1890 by Henry Ernest Hollins. It consists of 55 percent Merino wool and 45 percent long-staple cotton. Viyella is used above all for making Tattersall check shirts.

W

Waist Pleats

Pleats inserted under the waistband make pants look fuller at the front and hide the bulges caused by the contents of the pockets. One classic pants style has two waist pleats on each side of the pants, one that merges into the leg crease, another between this and the side pocket.

Waxed Jacket

A cotton jacket impregnated with wax for protection against the rain. The most famous waxed jacket is the one made by Barbour.

Whipcord

A flecked woolen fabric that makes hard-wearing casual suits and pants to go with sports jackets.

Windsor Knot

The necktie knot supposedly worn by the Duke of Windsor, though experts keep trying to prove that the abdicated king wore a four-in-hand knot that only had so much volume because his neckties were thickly padded. The Windsor knot is still the best knot to use if you are wearing a shirt with a cutaway collar. However, the slimmer, slightly asymmetrical four-in-hand usually looks better.

Wingtip

The curved toe cap of a man's shoe. A shoe with a wingtip is called a brogue.

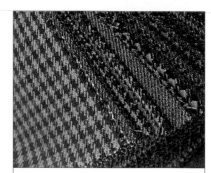

Tweed

Bibliography – a Selection

Alison Adburgham: *Shopping in Style: London from the Restoration to Edwardian Elegance*; London, 1979.

Hardie Amies: *The Englishman's Suit*; London, 1994.

Ann Barr, Peter York: *The Official Sloane Ranger Directory*; London, 1984.

Ann Barr, Peter York: *The Official Sloane Ranger Diary*; London, 1983.

Ann Barr, Peter York: *The Official Sloane Ranger Handbook*; London, 1982.

François Chaille: *Tradition und Trend. Krawatten*; Paris, Niedernhausen, 1997.

Nicholas Courtney: *The Very Best of British*; London, 1985.

John Crawshaw: *Made to Last: The History of Church's Shoes*; Eastbourne, East Sussex, 1998.

Brian Dobbs: *The Last Shall Be First: The Colourful Story of John Lobb, the St. James's Bootmakers*; London, 1972.

Fachzeitschrift Der Schneidermeister (specialist journal), *Die Zuschneidekunst "Herrenkleidung"* ; Hanover, 1934.

Alan Flusser: *Style and the Man* ; New York, 1996.

Sarah Gibbings: *The Tie: Trends and Traditions*; London, 1990.

Sarah Giles: *Fred Astaire: His Friends Talk*; New York, 1988.

Christina Giorgetti et al.: *Brioni: Fifty Years of Style*; Florence, 1995.

Wolfgang Glöss (ed.): *The H & R Book of Perfume*; Hamburg, 1992.

Wolfgang Glöss (ed.): *Fragrance Guide: Feminine Notes, Masculine Notes*; Hamburg, 1991.

Hugo Janistyn: *Taschenbuch der modernen Parfümerie und Kosmetik*; Stuttgart, 1966.

Charles Jennings: *People Like Us: A Season Among the Upper Classes*; London, 1997.

Paul Keers: *A Gentleman's Wardrobe*; London, 1987.

Jay McInerney et al.: *Dressed to Kill: James Bond, The Suited Hero*; Paris, New York, 1996.

Suzy Menkes: *The Windsor Style*; London, Glasgow, 1987.

George Michael, Rae Lindsay: *George Michael's Complete Hair Care for Men*; New York, 1983.

Caroline Rennolds Millbank: *Couture: Glanz und Geschichte der großen Modeschöpfer und ihrer Creationen*;

Property from the Collection of the Duke and the Duchess of Windsor (Sotheby's Catalogue); New York, 1997.

Sybil Gräfin Schönfeldt: *1x1 des guten Tons. Das neue Benimmbuch*; Hamburg, 1991.

Geraldine Trembath: *The Connaisseur's Guide to English Style*; Honiton, Devon, 1996.

Hugo Vickers: *The Private World of the Duke and Duchess of Windsor*; London, 1995.

Richard Walker: *The Savile Row Story: An Illustrated History*; London, 1988.

A. A. Whife: *The Modern Tailor, Outfitter, and Clothier*; London, 1928.

Frank Whitbourn: *Mr. Lock of St. James's Street*; London, 1971.

Acknowledgments

We would like to thank the following for patient explanations, expert advice, illuminating conversations, and warm hospitality:

John Balcombe, Peter J. M. Beerens, Jeremy Carrington Hull, John Coggin, Joanna Comfort, Angus Cundey, John Davis, Michael J. Drake, Richard C. Elliott, John R. Farrant, Robert Gieve, Jeremy Gledhill, Robert Godley, Geoffrey P. H. Grainger, Heinz Hagen, Neil B. Harrison, Patrick Jenkinson, Adam Keith, Peter-W. Klein, John Hunter Lobb, Jonathan Lobb, Maurizio Marinella, Paul Maskell, Peter O'Neil, Alan Pope, Christopher R. Pringle, Peter Pütz, Heinz-Josef Radermacher, Hellmut Rondholz, Richard Shaw, Ernst Sobotta, Janet Taylor, Ruth Warborn, Kenneth Williams.

We would also like to thank the following companies and institutions for their kind support:

Alden Shoe Company, Middleborough, Massachusetts; Apollo-Optik GmbH, Cologne; J. Barbour & Sons Ltd., Simonside; Bertram & Frank, Cologne; Boutique de la Peluco, Barcelona; Braun AG, Kronberg im Taunus; Brioni, Rome; British Menswear Guild, London; Brooks Brothers Clothiers, Madison Avenue, New York; Burberrys (Deutschland) GmbH, Düsseldorf; Cartier, Paris; Cheaney & Sons Ltd., Desborough, Kettering; Chester Barrie, Savile Row, London; Christy & Co. Ltd., Stockport, Cheshire; Church & Co. (Footwear) Ltd., Northampton; John Comfort Ltd., London; J. C. Cordings & Co. Ltd., London; D'Avenza Fashion spa, Avenza; Deutsches Textilmuseum, Krefeld; Deutsches Wollforschungsinstitut der RWTH, Aachen; Douglas Parfümerien, Hagen, Düsseldorf; Drake's Fine English Silks, Carrington Hull Associates Limited, London; Alfred Dunhill, Hamburg; Filofax, London; Filofax Deutschland GmbH, Schwalbach/Taunus; Kay Geffers Textilagentur, Linau; Gieves & Hawkes, 1 Savile Row, London; Gimeno, Barcelona; H. Greve, Schoenfabriek, Waalwijk; Hermès, Paris; Holland & Sherry, Savile Row, London; Hotel Havana, Barcelona; Internationales Wollsekretariat, Düsseldorf; Jockey/VOLMA Wirkwaren GmbH, Hechingen; John Crocket, Cologne; Kassuba Vertriebsgesellschaft mbH, Leinfelden-Echterdingen; G. B. Kent & Sons PLC., Hertfordshire; Eduard Kettner, Cologne; Nessrin Königsegg, Marketing, Contact, Public Relations, Hamburg; T. M. Lewin & Sons Ltd., London; Henri Lloyd, Manchester; John Lobb, London; James Lock & Co. Ltd., London; Maison de Chapeau, Cologne; Eugenio Marinella S.N.C., Shirtmaker and Outfitter, Naples; Marks & Spencer, Cologne; Mil, Sombreria, Barcelona; Missoni S.P.A., Sumirago (Varese); Moos + Co, Küsnacht; Ciro Paone S.p.A., Arzano (Naples); Philips GmbH, Hamburg; Henry Poole & Co., London; Peter Pütz Jewelier, Cologne; Heinz-Josef Radermacher, Maßschneider und Hemdenmacher, Düsseldorf; Regent GmbH, Weißenburg; Rimowa Kofferfabrik, Cologne; J. u. H. Rondholz, Cologne; Derek Rose Pyjamas Ltd., Savile Row, London; Samsonite GmbH, Cologne; Franz Sauer, Cologne; Schiesser AG, Radolfzell; Schuhhaus Herkenrath, Cologne; Swaine Adeney Brigg, London; Levi Strauss Germany GmbH, Heusenstamm; The London Badge & Button Company, London; Tibbett PLC, Wellingborough; Tobias Tailors of Savile Row, London; R. E. Tricker Limited, Northampton; Geo. F. Trumper, London; Turnbull & Asser Ltd., London; Variations, Hair & Beauty Salon at Fortnum & Mason, London; Verband der Zigarettenindustrie, Bonn; Louis Vuitton, Paris; Wilkinson Sword GmbH, Solingen.

The publishers would also like to thank Dr. Claudia Piras and Bernhard Roetzel for their energy and commitment looking at this English edition.

Index

Pages with detailed entries on subject are in bold.

A

Aaltsz, Tony 19
accessories **220-279**
Ackermann, Myron 102, 109
Acqua di Parma 22
'action-man' sweater 295
Adenauer, Konrad 138, 223
adjustable waistband 140, 143, 352
aftershave 15
Agnelli, Gianni 35, 65, 227
Alden (firm) 65, 116, 153, 154, 155, 158, 163, 178, 179, 181
Allen, Woody 127, 214, 267
Allen-Edmonds (firm) 153, 154, 158
Altman & Co., B. (firm) 111
Anderson & Sheppard (firm) 94, 101, 104
Angelo (firm) 109
  angling, see fishing
Anne, Princess 201
aran sweater 291, 295
Armani 113
Armstrong, Neil 228
Asprey (firm) 256
Astaire, Fred 37, 133, 214, 327
Audemars Piguet (firm) 228, 229

B

Babers (firm) 171, 177
Badge & Button Company (firm) 149
Balmoral Oxfords 158, 348
bandanna 72
Barbera (firm) 128, 297
Barbour (firm) 201
Barbour jacket **200-203**, 305
Barbour, John 201
baseball cap 213
Bass (firm) 65, 154, 162
Bass Weejuns 162, 317
bathrobe
  see also dressing gown 337
Battistoni (firm) 109
Baume & Mercier (firm) 228, 229
Baume, William 228
Bausch & Lomb (firm) 268, 269
beard care 21
beard styles 20
Bedford cord 125, 305, 348

beefroll loafer 162, 348
Belcher, James 72
belt 96, **144-145**, 349
Belvest (firm) 109
Bemberg rayon/silk 129, 348
Benetton, Luciano 267
Bengal stripes 348
Bennett, Tony 37, 113
beret 213
Berluti (firm) 157
Bernhard, Prince of the Netherlands 18
bill clip 225
bill pocket 225
Billings & Edmonds (firm) 104
blazer **146-149**, 318, 348
Blucher 160, 161, 179, 348
Blücher, Gebhard Leberecht 160
boat shoes 163, 186, 319, 348
boater 212, 348
Bogart, Humphrey 37
Boothby, Sir Brooke 277
boots 305, 308, 312, 313
Borotra, Jean 316
Borsalino 213
bow tie **85, 86**, 325, 327
Bowler & Son (firm) 211, 348
bowler hat **210-211**, 213, 348
Box, Joseph 169
boxcloth 142, 143
boxer shorts 42, 44
Braun (firm) 19
breeches 348
Breguet (firm) 228, 229
Breguet, Abraham-Louis 228
Breitling (firm) 228, 229
briefcase **250-251**
Brigg & Sons 264
Brigg, see Swaine, Adeney, Brigg
Brioni (firm), 109, **110-113**, 128
British warm 195, 348
brogue **158**, 159, 160, 161, 165, 181
Brooks Brothers (firm) 65, 116, 127, 142, 143, 179, 182, 214, 297
Brooks Brothers shirt 65
Brooks, John 65
Brown, Davies & Co. (firm) 50
Brugnon, Jacques 316
Brummell, George Bryan 72
Brun, Henrik 45
brushes,
  see hairbrushes; clothes brushes
Budapests 159, 165, 348
buffalo horn 348
Burberry, Thomas 198
Burberrys (firm) 198
Burlington (firm) 187

Burton, Richard 113
Bush, George 80
button-down shirt 64, 65, 249, 297
buttonhole 96
buttons 51, 96, 123, 129, 149

C

Cagney, James 213
Calcani, Armando 110
camelhair cloth 189
canvas 101, 129, 348
Caraceni (firm) 109
Caraceni, Domenico 109
Cardoso, Lopez 18
care of clothes **57, 68-69, 344-347**
Carré, John le 130
Carreras, José Joaquin 236
Cartier (firm) 228, 229, 233, 237
cashmere 348
  jacket 128, 314
  necktie 75, 76
  production 284
  scarf 278, 279
  suit 114, 115
cavalry twill 130, 131, 148, 195, 348
chalkstripes 97, 189, 348
chambray 64, 65
Chameau, Le (firm) 305
Charles II, King of Great Britain 72
Charles, Prince of Wales 35, 53, 94, 104, 143, 201, 209
Charvet (firm) 74, 339
Cheaney & Sons, Joseph (firm) 153, 154, 167, 170
checks 189, 314, 348, 350
see also gingham; house check; Prince of Wales check; shepherd's check
chest hair 37
Chester Barrie (firm) 102–103, 141
Chesterfield (coat) 194, 348
Cheviot 125, 189, 348
chinos 65, 134, 149
Church, Thomas 171
Church's (firm) 153, 154, 155, 159, 162, 166, 170-171, 175
Churchill, Randolph 237
Churchill, Winston 84, 183, 215, 228, 237
Cifonelli (firm) 109
cigar 242-245
cigarette 236-237
cigarette case 222, 237
cigarette lighter 222, 237
Clapton, Eric 104

Cleverly, George (firm) 165
clothes brush 344, 345
clothes hanger 344, 345
club jacket 146
club necktie 72, 73, 348
coat **192-199**, 304
coat maker 92, 100, 348
Cochet, Henri 316
Coggin, John 95
Coke, William 211
Colacello, Bob 137
collar, see shirt collar
college scarf 279
Collischon, David 252
Collischon, Lesley 252
Comfort, John (firm) 79
Connery, Sean 36, 75, 104
Cooper (firm) 46
Cooper, Gary 113, 139
Cordings of Piccadilly (firm) 107, 148, 205, 247, 304, **306-307**
cordovan **178-179**, 348
corduroy 125, 130, 131, 148, 189
cotton 348
  manufacture **54-55**
  piqué shirt 317
  pajamas 339
  shirts 56
  suits 114-115
  sweaters 291
  wadding 101
court shoes 349
covert cloth 125, 189
covert coat 195, 307, 348
cravat **87**
Craven, Earl of 236
credit card holder 225
cricket sweater 294
Crockett & Jones (firm) 153, 154, 170, 171
Crockett, John (firm) 305
Crombie coat 194, 348
cuff links **248-249**, 325, 350
cummerbund 325
Cundey, Angus 95, 325
custom-made
  hats 213
  shirts **62-63**
  shoes **156-157**
  sports jackets 128-129
  suits 80, **92-93, 99-103**, 111
  tailoring 102, 348
cutaway collar 52, 53, 67, 83, 348
Cutler & Gross (firm) 269
Cutler, Graham 269
cutter 92, 99–101, 348

D

D'Avenza (firm) 109
Dalí, Salvador 20

Davis, John 95
deerstalker 349
Dege & Sons, J. (firm) 94
Della Valle, Diego 22, **184**, 185
Delon, Alain 214
denim 349
Derbys 160, 161, 165, 349
detachable collar 52, 53
Dietrich, Marlene 23, 104
Dior, Christian 22
Disney, Colonel 252
diver's watch 231
dog tooth 125, 349
Donegal tweed 124, 349
double cuffs 249, 350
double-breasted coat 96, 352
Douglas, Michael 143, 185
Drake, Michael J. 75, 278
Drake's (firm) 74, 80
dress handkerchief **270-275**, 325
dressing gown 334, 336, **337**, **341**
dry cleaning 344, 347, 351
duffel coat **199**, 349
Dunhill (firm) 237, 238
Dupont (firm) 237
Dusty Madder 349

E
Eau de Hermès 22
eau de toilette 15, **22-23**
Eau Sauvage 22
Edinburgh, Duke of, see Philip, Prince
Edmonds, Colin 104
Edward VII, King of Great Britain and Ireland 105, 139, 212
Edward VIII, King of Great Britain and Northern Ireland, see Windsor, Duke of
Einstein, Albert 35
electric shaver 14, **18-19**
Elizabeth I, Queen of England 238, 288
Emanuele Filiberto, Prince of Savoy 20
equestrianism 302-303, **308-311**
espadrilles 183, 319
Evans, David (firm) 349
evening dress 323
Extract of Limes (eau de toilette) 22

F
fabrics
see also individual fabrics **56**, **58**, 97, 114, 117, **124-125**
Fair Isle pullover 105
Fay (firm) 183

fedora 212
felt 101, 123
Filofax **252-253**
finger nails, care of 39
fish tail 349
fishing 302-33, **312-313**
fitting 348
see also custom-made
flannel 117, 120, 130, 131, 133, 146, 148, 189, 349
flask **246-247**
fleur de lys sweater 295
Florsheim (firm) 154
Fonda, Henry 113
Fonticoli, Nazareno 110, 111
Foster & Son (firm) 157
fountain pen 222
four in hand knot 82, 83, 349
Fox, Samuel 263, 265
fragrance notes 24
fragrances 22-25
Fremont, Vincent 137
french cuffs 249, 350
Friday shirt 65
Frisch, Max 192
frock coat 331

G
gabardine 197, 198, 349
Gable, Clark 113
Galliano, John 214
galloon 326, 349
galoshes 185, 349
gentlemen's outfitters, see individual firms; Jermyn Street; Savile Row
George VI, King of Great Britain and Northern Ireland 224
Gidden, W. & H. (firm) 308
Gieve, Robert 96, 350
Gieves & Hawkes (firm) 74, **98-101**, 147, 195, 290, 351
gingham 349
Giorgio of Beverly Hills (eau de toilette) 23
glasses **266-269**
glen check 97, 105
gloves 276-277, 327, 331
Godley, Robert 75
golf **314-315**
Goodyear, Charles 171
Gorbachev, Mikhail 80
Gravati (firm) 154
Green, Edward (firm) 153, 154, 171
Grey Flannel (eau de toilette) 23
Gross, Tony 269
Gucci (firm) 154, 164, 165, 329
Guerlain (firm) 23
Guernsey pullover **288-289**,

319, 349
Guylas, Stephen 205

H
Hackett (firm) 140, 171
hacking jacket 309, 349
hair brush **38**
hair-care products **30-31**
hairstyles **34-35**, 208-209
hairwashing **32-33**
Halston (designer) 14, 22
Hamilton (firm) 228, 229
handkerchief, see dress handkerchief
Hanway, Jonas 263
Harai (firm) 154, 157
Hardy, Oliver 211
Harris, D. R. (firm) 30
Harris tweed 124, 349
Harrods 338
Harvie & Hudson (firm) 61
hats **208-217**, **310-311**, 312, 314
see also individual styles
Hawes & Curtis (firm) 82, 96, 104, 327
Hayward, Douglas 104
Hefner, Hugh 337
Hemingway, Ernest 20
Hepburn, Audrey 133
Hermès (firm) 76, **77**, 83, 273, 308
Hermès, Emile-Charles 77
Hermès, Thierry 77
herringbone 117, 124, 125, 194, 349
herringbone twill 56
Herriot, James 64, 329
Hetherington, John 212
Heuer, Edouard 228
Hilditch & Key (firm) 61, 74
Hill, Charles (firm) 74
Hockney, David 35
Holliday & Brown (firm) 74
homburg hat 212, 349
hopsack 146
horsehair 101, 123, 129, 351
Horween (firm) 169, 178, 179
Horwitz, Alexandre 18
houndstooth 125, 349
house check 349
house style 349
Hughes, Fred 137
Hunter wellies 305
hunting 201, **302-303**, **304-305**
Huntsman & Sons (firm) 93, **94**, 103, 308
Hurd, Douglas 267
husky jacket 205, 305, 308

I
International Watch Co 228, 229
ironing **68-69**, 344

J
jacket, see blazer; club jacket; evening dress; fishing; golf; husky jacket; knitted garments; morning coat; packing a suitcase; quilted jacket; riding; sailing; sheepskin jacket; smoking jacket; sports jacket; suit; tails; waxed jacket
Jaeger-Le-Coultre (firm) 229
Jagger, Bianca 104
Jagger, Mick 104
Jaime, Don 20
jeans 134, **136-137**, 149, 189
Jermyn Street **59-61**, 350
jewelry **232-233**
Jockey (briefs) 42, 44, **46-47**
John, Elton 37, 104
Johns & Pegg (firm) 104
Johnson, Herbert (firm) 213
Johnson, Philip 267

K
Kent & Sons, G.B. (firm) 38
Kent, John 96
key holder 222
Kilgour, French & Stanbury (firm) 95, 327
King, Larry 142
kipper necktie 82, 350
Kiton (firm) 104, **109**, 128, 141, 297
Klemann, Benjamin 157
knitwear **282-297**
Knize (firm) 23
Knize Ten (eau de toilette) 23
Kohl, Helmut 80

L
Lacoste (firm) **316-317**
Lacoste, René 316
Lagerfeld, Karl 35
Lange & Söhne, A. (firm) 228, 229
Lange, Ferdinand Adolph 228
Langsdorf, Jesse 72
lap robe **261**, 351
last 175, 350
Lauren, Ralph 22, 64, 116, 141, 171, 182, 297, 317
lavender 25
leather 144, 168-169, 178-179, 277
Levi's 65, **136**, 149, 297, 317
Lewin, T. M. (firm) 60
Lewin, Thomas Mayes 60

Liebeneiner, Wolfgang 182
Lincoln, Abraham 116
Lindbergh, Charles 228
linen 114, 115, 271
lining 79, 123, 129, 141, 349
Lloyd, Henri (firm) 205, 318
loafer **162-164**, 165, 179, 181, 184-185, 186, 189, 329, 331
Lobb, John (firm) 153, 155, **156-157**, 165, 171, 173
Lock & Co. (firm) 211, 310
loden 196, 303, 304, 350
Loewy, Raymond 19
Longines (firm) 228, 229
Lorillard, Griswold 325
Lotusse (firm) 153, 155
Lumsden, Sir Harry 134

M

Macclesfield tie 72
macintosh 197, 350
Macintosh, Charles 197
MacNee, Patrick 210
Madras check 314, 350
Major, Dimi 104
manicure **39**
Mann, Thomas 208, 234, 261
Marie-Antoinette, Queen of France 228
Marinella (firm) **80–81**
Marinella, Eugenio 80
Marinella, Maurizio 80
Marlboro 236-237
Mary I, Queen of England 288
Mary, Queen of Scots 288
master tailor 350
Mastroianni, Marcello 278
Materna, Georg (firm) 157
McCartney, Paul 104
Menkes, Suzy 82
Mercier, Paul 228
merino wool 133, 284, 350
Michael, Dr. George 38
Michael, Prince, of Kent 82
Missoni (firm) **296-297**
Missoni, Angela 297
Missoni, Octavio 296, 297
Missoni, Rosita 296, 297
Mitterand, François 80
mixture of patterns 274-275
mobile phone 222
moccasins 154, 162, 163, **165**, 350
mohair 114, 115, 284, 350
moleskin 130, 131, 350
money 224-225
monkstrap shoes **166**, 331, 350
Montezemolo, Luca di 22
Montgomery, Bernard Law 199
Moore, Roger 104

Moreschi (firm) 154
morning coat 209, 331, 348
morning dress **330-331**
Morris, Philip 236, 237
mufti 350

N

nailhead 97, 189
Napoleon Bonaparte 228
neckcloth 72, 85, 331
necktie 66, **72–87**, 148, 274–275, 313, 331, 350
    black 323, **324-325**
    business 81
    buying 74
    care of 347
    Hermès 77, 148
    history of 72, 85
    knitted 75
    making 79, 81
    Marinella 80
    striped 73
    tying 82–83
    see also bow tie; cravat; individual firms; neckcloth
necktie knots **82–83**
Nelson, Albert 101
Nelson, Horatio 288
New & Lingwood (firm) 60
Nicky (firm) 75
Nicoletto, Aldo 109
nightshirt 338
Niven, David 20
Norfolk jacket 120, 350
Norman & Hill (firm) 252
Nutter, Tommy 104

O

Ogilvy, David 239
Omega (firm) 228, 229
O'Neil, Peter 99
open (cutthroat) razor 14, 17
ostrich leather 351
overshirt **50-69**
Oxford cloth 56, 65, 350
Oxford shoes 158, 159, 163, 165, 331, 350

P

packing a suitcase 258-259
Paco Rabanne pour Homme 23
pajamas 334, **338-339**, 351
Panama hat **216-217**, 314
pants 120, **130–141**, 148-149
    see also evening dress; golf; jeans; riding; sailing; shorts; suit; tails; trouser makers etc
Paone, Ciro 109
Partridge, John (firm) 205
Patek Philippe (firm) 228, 229

patent shoes 329
penny loafers 162, 179, 351
Pepita 124
perfumer **24**
perfumes **22-25**
Philip, Prince 96, 104, 201
Philips (firm) 18-19
Philishave 18
Piaget (firm) 228
Picasso, Pablo 215, 237
pigskin 351
Pink, Thomas (firm) 61
pinpoint 56
pinstripes 97, 189, 350
pipes **238-241**
pleated-front trousers 46, 138–139, 140, 141, 348
plus fours 351
pocket flask **246-247**
pocketknife 222, **307**
Poco briefs 44
Poitier, Sidney 113
Polo (eau de toilette) 22
polo coat 196
polo shirt 314, **316-317**, 351
Poole & Co., Henry (firm) 95
poplin 56, 351
pork-pie hat 214
portfolio 251
Prince of Wales check 97, 105, 117, 189, 351
profiled soles 184
pure wool
    blazer 146
    necktie 75
    suit 114, 115
    trousers 131
    see also knitted garments
purse 225

R

Rabanne, Paco 23
Radermacher, Heinz-Josef 62
Raft, George 213
Raglan sleeve 197, 351
Raleigh, Sir Walter 235, 238
Ray Ban 268, 269
ready-to-wear garments 93, 111, 350
Reagan, Ronald 53
Regent (firm) 102
regimental necktie 73, 351
Reiter, Ludwig (firm) 153, 155
ribbed twill 56
riding mac 197, 309
riding, see equestrianism
Rockwell, Norman Perceval 334
Roden, Geroge 95
Rogers & Co. (firm) 94
Rolex (firm) 228, 229

Rose, Derek (firm) 337, 338
Rosetti, Fratelli (firm) 154
Rothmans, Louis 236
Roudnitska, Edmond 23
Rubinstein, Arthur 228

S

saddle shoes **182**, 351
sailing **318-319**
Saint Laurent, Yves 237
Samsonite (firm) 256
Santos 110
Savile Row **92-95**, 96, 99, 102-103, 104, 128, 351
Savini, Gaetano 110, 111
Scalfaro, Oscar Luigi 80
scarf **278-279**, 326
school neckties 73, 351
Schweitzer, Albert 20
Scurr, Grace 252
Sea Island cotton 56, 351
Seafield, Countess of 97
Sebago (firm) 154, 162
seersucker 117
Segal, Fred 136
Sellers, Peter 113, 316
serge 146
seven-fold tie 76
shaving **14-21**
shaving brush 14, 17
shaving cream 14
shepherd's check 124
Shetland wool 291, 351
shirt collar 50, 51, **52-53**, 66-67
shirts, care of 57, **68-69**
shirts, see nightshirt; overshirt; poloshirt, smoking jacket; tailcoat; underwear
shoe trees 347, 351
shoes: **152-203**, 305, 308, 315, 319, 329, 331, 334
    buckled 166
    buying 152-155
    care 346-347
    lace-up **158-161**, 181, 182, 189
    manufacture 165, 172-177
    repair 346
    see also boots; individual firms; individual models
shorts 135
shoulders 96, 128
Shwayder, Jesse 256
silk 351
    cravat 87
    necktie 75, 76
    origins of 78
    pajamas 339
    production 284-285
    shirt 56

suit 114, 115
Simenon, Georges 238
Simpson (firm) 338
Sinatra, Frank 37, 113, 143, 214
Sinclair, Anthony 104
single-breasted coat 349
slip-on coat 197, 351
slippers **183**, 334
Smith & Son, James (firm) 263
Smith, Peter 99
smoking 235
see also cigar; cigarette; pipe
smoking jacket 323, **324-325**,
328, 329
socks **186-187**, 325
soft roll collar 52, 53, 65, 249
Sperry Topsiders 319
sport **300-319**
see also individual sports
sports jacket **120-129**, 351
spread collar (cutaway collar)
52, 53
Stokowski, Leopold 255
Strauss, Levi 136
straw hat 212
suede shoes **180-181**
suit 90–117, 348
  care of 344–345
  casual 351
  double-breasted 96, 352
  English 96, 108
  history 91
  in general 90–91
  Italian 108
  summer 115
  see also individual fabrics,
  individual firms; made to
  measure; morning dress;
  packing a suitcase; Savile
  Row; tails; tuxedo
suitcases 251, **254-259**
Super 100 (wool) 114, 351
suspenders 96, 116, 138, 139,
140, **142-143**, 349
Swaine, Adeney, Brigg & Sons
(firm) 251, 263, **264-265**
sweater, see individual models;
knitwear
Swiss batiste 56

T
tab collar 52, 53
TAG Heuer (firm) 228, 229
tailcoat 209, 323, **326-327**, 329,
349
tailor 92, 93, 95, 102, 350
Tailors, Tobias (firm) 74, **95**
tartan 352
tassel loafers 162, 163, 179, 352
Tattersall check 56, **64**, 75, 352

Tattersall, Richard 64
Telerie Spadari (firm) 58
Thurston, Albert (firm) 143
Tibbett (firm) 194
ticket pocket 348
Timberland 154
tobacco processing 235
Tod's, J. P. (firm) 154, 184-185,
297
top hat 209, 212, 327, 331, 352
toupee **36-37**
trench coat 198, 352
Tricker's (firm) 153, 154, 167,
170, 171, 183, 305
trilby hat 209, 212, **310-311**,
352
trimmer 352
trouser maker 92, 100, 352
trousers, see pants
Trumper's (firm) 22, 30, 33
Tumi (firm) 256
Turnbull & Asser (firm) 53, 58,
60, 74, 104, 196
turndown collar 52, 53
tuxedo 323, 324-325, 328, 329,
349, 352
tweed
  caps 213, 312
  fabrics 75, **124-125**, 352
  hats 212, 312
  jackets 120, **126-127**, 128,
  205, 311
  suits 96, **106-107**, 304, 311

U
umbrella **262-265**, 313, 315
underwear **42-47**

V
Vass, László 157
vest 203, 285, 308, 312, 326,
331, 352
vest maker 92, 100, 352
vetiver 23
Victoria, Queen of Great Britain
and Ireland 147
vicuña 284, 352
Villemin, Jean Nicot 235
Vitucci, Angelo 109
Viyella 56, 339, 352
Vuitton, Georges 254
Vuitton, Louis (firm) 250, **254-
255**, 256

W
Wagner, Robert 113
waistband
  adjustable 140, 143, 352
  elasticized 349
waist-pleat trousers 46, 138-

139, 140, 141, 348
walking cane **260**
wallet 222, 225
Warhol, Andy 37, 42, 116, 137
watch **226-231**
see also individual
manufacturers
Watson, Teddy 96, 104
waxed jacket 200-203, 352
Wayne, John 113
Weatherill, Bernard 95
Wellington, Duke of 228
Welsh & Jeffries (firm) 104
Weston, J. B. (firm) 154
wet shaving **17**
whipcord 352
Wilde, Oscar 341
Wildsmith (firm) 154
Wilkinson & Sons (firm) 94
windcheater 314
Windsor knot **83**
Windsor, Duke of 53, 82, 97,
105, 143, 239, 304, 306, 325, 352
wingtips 158, 161, 179, 348
Wolfe, Tom 50, 53
wool
  blazer 146
  coat 194-196
  knitwear 282-297
  necktie 75
  pants 133
  scarf 279
  suit 114, 115
see also cashmere; flannel;
merino wool; mohair; pure new
wool; worsted
worsted 97, 125, 128, 146, 288
Wright of Derby, Joseph 277

Y
Young, Terence 104

Z
Zola, Emile 16

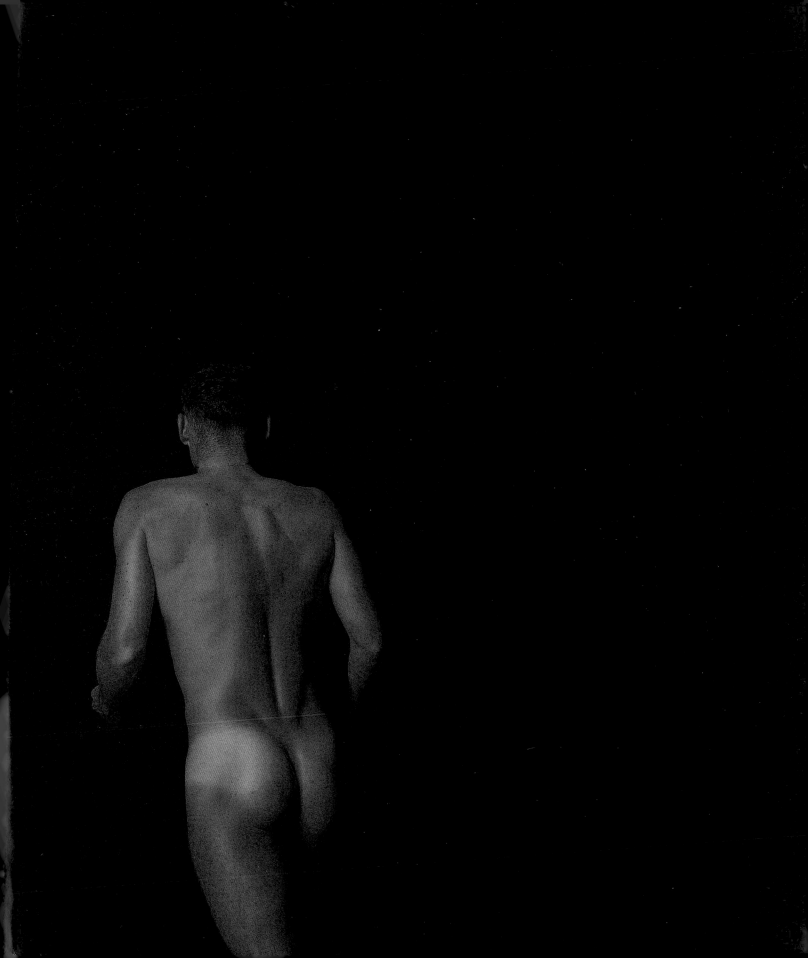

Picture Credits